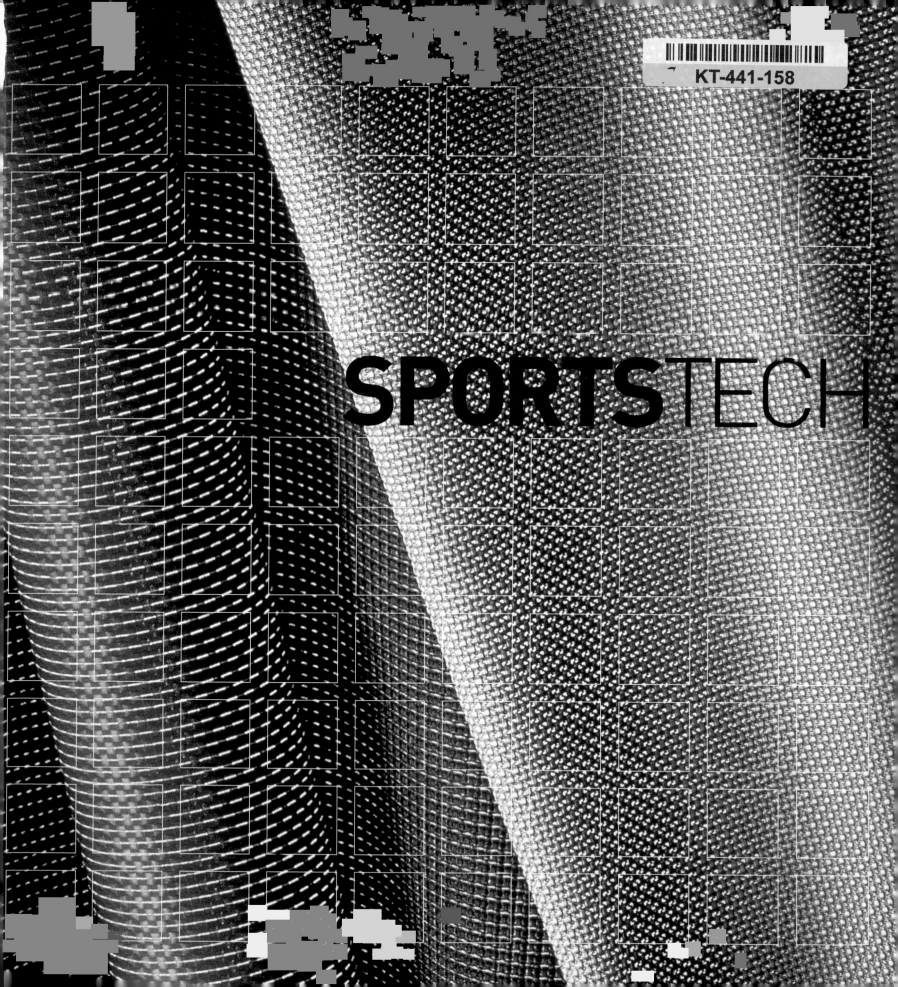

SPORTSTECH

KT-441-158

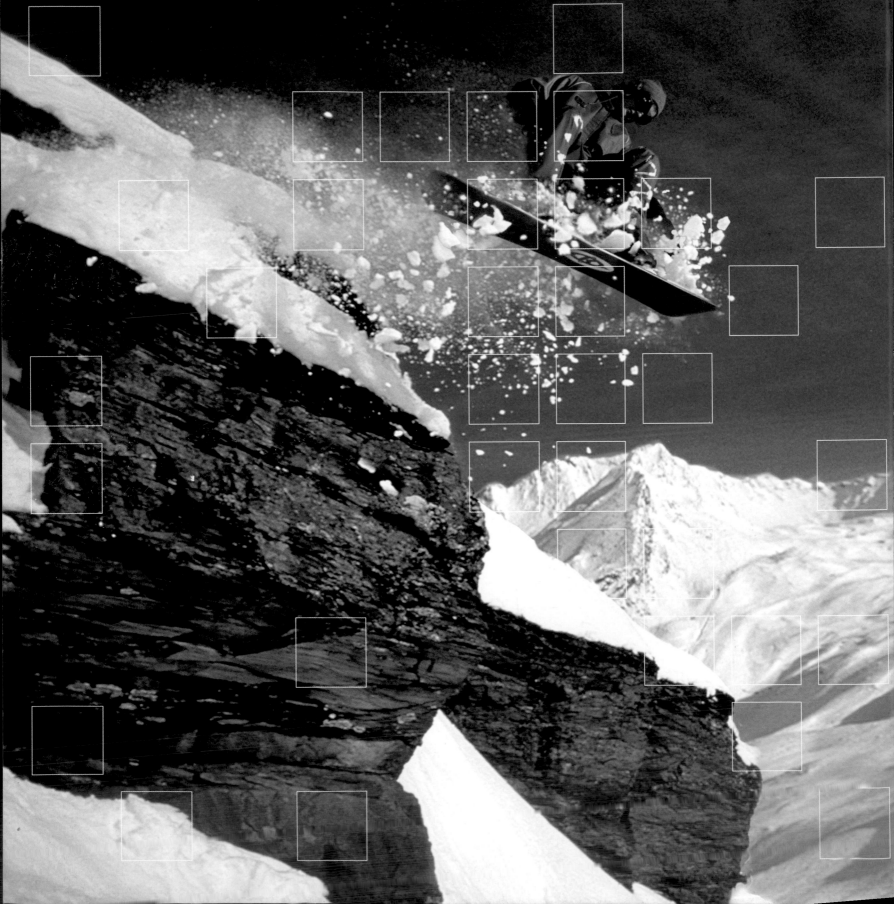

TOWER HAMLETS COLLEGE
Learning Centre

079536

NEW CITY COLLEGE LIBRARY
REDBRIDGE CAMPUS

WITHDRAWN FROM HAVERING COLLEGES
SIXTH FORM LIBRARY

THE LEARNING CENTRE
TOWER HAMLETS COLLEGE
POPLAR CENTRE
POPLAR HIGH STREET
LONDON E14 0AF

MARIE O'MAHONY AND SARAH E. BRADDOCK

SPORTSTECH
REVOLUTIONARY FABRICS, FASHION AND DESIGN

WITH 262 ILLUSTRATIONS, 239 IN COLOUR

Thames & Hudson

Page 1: schoeller-reflex,
a reflective textile by the
Swiss company Schoeller,
made from Cordura (DuPont)
and Scotchlite (3M).
Pages 2–3: Philips Design,
Techno Surfer. The snowboarder
in action, wearing protective
clothing and proximity sensors
to avoid collisions. Copyright
Philips Design.
This page: The Korean-based
Wooda Corporation Ltd have
produced a range of fine
synthetic fabrics treated with
a holographic print, such as
the stipple pattern shown here.

Order No: 746.92 OMA
Class: ~~CAMOUFLA~~
Accession No: 079536
Type: STL

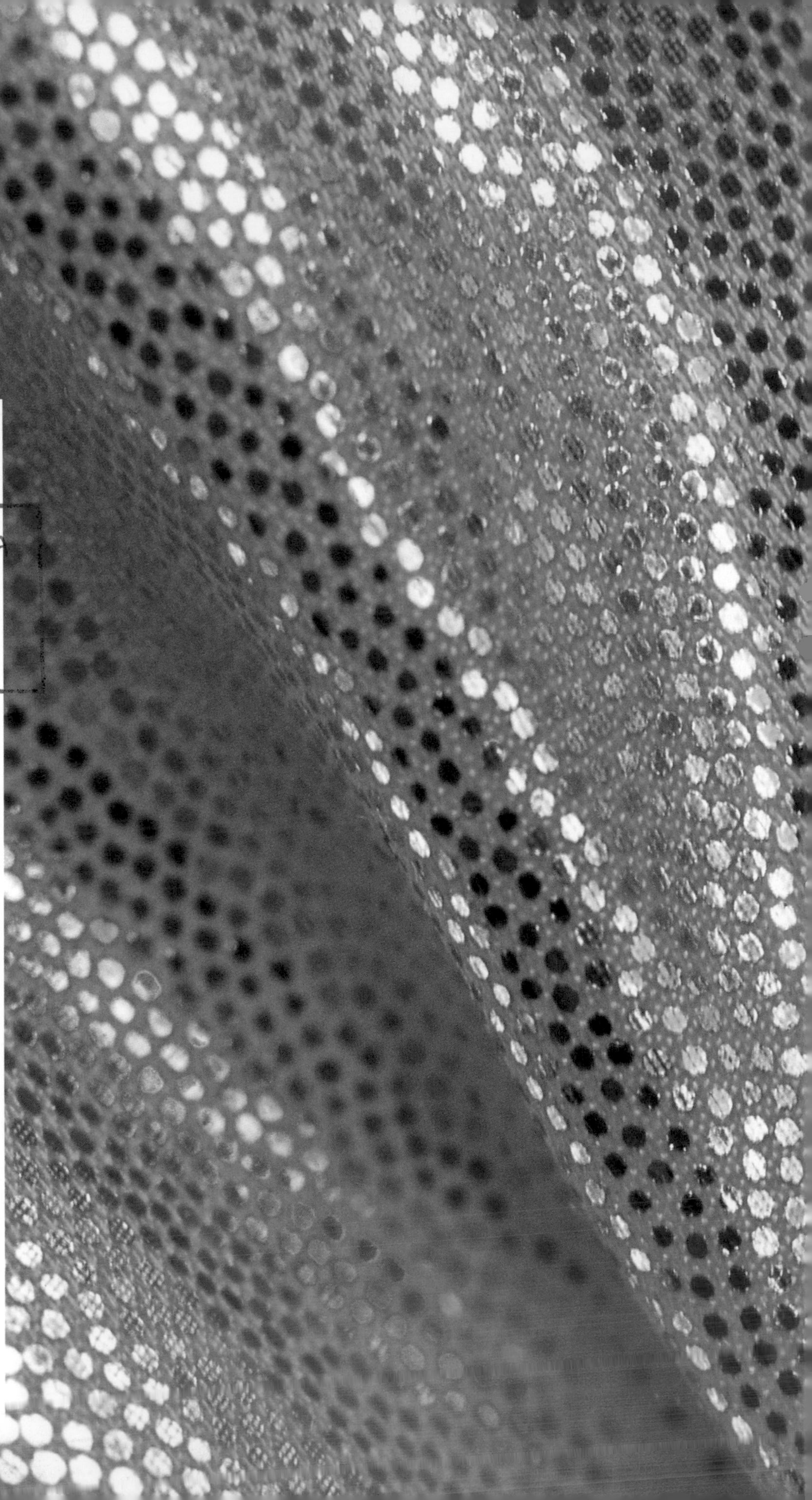

Any copy of this book issued by the publisher as a paperback
is sold subject to the condition that it shall not by way of trade
or otherwise be lent, resold, hired out or otherwise circulated
without the publisher's prior consent in any form of binding or
cover other than that in which it is published and without a
similar condition including these words being imposed on a
subsequent purchaser.

First published in the United Kingdom in 2002 by
Thames & Hudson Ltd,
181A High Holborn, London WC1V 7QX

www.thamesandhudson.com

© 2002 Marie O'Mahony and Sarah E. Braddock

All Rights Reserved. No part of this publication may be
reproduced or transmitted in any form or by any means,
electronic or mechanical, including photocopy, recording or
any other information storage and retrieval system, without
prior permission in writing from the publisher.

British Library Cataloguing-in-Publication Data
A catalogue record for this book is available from the British
Library

ISBN 0-500-51086-5

Printed and bound in Hong Kong by
C & C Offset Printing Co. Limited

Order No:
Class:
Accession No:
Type:

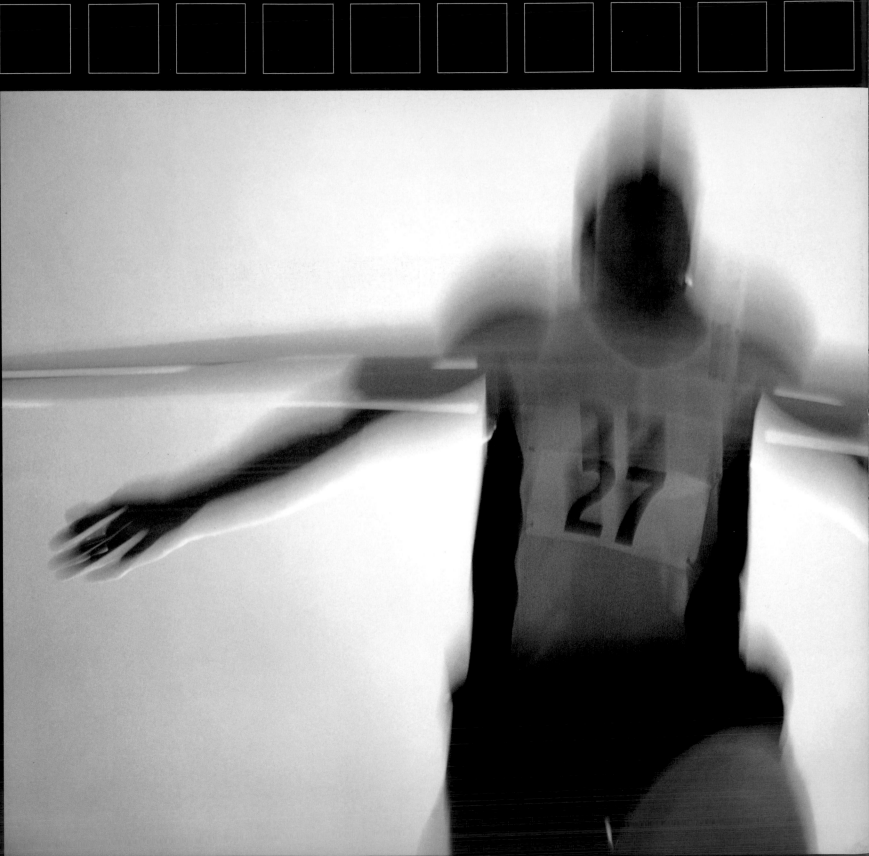

INTRODUCTION
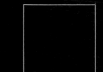

Sport is arguably the most dominant cultural influence in the world today. It percolates into almost every aspect of our lives, from fashion and entertainment to business and health. For some it is the new religion, which is interesting in view of the fact that many games and displays of athletic prowess were part of religious festivals in the ancient world – the *Iliad* describes the funeral games following the death of Hector. The basis for all sporting activities is social, a way for people to interact with one another, and this aspect remains central; it has developed as a communal activity through team sports and events. This is evident even in such apparently solitary activities as swimming or jogging, which many people choose to do in clubs or in the company of fellow enthusiasts.

Sports clothes perform a dual function, providing not only protection for the body but also a means of communication Graphics, colour and pattern have become both an aesthetic and a sign system. The advent of television, and colour television in particular, has served to bring sport before a mass public. New variations, and even new sports, develop to suit new needs, and this state of flux prevents any complacency among sportswear designers. The result is a vibrant and energetic industry.

Advances in science and engineering have been taken up by fibre and fabric manufacturers, and have transformed sports clothing and accessories – the new sports textiles provide protection and comfort while allowing competitors to give of their best. Textiles are constantly developed with improved or new functions for sports, and this is a growing market in an important industry.

Innovative technical fabrics also provide a new aesthetic and different tactile qualities that streetstyle and fashion designers are quick to take up. Synthetics have made an astonishing difference in high-performance sports clothing and accessories, but there is also increasing use of the new 'techno-naturals', usually blends of natural fibres with technical textiles or naturals given sophisticated finishing treatments. Rubber, foam, ceramics and glass can also all be successfully used in conjunction with traditional or high-tech textiles. Digital circuitry and micro electronics mean that new interactive textiles can monitor heart and pulse rates and body temperature, and can also incorporate information and communication systems. All of these have useful sports applications, but are also full of potential for more general use.

Just as sports clothes permeate every aspect of our culture and society, the converse is also true. The sports designer can be compared to a magpie, continually looking for bright, shiny things that catch the eye, but, unlike the bird, the designer does not simply hoard – instead the various influences are carefully analysed before being utilized. It is this ability to change the context that makes this design discipline so exciting and also very much of the moment. As the pace of technological development shows no sign of slowing down, multidisciplinary design is becoming a necessity. It is no longer possible for one person to hold in his or her head all

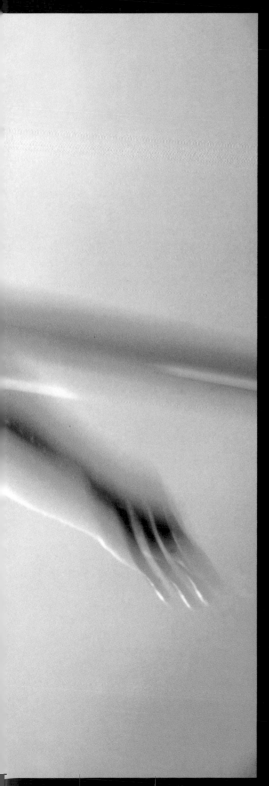

Going for gold. The professional and leisure sports enthusiast both demand, and receive, the highest quality of performance, comfort and style in their clothing.

Julien Macdonald, Spring/
Summer 2000 Collection.
Sponsored by Acordis, this
sports-inspired collection,
shown at London Fashion Week
September 1999, featured the
company's antimicrobial fibre
Amicor, which was originally
developed for sports clothes.

This unisex track spike shoe from
Mizuno has seven strategically
positioned spikes for greater
traction and speed. The company's
Bio-Lock technology uses internal
straps to lock the foot in place to
provide a well-fitting shoe.

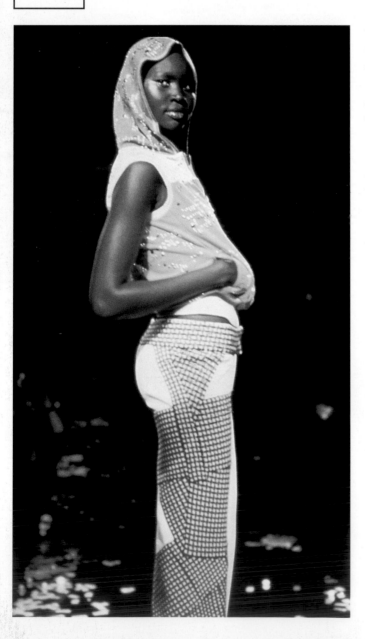

the necessary information about aesthetics, new material developments, changes in ergonomic theory, marketing and design. Each of these areas has become a speciality, and this brings with it a different way of thinking, enriching the design culture.

Fashion designers, always on the lookout for a new look and a better handling quality, have turned with whole-hearted enthusiasm to the new textiles developed for sports, and wearers of these high-performance fabrics appreciate the association with a healthy and active lifestyle. Fashion, in turn, has influenced performance sports attire, which can now be aesthetically pleasing as well as technically sophisticated. Fashion used to concentrate on silhouette, proportion, styling, hem-length and colour, but now function plays a major role. Previously prohibitively expensive, highly technological materials now cost less and are widely available. In the late 1990s, many of these innovations were still in the protoype-stage; they have progressed so rapidly that most are now in production, from ready-to-wear to haute couture. The choice of textile is paramount, and is often the starting-point for a fashion design, while more relaxed styling and functional detailing completes the look. Many international fashion designers now offer 'de luxe sportswear' collections – casual, comfortable clothing using advanced fabrics and offering functional features. Separates

from these collections are as readily included in the wardrobe of the fashion-aware as are the fashion classics.

In spite of the omnipresent nature of sport, this does not mean that the language is universal. In the United States, for instance, people speak of sports rather than sport, and there sportswear generally means casual leisure clothing. In the UK the term sportswear is taken to mean active and performance clothing usually designed and manufactured specifically for sports, and in this book we have followed the British definition of sportswear – this should be self-evident from the examples we illustrate. The ubiquitous British term 'trainer' describes the footwear known in the United States as sports shoes, sneakers or training shoes, so we have tried to use this term as sparingly as possible to avoid confusion with the US 'person who trains'. The Glossary, however, will help readers confused by any of this terminology.

Sport in its various guises has become as familiar as Coca-Cola, and, gradually over the last hundred years, has become a multibillion-dollar and multinational industry. In recent years, some of the business and employment practices of the major manufacturers have come under fierce media scrutiny. The focus of this book, however, is not political, but is concerned rather with design and the cultural impact of the sports industry.

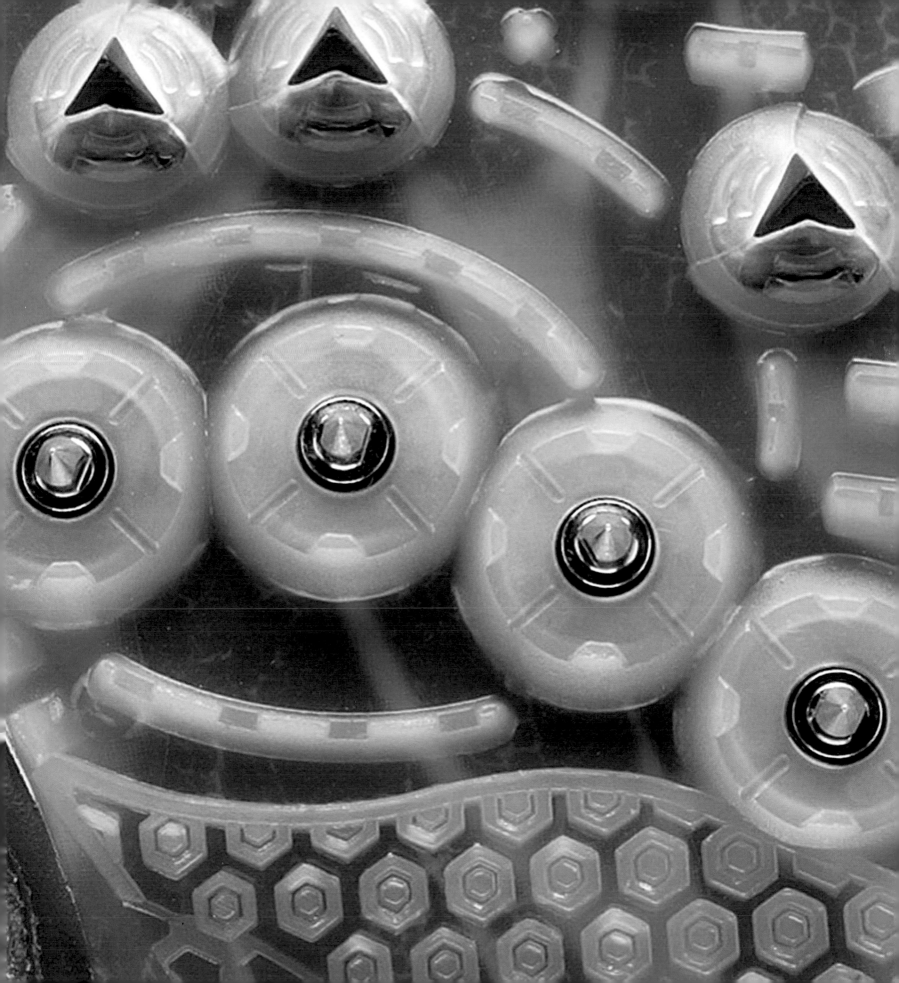

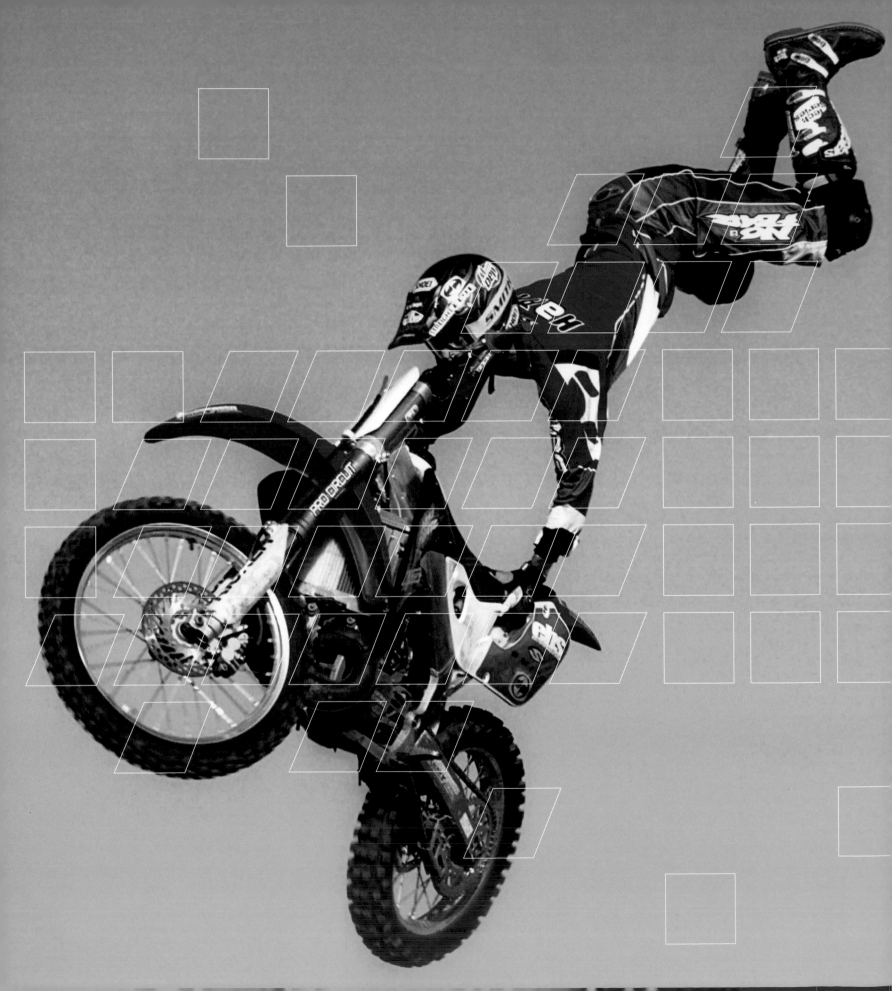

CHAPTER ONE
THE
SPORTING
CULTURE

Sports, and the clothes associated
with them, have become one of the
most significant influences on
the modern world. Gary Hart
from the USA is shown here
in action during the Freestyle
Motocross competition at the
December 1999 Extreme Games
in Brisbane, Australia.

Tom Wolfe, a barometer of American popular
culture, wrote a series of vignettes for *Harper's*
magazine. The first of these was entitled
'The down-filled people', and the year was
1980: 'They wear down-filled coats in public,'
he wrote. 'Out on the ski slopes they look like
hand grenades.' But the down-filled people
were not so easily dissuaded, and they are
still around today, accessorizing with a Louis
Vuitton handbag or a Gucci belt. The loafers
have been superseded by sneakers, adding
to the mirth of Mr Wolfe. But how did we arrive
at a point where sports clothing has become
such a significant part of global culture?

The German filmmaker Leni Riefenstahl's *Olympia* (right) was a paean to the 'body beautiful' in the guise of a record of the 1936 Berlin Olympics. The occasion was intended as Nazi propaganda, but, ironically, the African-American track star Jesse Owens was undisputed hero of the games.

Following Coco Chanel in the 1920s, movie stars like Katharine Hepburn (far right in a publicity shot) wore trousers with exceptional panache before this was socially acceptable for women.

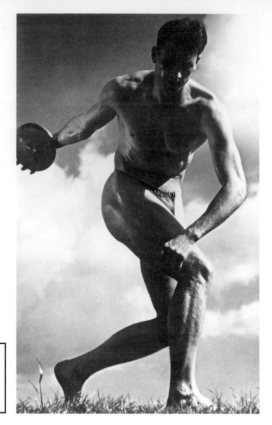

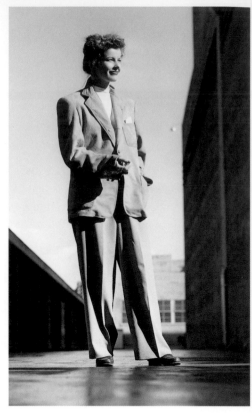

THE DEVELOPMENT OF SPORTS CLOTHING

At the first Olympic Games in the eighth century BC, the athletes took part naked. When the modern Olympics were introduced in 1896, participants were clothed, though this clothing amounted to little more than comfortable leisure wear that allowed ease of movement while protecting modesty. Sports clothing as we know it today emerged slowly over the course of the twentieth century, influenced by changing social, political and cultural circumstances as much as by new material developments.

One of the most dramatic of recent social upheavals was the Industrial Revolution, which in the West saw the nineteenth-century shift from predominantly agricultural to industrial employment, moving large sectors of the population from a rural to an urban environment. People formerly involved in physically active employment found themselves confined to factories and offices, and organized sports met their need for exercise. Equally important were the social interactions, especially the team activities. Sport became a way of identifying not only a common interest, but often a shared geographical origin – vital for people who felt themselves displaced by the move

to cities where they no longer knew all their neighbours. Organized sports also became a strong feature of British public school education, advocated by Dr Thomas Arnold, the head of Rugby School (where Rugby football was born), for a healthy mind in a healthy body. While all these changes established a popular demand for sports, it would take another century before the manufacture of sports clothes became a thriving industry.

The 1914–18 war highlighted the importance of the right clothing for servicemen. Pilots who had to contend with extreme cold and chill winds were given layers made from various fabrics, including wool, silk and leather. This provided some thermal insulation, but was bulky, making movement difficult. Sidney Cotton, a British pilot and a man of independent means, was unhappy with his Royal Air Force clothing and decided to take matters into his own hands. He commissioned from his tailor in London's Savile Row clothing specifically designed for a pilot's needs. The result was the Sidcot, an amalgamation of his first name and surname. This had a thin fur lining, followed by a layer of air-resistant silk with an outer

layer of checked Burberry fabric. The one-piece garment was further insulated at the neck and cuffs with a draught-proof fur trim.

Meanwhile, social changes and a new interest in sporting activities were gradually beginning to affect the way that women dressed. Amelia Jenks Bloomer, the American campaigner for Rational Dress, had caused a great deal of controversy in 1849 by wearing ankle-length knickerbockers, but 'bloomers' didn't catch on in Britain until the 1880s when women in their bid for independence took up outdoor sports and cycling. It was not until the First World War, however, that Western women in general began to wear trousers as they took over conscripted men's work in munitions factories and the fields – boiler suits or knee-breeches were more practical than skirts.

One of the most famous fashion designers to show sports influences in her work was Paris-based Coco Chanel. Her look was relaxed and comfortable yet elegant, and revolutionized women's fashion. In 1914, she had made the first sporty bathing costume for women, and started the vogue for the open-air healthy look by making the suntan fashionable. In the early 1920s, the young smart set disported themselves on summer beaches, wearing the loose 'beach pyjamas' and 'lounging pyjamas' that Chanel had pioneered, and taking up the softer, freer clothes that Chanel had been cutting from the jersey fabrics associated with sports attire. In 1927 several women wore men's tennis trousers to play on court, and a few women began to adopt men's suits off the court, too, sometimes with the whole male look – shirt and tie and Eton crop.

Hollywood in the 1930s and 1940s glamorized the new liberal clothing for women, and Marlene Dietrich, Greta Garbo, Katharine

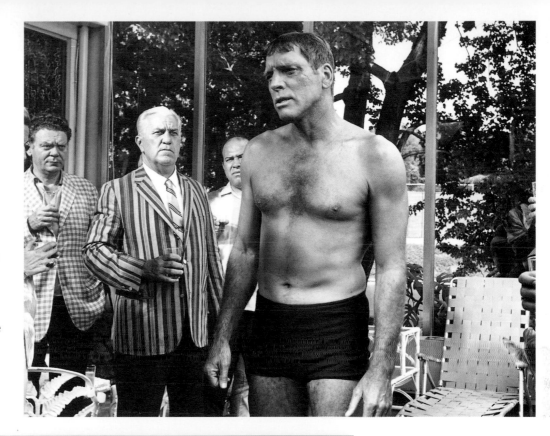

Burt Lancaster stars in this adaptation of John Cheever's dreamlike short story that first appeared in the *New Yorker* about one man's attempt to find meaning in his life. The film involved Lancaster swimming his way home through the neighbourhood pools of his friends. The actor was rumoured to have a secret fear of water.

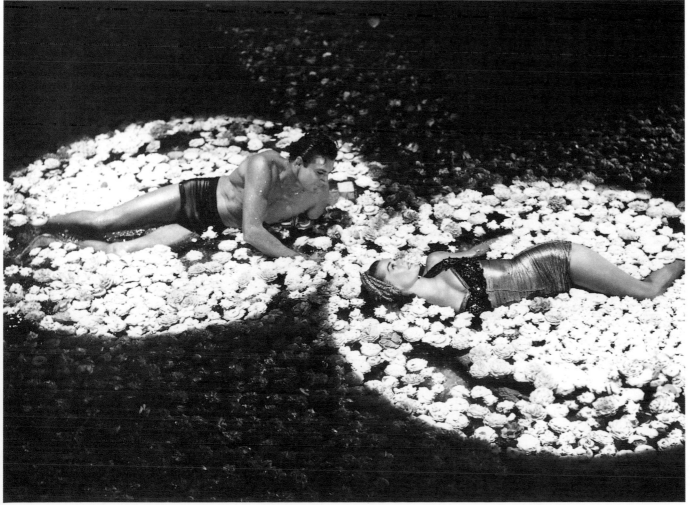

When the 1940 Olympic Games were cancelled it seemed to be the end of Esther Williams's plans for a glittering career. She was talent-spotted and given the female lead opposite Olympic hero and screen star Johnny Weismuller in his San Francisco *Aquacade* review. The two are shown here in a typically glamorous publicity shot.

Glitter prints from i.e. Uniform,
the fashion designers. This design
duo reflects a growing interest in
glamour from the 1940s and
1950s. Its designs often combine
functional or plain fabrics that
are transformed by the addition
of glitter and reflective prints
or beading.

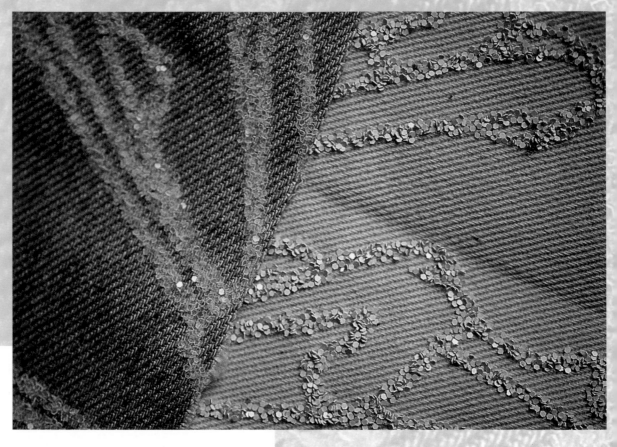

Hepburn and other icons of glamour were regularly seen wearing trousers both on and off screen. Many of the studio promotional photographs of the time depicted stars looking as glamorous in trousers or tuxedo as in evening gown. In the 1930s the fashion for 'slacks', tailored like men's trousers rather than Chanel's leisure pyjamas, had arrived for everyday wear. And during the Second World War, women workers, as in 1914–18, found trousers and overalls more practical.

The most dramatic changes in the development of sports clothes and accessories also came about through the Second World War. New materials developed for military purposes were used commercially after the war. Equipment manufacturers began to adopt carbon and glass fibre because these materials combined high strength with low weight. These were, and remain, relatively expensive, although this is offset by their high performance. Garment manufacturers were more

fortunate in the materials suited to their needs: synthetics offered man-made alternatives to natural fibres, and these nylons and polyesters could provide rough simulations of such natural materials as silk and cotton. They had the benefit of being robust, easy to maintain and – most importantly for their mass-market appeal – cheap. Less attractive was their lack of breathability and unappealing tactile quality. But in a depressed postwar economy, the availability and cost factors far outweighed any aesthetic considerations, and these materials became very popular for the mass production of low-cost, functional clothing.

It was in the USA in the mid-1940s that interest in sports-related, casual, robust yet elegant clothing was renewed by fashion sports-clothing designer, Claire McCardell. Her use of knitted fabrics, and simple, practical cutting and relaxed styling, with a slightly masculine feel, inspired the whole sports look as fashion started to use new

fabrics such as nylon and stretch textiles. McCardell was the precursor of several of today's designers in the United States. It was also McCardell who linked dancewear to fashion by putting flat 'ballerina' shoes in her 1941 collection.

In the 1950s sport itself was glamorized in Hollywood. Particularly popular was a series of musicals with the swimming star Esther Williams. Synchronized swimming proved an ideal vehicle for combining the new interest in fitness with spectacle. Hollywood glamour fed back into the sport, and today, in comparison with speed-swimmers, synchronized swimmers wear very exotic swimming costumes. Textile manufacturers are now starting to introduce decorative finishes and embellishments in their sports fabric ranges.

Sports gear companies have long recognized the importance of advice from sports people. Speedo employed the services of swimmers in the late 1950s, while other practitioners have

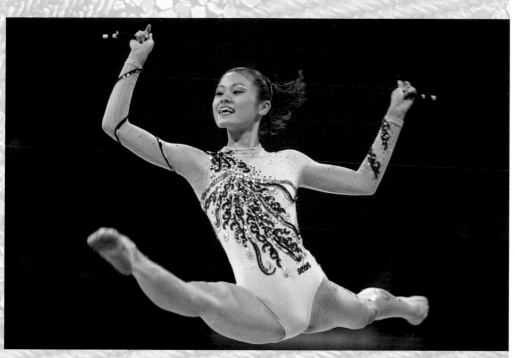

Glamour has become an essential ingredient in certain sports, such as gymnastics and figure-skating. The Japanese gymnast, Reiko Matsunaga, is shown here performing at a Rhythmic Gymnastics event at the 2000 Olympic Games in Sydney, Australia.

In recognition of the appeal of sports fabrics outside the industry, manufacturers have begun to add more aesthetic and tactile finishes to synthetic fabrics. The Taiwanese company China Lush has designed a range of these materials, such as this nylon fabric with silicone rubber print.

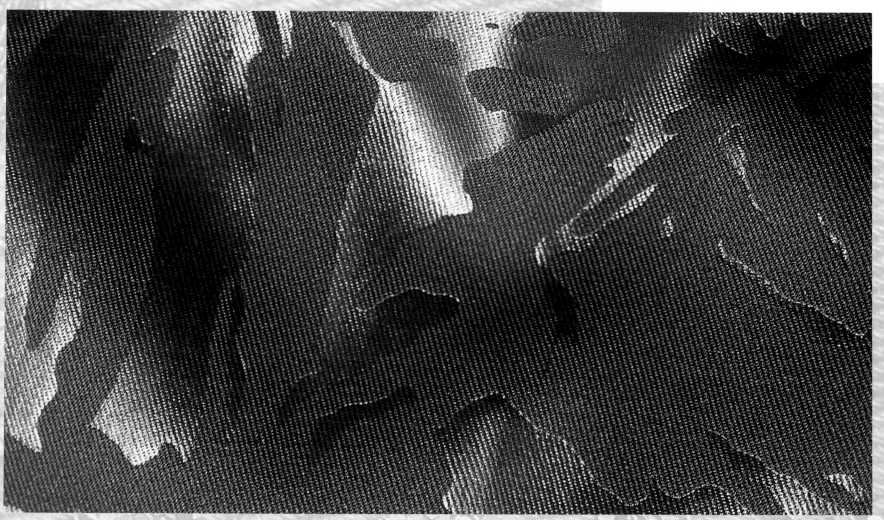

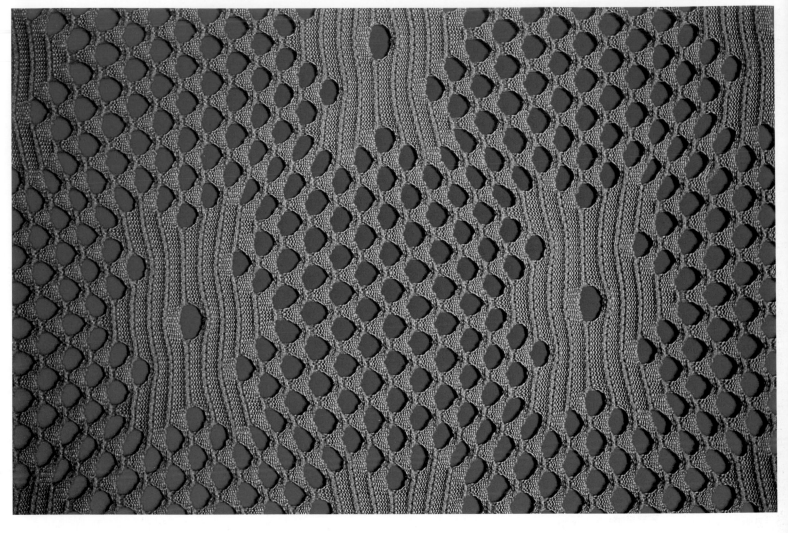

gone on to design their own clothing label. US companies such as OP (OceanPacific) and O'Neill were set up by sports people dissatisfied with the performance of commercially available clothing. OP began when two surfers, Jim Jenks and Chuck Buttner, made stronger swimming costumes out of a heavy tablecloth belonging to the mother of one of them. When Jack O'Neill first opened his surf shop in California in the 1950s, he sold mainly surfboards. Contrary to popular mythology, Californian beaches can be chilly, and from his own experience O'Neill was aware of the need to keep warm in the water and when standing around waiting for the surf. He began experimenting with sheets of unicellular foam, but it was his use of neoprene, an industrial textile, that led to the evolution of the contemporary wetsuit.

In 1952 he invented the basic all-in-one wetsuit with a high neck and long zip, and the O'Neill company continues to refine its wetsuit designs, remaining the leading manufacturer in this area.

The use of neoprene by Jack O'Neill is not an isolated instance of the appropriation of materials from other industries. The sports industry has always been quick to recognize suitable materials as well as developing its own materials and technologies.

In the early 1970s, sports of all kinds were becoming increasingly popular and were seen as fashionable. Several factors contributed to this change in perception. The introduction of a stretch fabric, DuPont's Lycra, developed back in the 1950s, allowed for the design of

garments that provided ease of movement, comfort and style. Synthetics had previously afforded little inherent elasticity, relying instead on the fabric structure to provide this. Knit rather than weave was the preferred process for producing garments where stretch was needed. However, knitted structures were not appropriate for all sports attire, so a fibre with inherent elasticity was welcomed by designers and consumers alike for the new design potential it offered.

The 1960s had seen the development of another fashion for active wear – the catsuit, a futuristic body-clinging version of the flying-suit. It was designed for Diana Rigg who played one of the leads in a British TV programme called *The Avengers*, and was usually made of stretch jersey. Cool, witty, ruthless, skilled

Most fabric structures can take the addition of a decorative surface or structure. This knitted mesh from China Lush uses a subtle floral pattern combined with a lively mint green to create a more interesting mesh.

Pharetra produces a range of foam-padded fabrics for many applications, including medical bandages, car baby-seats and sports. The foam inserts can be varied in thickness, and new patterns for the outer fabric are regularly introduced. The ridges between the foam are heat-bonded rather than stitched into place.

Manufacturers do not rely solely on pattern for dramatic effect. This fabric from Palmhive combines striking hues of electric blue and custard yellow to create an eye-catching material.

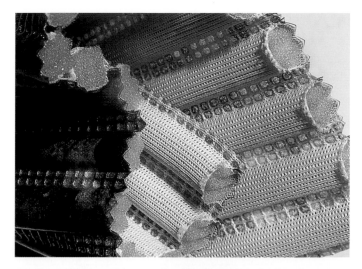

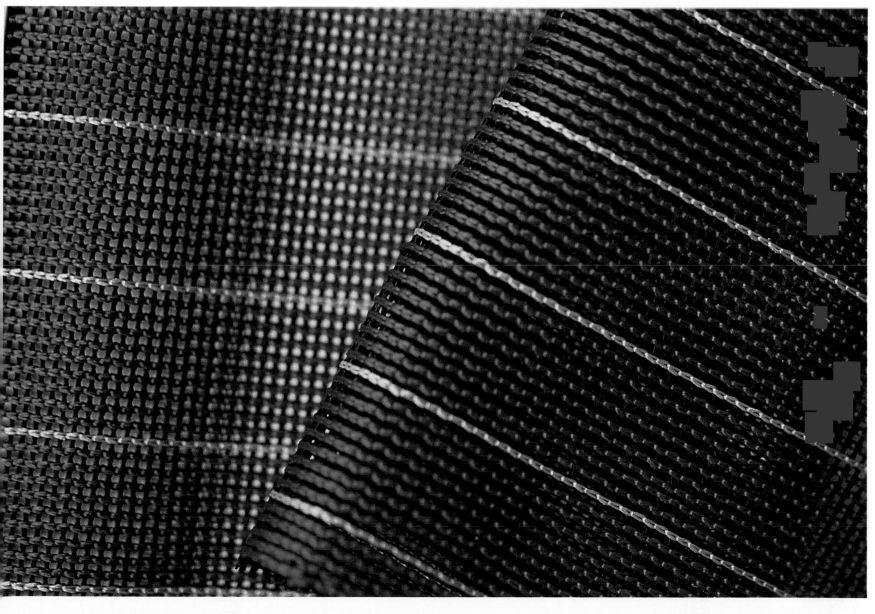

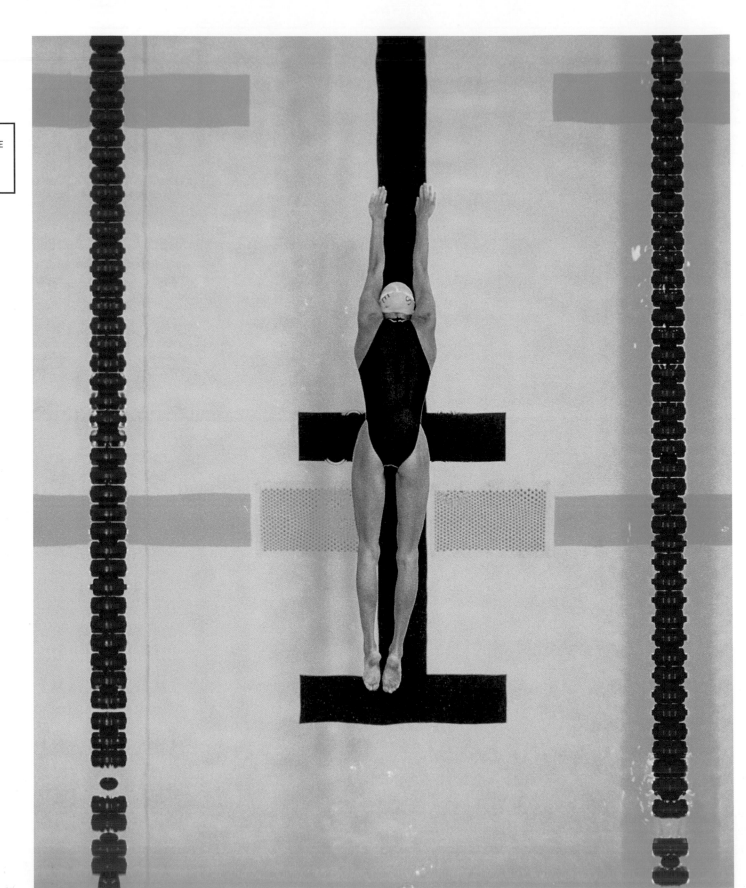

The start of a competitive swimming event (left). Today's sports stars can look forward to careers after their competition years. Many have even gone on to become household names as film or TV personalities, or to launch their own sports brand. Business acumen is becoming as essential as fitness.

The sports stars who made the transition to small and large screen with varying degrees of success include former Mr Universe contender, Lou Ferriago (right), who was offered the role of the Incredible Hulk in the 1970s TV series. Bruce Lee (below in *Enter the Dragon*) was more successful, though his death in 1973 meant that he did not live to see the cult following that grew around his short film career.

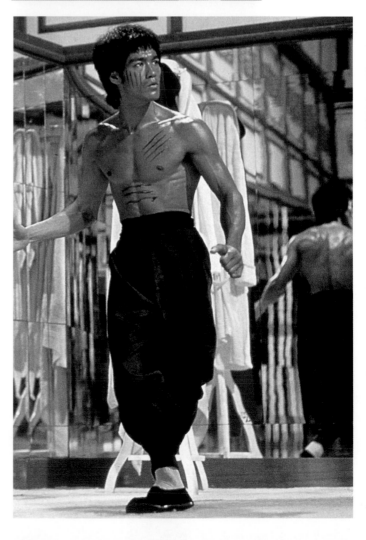

in the martial arts, her character Emma Peel always remained a cool and glamorous image.

In the 1970s colour television sets began to replace the black-and-white screens that had previously dominated living rooms. The 1972 Munich Olympic Games, which many people would have watched in colour, saw the launch of Lycra-based swimwear. Colour made it easier to distinguish participants, and added an element of style to the proceedings. The growing popularity of sports activities did not go unnoticed by Hollywood filmmakers, who were looking for new symbols of glamour, and this was an ideal vehicle, providing an antithesis to the hedonistic excesses of the 1960s, promoting instead fit, healthy bodies and the associated lifestyle.

Sports stars turned to the film and television industry as an alternative to setting up sports and fitness centres or lending their names to sports brands when they retired from competition. Some, like Bruce Lee, even managed to do both. Lee had a successful film career in Hollywood and Hong Kong while running his own martial arts centres on the West Coast of the USA. Former Mr Universe winner, Arnold Schwarzenegger, became a cult figure, beginning his film career in strong-man roles such as *Conan the Barbarian* and the *Terminator* films. His fellow Mr Universe competitor, Lou Ferriago, had less success as the television character

the Incredible Hulk. It was not a speaking part, and Ferriago was confined to growling and flexing his biceps. Interest in the martial arts and bodybuilding both peaked in the 1970s when Bruce Lee and Arnold Schwarzenegger were at their most popular.

The modern sports industry has an impact on almost every aspect of our lives, permeating fashion, advertising, tourism, and even food and drink. This has brought about a greater awareness of the importance of health and fitness. The form this takes varies dramatically in different cultures, with the result that levels of fitness fluctuate, and certain sports have become associated with particular areas of the world. Forty per cent of the international honours in men's long-distance running have gone to a single tribe in Kenya, the Kalenjin. Experts disagree on the reason, with some attributing it to a genetic disposition, and some to environmental or social factors. Baseball is almost exclusively an American sport, attracting a huge following in the USA but little interest elsewhere, while American football is not at all the same game as the football played in most of the rest of the world. Not all sport is competitive. Jogging and fitness clubs are a popular recreation, and, although manufacturers were initially slow to embrace this market, it has now become an important part of the sports industry.

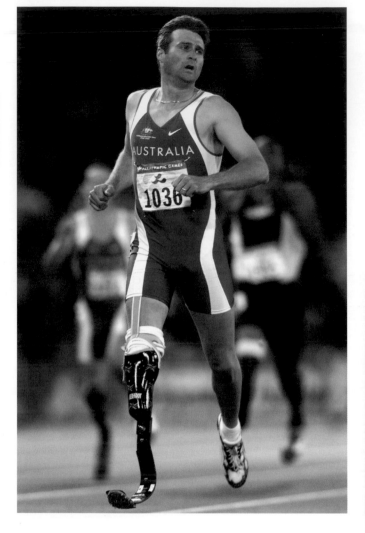

The Paralympic Games take place at the same time as the Olympic Games. Shown (left) at the 2000 Paralympics in Sydney is Neil Fuller of Australia taking part in the Men's 400m T44 Final. The design of his carbon-fibre lower-leg prosthesis is based on the hind leg of the cheetah, the fastest animal on earth.

Joey Johnson of Canada (below) takes an off-balance shot during The Netherlands v Canada Men's Wheelchair Basketball match during the 2000 Paralympic Games.

New sports continue to emerge with many, such as sky-diving (shown opposite), derived from more conventional sporting or recreational activities. These can take time to be accepted into the traditional sporting calendar with the result that alternative events are often set up, such as the Extreme Games, ESPN X Games and ChamJam.

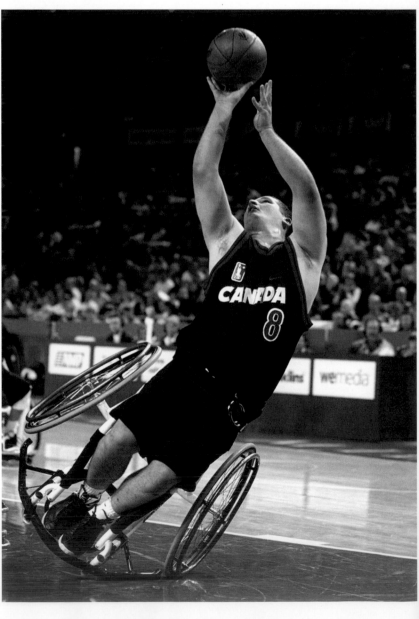

It is estimated that between 80 and 90 per cent of training shoes are used for non-sporting activities, and as fashion accessories – a lifestyle purchase. Many people, however, regard sport as an integral part of their lives, as the number of fitness centres and the popularity of sports-orientated holidays testifies. In some instances, new sports or sporting events may emerge that incorporate elements of an existing sport but are sufficiently different to infuse the industry with renewed energy. Initially born to occupy an unfulfilled need, many have now launched their own international competitions. The Paralympics, X Games and Ironman Triathlon are all examples of events that have emerged as the result of interest from focused segments of society, and, as such, can be considered popular movements within sport.

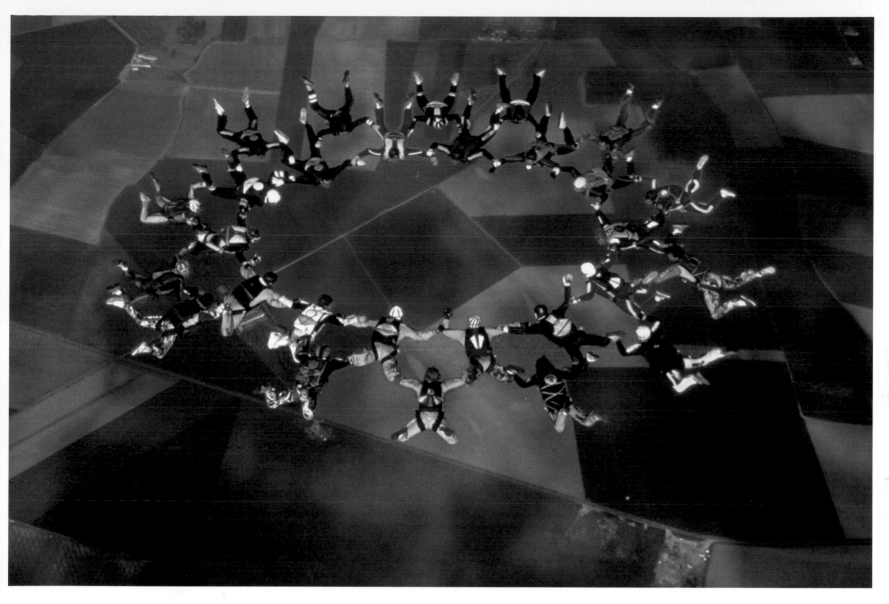

In 1948, Sir Ludwig Guttmann decided to organize a sports competition for Second World War veterans suffering from spinal cord injuries. The event took place in Stoke Mandeville, England, the British centre for the treatment of spinal injuries.

The games grew when competitors from The Netherlands joined in, and the first Olympic-style games for athletes with disabilities, the Paralympics, were held just twelve years later in Rome. As its popularity increased, the first Paralympic Winter Games were held in Sweden in 1976. The Rome games saw four hundred participants, but for the Sydney Paralympics in 2000 those who took part numbered around four thousand. The games are always held to coincide with the Olympic Games.

Each event has its own particular style, with rules especially adapted for it. Wheelchair basketball is one of the most popular events, and its rules are set out by the International Wheelchair Basketball Federation (IWBF). As with the Olympic Games, it is the track and field events that attract the greatest interest, and athletics have been central to the Paralympics from the beginning. The events are open to participants from six different disability groups to include competitors in wheelchairs, those using prostheses and the visually impaired and blind who compete with the guidance of a sighted companion. The Paralympics organizers emphasize, however, that the focus of the events is on the participants' athletic achievements rather than on their disability.

Extreme sports emerged in the 1990s. The term refers to such diverse activities as snowboarding, wakeboarding, bungee jumping, BASE jumping, trial-riding and freestyle motocross. Many of the sports classed as extreme have their basis in more conventional sports and (sometimes controversially) share the same terrain. Snowboarding marries water, street and mountain sports, using a board similar in shape and size to a skateboard, but the technique lies somewhere between skiing, surfing and skateboarding. Wakeboarding returns to the water, bringing together elements from surfing, snowboarding and water-skiing. The rider is positioned sideways on the board, which differs from the surfboard mainly in that it has boots attached. The wakeboarder is towed by a specially weighted

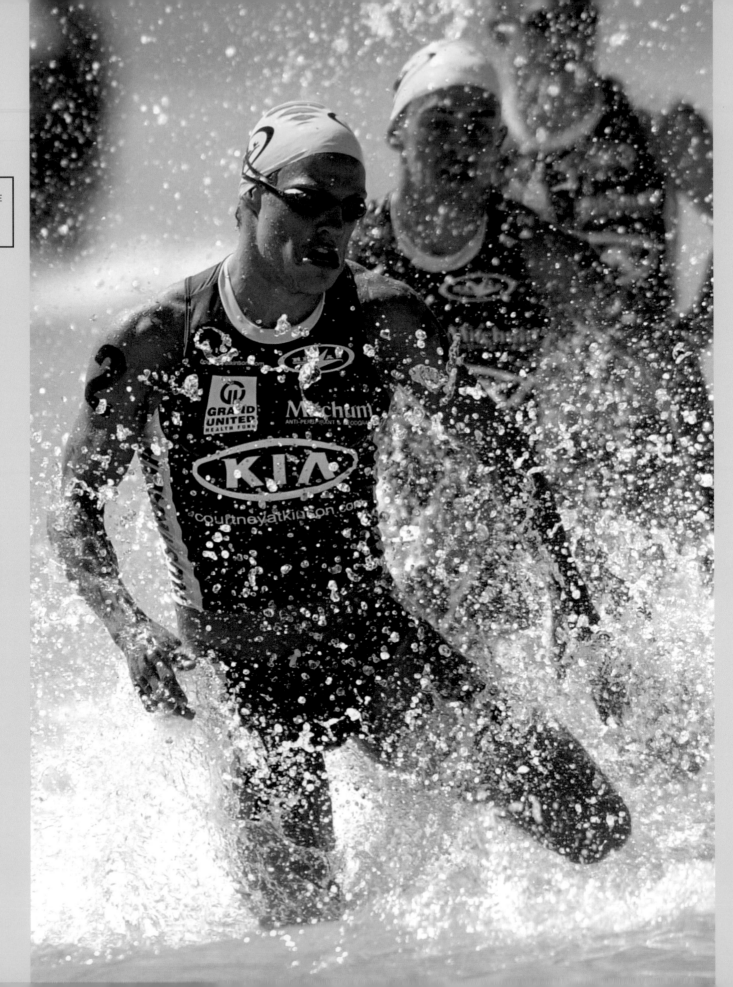

Triathlon competitors led by
Courtney Atkinson of Australia
in action during at round three
of the Kia Formula One Triathlon
series held in February 2001
on the Gold Coast, Australia.
The triathlon is a combination
of all-round fitness and sheer
endurance, combining swimming,
cycling and athletics.

speedboat, and uses the wake of the boat to perform spectacular tricks and jumps. Surfers have also been known to use speedboats to gain sufficient speed to ride big waves that would otherwise drag them under. Extreme sports have transformed their allied sports, turning the genteel world of ice- and roller-skating into a more forceful activity – the hybrid in-line skating, with wheels placed in the centre of the skating shoe, allowing enthusiasts to perform outrageous stunts. Relatively new on the scene are land lugeing – lying on a large skateboard close to the ground – and zorbing – rolling down a hill in a giant plastic ball. Snowblading, inspired by snowboarding, uses shorter skis for greater manoeuvrability. Besides the so-called extreme sports, there are other activities that stretch the capabilities of participants and their equipment, such as mountaineering, diving, pot-holing, mountain-biking, heli-skiing, tow-surfing and kite-surfing.

Extreme sports have a strong element of reaction against the formal constraints of conventional sports. Entertainment Sports Programming Network (ESPN), recognizing their viewers' interest in games with a high level of risk, organized the Extreme Games in North America. The ESPN X Games were envisaged as a showcase for alternative sports, with the first event held at locations in Newport and Providence, Rhode Island, as well as Mount Snow in Vermont in 1995. What was intended to be a biennial event quickly become annual and was followed in 1997 by the Winter X Games.

The main difference between extreme and conventional sports is one of attitude. For the extreme sports enthusiasts it is not simply a matter of training and competing – their sport is about a whole way of life that seeks to push the body to its limits. Describing the party-like atmosphere at ChamJam mountain festival at Chamonix near Geneva, DJ Eddy Temple-Morris spoke of it as 'like Woodstock on a mountain' (*Guardian*, 9 March 2002). The choice of clothing is driven in part by performance, but it also places the emphasis on the personal style of the individual rather than the manufacturer's branding. It has directly and indirectly revitalized an industry where the money spent on marketing can often exceed that of production. Essentially born as an underground movement, its spending power is such that industry cannot ignore it.

The Triathlon now equals the marathon as the most important endurance race. Combining swimming, cycling and athletics, it has become the ultimate challenge. Hawaii hosts the Ironman Triathlon World Championships, with additional events held in Japan, New Zealand and Australia. The New South Wales (NSW) Triathlon Association modelled its triathlon on the Hawaii event, and was granted Ironman status by officials from the Hawaii race in 1988, and it is now an official qualifying race for the world championships. The Australian race is held at the twin coastal towns of Forster and Toncurry 200 kilometres (125 miles) north of Sydney.

The Australian Triathlon consists of the Seal Mask Swim of just under 4 kilometres (2½ miles) in sheltered waters over a two-lap rectangular course. This is followed by the Avanti Cycle over a gruelling 180 kilometres (112 miles) on a sealed but granular road surface with climbs described by the course organizers as 'moderate'. The final Asics Run is two laps of generally flat terrain amounting to a further 42.2 kilometres (26 miles). Temperatures in the late summer/early autumn when the event is held range between 17°C (62°F) and 25°C (77°F).

The Bearskin parka from Griffin (right and below) prepares the wearer for any environment. The jacket can be a parka, a poncho or even, as the name suggests, a rug. It can be unzipped along the seams to become a poncho, while underarm zips release extra fabric to spread out as a flat rug.

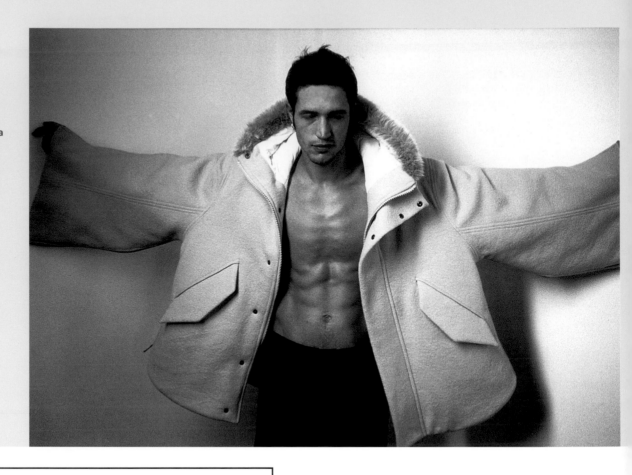

MARKETING

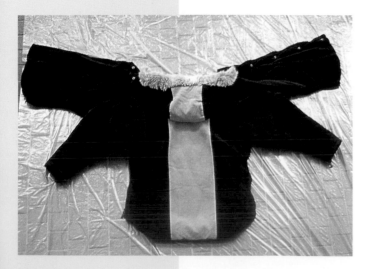

A 1997 study at the Georgia Institute of Technology concluded that the sports industry in America was bigger than the motion picture, radio, television and educational services combined. This dominance has not emerged through natural public demand – marketing lies at the heart of it.

As with all products, quality, brand recognition and loyalty play an important role in the success of sports clothes manufacturers. The companies who do best build up a following of loyal, sometimes fanatical, customers who repeat-purchase their products. This type of company is attentive to the needs of its customer, and constantly strives to improve on existing products and innovate. Although ultimately many of the products will not be used for sports activities,

it is vital that each product has the potential to perform well. It is the idea of sport that the customers are buying, but whether they ever intend being involved in any form of sporting activity is another matter.

In terms of sports clothes and accessories, the area of greatest global impact is undoubtedly footwear and specifically training shoes known in the UK as 'trainers'. The American Sporting Goods Marketing Association estimated that manufacturers of training shoes spent an average of 9.7 per cent on sales and marketing in 1995. As an indication of how this figures as a proportion of the overall cost, *The Washington Post* in 1995 published an estimate of the cost breakdown of a pair of Nike Pegasus priced in the shops at $70.

The newspaper concluded that the amount spent on materials was $9, production labour $2.75, promotion and advertising $4, with research and development just 25 cents. The amount spent on marketing by manufacturers of sports shoes is almost 6 per cent more than the amount spent by non-athletic footwear companies. Although specifically marketed as non-fashion footwear, training shoes now account for around 18 per cent of all footwear being sold in the USA. Of these, the percentage actually being used for sport is estimated to be 20 per cent at best, though some would place the figure nearer 2 per cent.

Unlike the Hollywood film, sports offer a lifestyle that people can readily buy into. Few can afford a beach house in Malibu, but most can afford a T-shirt or a pair of sneakers. Marketing executives recognize this, and sell their products as personality-driven lifestyles. Product endorsement has never been so essential, and now consumers buy a pair of Air Jordans in the same way that they will buy a pair of Guccis. Largely aimed at the youth market, such purchases are usually a first experience of 'designer' goods. The performance aspect of the shoes and their association with sport (as opposed to fashion) is important to the consumer, so the sports star endorsing the product must be perceived as top of his or her profession and 'cool'.

Defining what is 'cool' is not an easy task. Furthermore, the youth market at which this type of marketing is largely aimed is notoriously fickle. Trend forecasters and marketing men are forced to tread a fine line between predicting what the youth market is likely to want in six months without being perceived as trying to influence it. The most accurate information on what is or is about to be cool comes from the young themselves. In an article for the *New Yorker* entitled 'The Coolhunt', Malcolm Gladwell describes how sports companies identify trend-leaders among teenagers who are referred to as 'innovators'. These are the small number of 'cool' kids to be found in every group whom the others follow and try to emulate – the people who have their own vision and are followed to some extent by virtue of the fact that they are doing what others are not. In copying this small group, their friends become 'early adopters' to be followed by the 'late majority'.

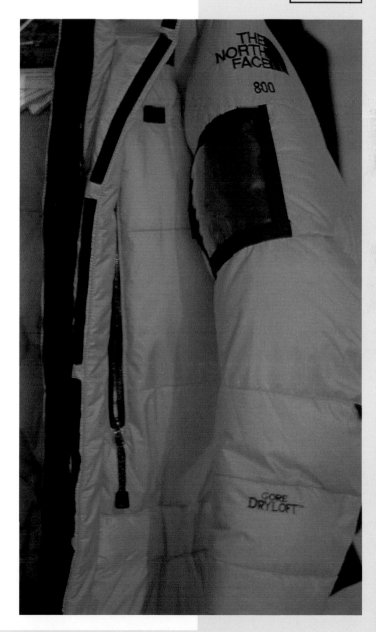

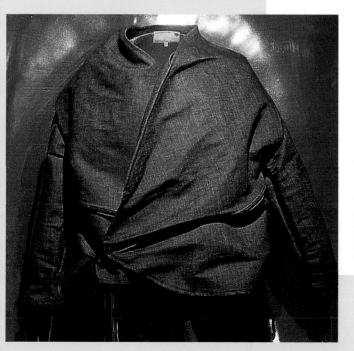

The same advanced textiles are being used by both fashion and sports designers, so the performance properties are the same, but the aesthetic is quite different. Both Vexed Generation in its Wrap Liberation jacket (left) and The North Face in its jacket (right) use water-resistant DryLoft fabric developed by Gore. The DryLoft membrane is laminated to the back of the face fabric, providing a barrier against moisture while keeping outer wear light and compressible.

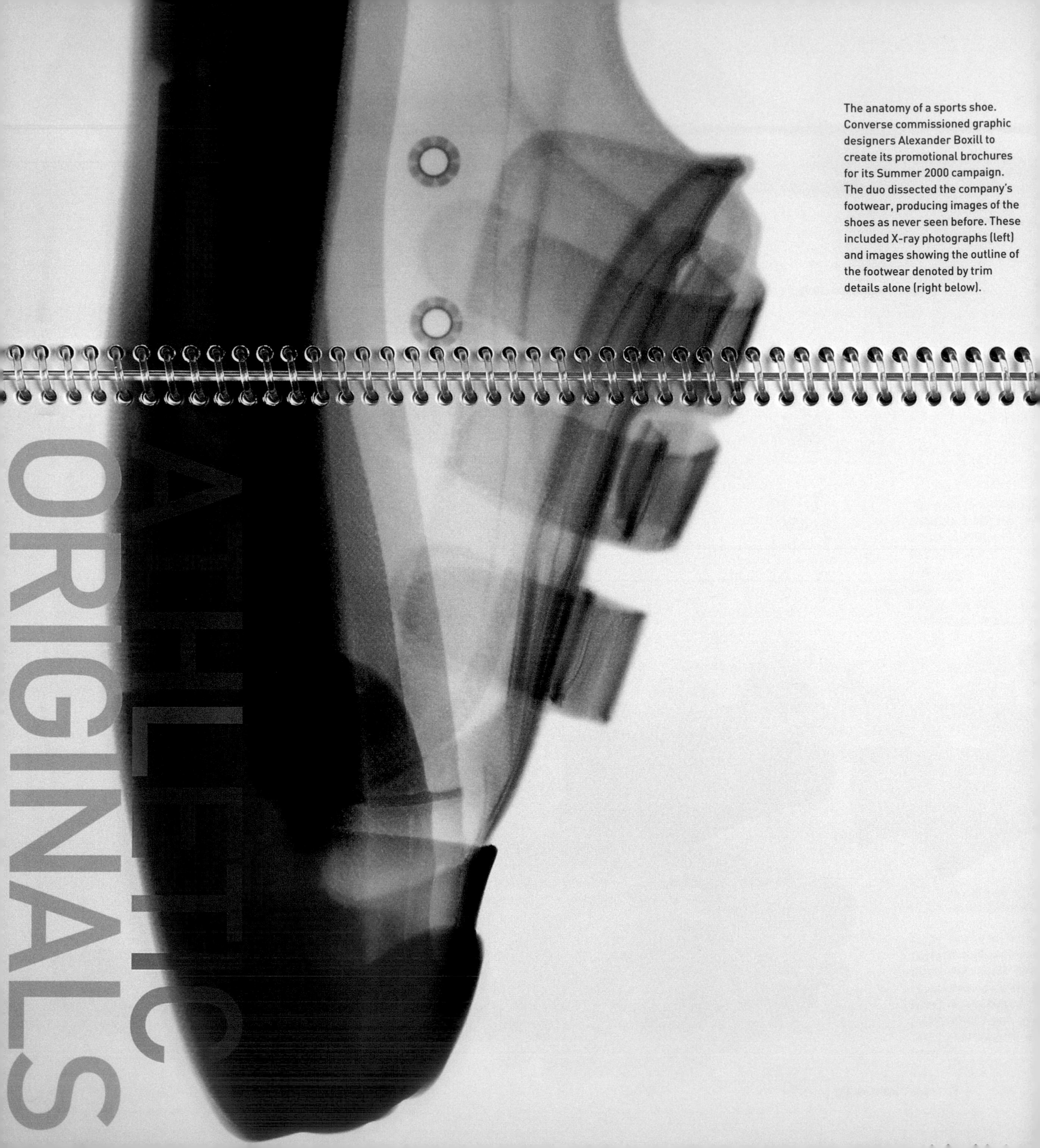

ORIGINALS

ATHLETIC

The anatomy of a sports shoe. Converse commissioned graphic designers Alexander Boxill to create its promotional brochures for its Summer 2000 campaign. The duo dissected the company's footwear, producing images of the shoes as never seen before. These included X-ray photographs (left) and images showing the outline of the footwear denoted by trim details alone (right below).

Prototype sports gear is sometimes given to schools and colleges for feedback. When Reebok gave a prototype of an Emmitt Smith shoe to members of the Boston College football team, it was returned to the company minus a piece of moulded rubber attached to the end of the tongue, cut away because it was seen as not cool. There are some examples of information gathered in this way being misinterpreted. In one instance where Nike looked to inner-city graffiti it considered naming a shoe Air Jack. This had a street reference to 'money' or 'success', but unfortunately it can also be taken to mean 'kill' or 'rob'. When launched, the shoe's name was altered to Air Raid.

Fortunes can change as brand names are perceived as trendy or not trendy, but such perceptions can extend to cover whole sporting disciplines or even individual items of clothing. In *The Sneaker Book*, author Tom Vanderbilt describes how Reebok CEO Paul Fireman transformed the company's fortunes on the basis of observation and a hunch. He noticed that aerobics were becoming a popular form of exercise with young women, a large shoe-purchasing sector of the market that had been largely ignored. This was not perceived as a fashionable area of the market with which to be aligned, yet Reebok took a chance. Its sales rocketed from $3.5 million in 1982 to $11 million the following year, which made it a serious market contender.

Times have changed for the anorak, which has gone from being the ultimate in uncool to being the pinnacle of cool. It is no longer the thin nylon or polyester jacket of before. It is now a high-tech piece of equipment that no self-respecting sports or pop star would be seen without. One of the most iconographic photographs of the 1960s is a David Bailey portrait of Mick Jagger. The image shows a close-up of the singer's face framed by the fur trim on the hood of a parka, part of the 'uniform' of the British Mod in the 1960s, who bought them in army surplus stores. What started as an anti-fashion statement has since been picked up by the fashion industry and transformed by innovative young designers such as Griffin and Vexed Generation.

Ironically, there is a strong element of anti fashion in the purchase of sports clothing. The result is a surge in popularity for companies previously regarded as conservative and

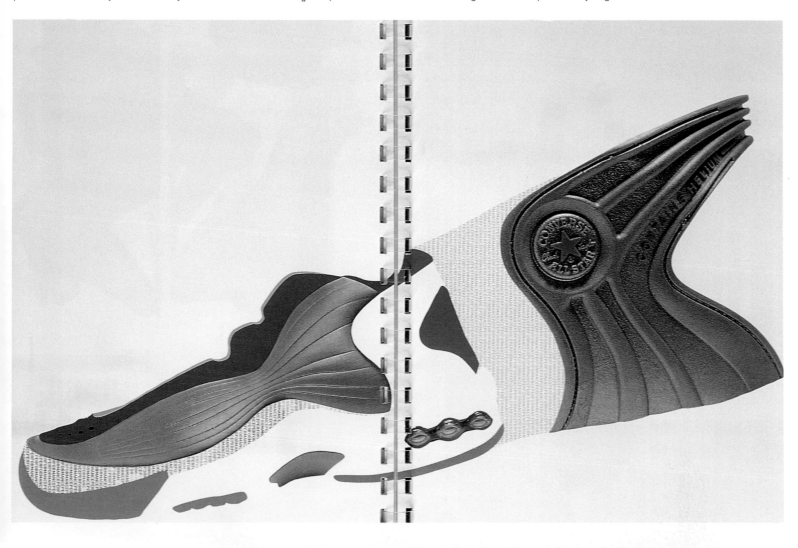

Nike's sponsorship of high-profile sports stars and their input into the design of the product range has proved a successful formula. But the right name endorsing the product is not enough, and the company tries to marry it with technological innovation, perhaps nowhere so successfully as the Air Jordan range (below).

Patagonia focuses its sponsorship on environmental causes. Clothing, such as the fleece tops manufactured out of recycled plastic bottles (opposite), is at the vanguard of this policy.

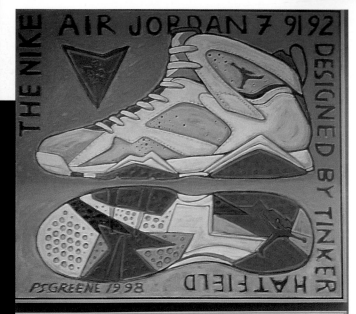

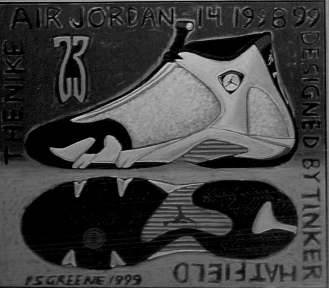

certainly not of interest to a younger market. Selling to a new generation, Fred Perry's range of sporting casuals has recently had a new lease of life, regularly featuring in fashion magazines, such as the UK's *i-D*. Similarly, Burberry, with its signature check pattern, had largely been associated in the UK with the American and Japanese tourist market, but has more recently become very popular with a youth market in Japan and elsewhere.

While customization is accepted as an inherent part of sports equipment, it is less commonly used for non-professionals. Manufacturers have begun to realize that the same people who ask for customized equipment would also like their clothes made to order as well. Mizuno USA have launched an Airfit Baseball Glove that can be personalized. The user's name embroidered along the thumb is just the start. The glove's main attraction is a built-in pump that can be inflated or deflated to provide a snug fit, effectively moulding the glove to suit the individual size and shape of the player's hand. Nike is also offering customization on-line. Part of the service offers the opportunity to have a word or phrase stitched on to the shoe just below the company logo. One potential customer requested that the word 'sweatshop' be emblazoned on his new trainers. The company rejected the order claiming that the customer had requested 'inappropriate slang'.

As with every industry the sports industry has its share of mavericks. The unsuccessful ones disappear without trace, but the more successful set new industry standards. Patagonia are an example of the latter. The California-based company was started by climber Yvon Chouinard who, having trained as a blacksmith, initially produced climbing-gear for his own use, but went on to make equipment for friends and colleagues. What makes Chouinard's approach distinctive is his concern for the environment. His core business was transformed when he found that the popularity of his own products was destroying the natural beauty of America's national parks. Patagonia prides itself in conducting its business in a sustainable manner. It has carried out an environmental audit on the T-shirt, and balances its use of polyester/cotton blended fabrics (difficult to recycle) with the use of organic cotton and fleece made from recycled plastic bottles. This has prompted other companies to consider the impact of their products on the environment. Several offer a repair service on waterproof jackets, for instance. As with many items of clothing it is often just one part that is damaged. Companies report, however, that customers have been slow to take advantage of this service, a clear illustration that environmental awareness is not simply an issue for designers and manufacturers but the responsibility of all.

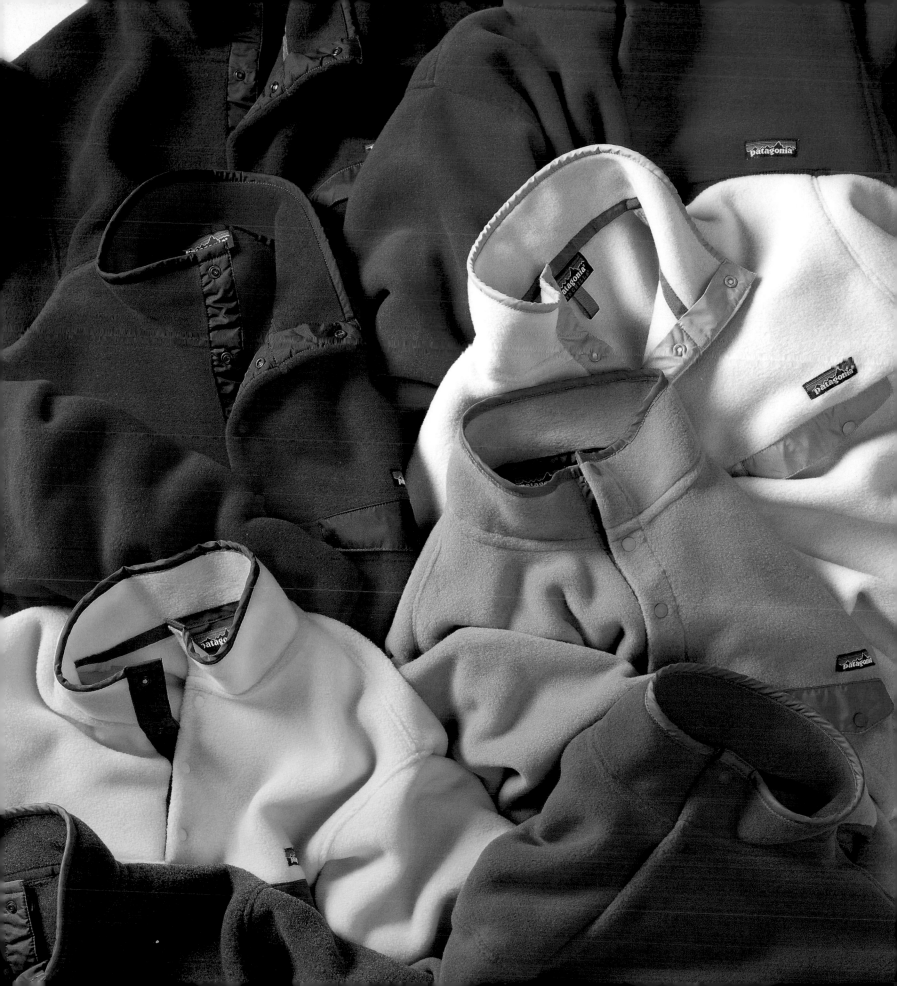

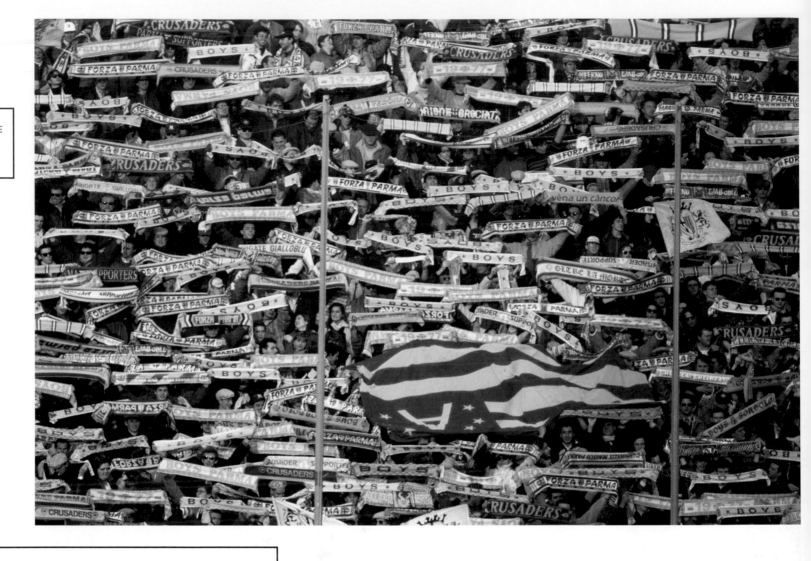

GRAPHICS, COLOUR AND PATTERN

Graphics have become synonymous with sports clothes in what has become a marketing executive's dream. Some sports clothes would appear incomplete without their assortment of team and sponsor's logos. It's hard to imagine a racing driver or football player without his logos, and in contrast the pristine white of the cricket or tennis player transformed by them. Whether in abundance or absent the spectator is always aware of the graphics.

Graphics were employed in an understated fashion at first, positioned on a top or jersey as a membership pin or button might be on the

top right or left 'lapel' area. Such signs took the place of other adornments, and had the advantage of being integrated more fully into the fabric of the garment. For many advertisers, sport was the ideal vehicle to promote their products to the youth market. Tobacco and drinks companies, and also sports equipment companies themselves, have been especially active in sponsorship. Both sponsor and sponsored have come to rely on one another not just financially but through the promotion of an associated image or lifestyle that neither can attain separately. These mutually beneficial arrangements are

now being questioned, and some forms of sponsorship are in the process of being banned because they not felt to be in the best interests of the general public. It is ironic that tobacco and alcohol, neither of which is an aid to fitness, are considered suitable products to help finance sports events. Even in the USA, where some states are 'dry', and others have a legal drinking age of twenty-one and over, sports events with a youth or family following are still alcohol-sponsored.

The advent of colour television in the 1970s highlighted the importance of colour in helping viewers to identify teams and players. As a result, some sports that are difficult to follow clearly on television have suffered in popularity. Table tennis is one example of a fast-moving game that is rarely featured on television – the ball used is both small and white, and, given the speed of play, it is almost impossible to follow the game. Ice-hockey overcame a similar problem when Fox Sports network developed the Fox Trax Hockey Puck in 1996. This is an electronically enhanced puck designed to make the white puck (moving at speed along white ice) easier to see. The Fox Trax appears on the television screen with a comet-like tail that can be adjusted in length or colour.

Patrick Burgoyne, writing in *Winning: The Design of Sports* (edited by Susan Andrew, 1998) finds a link between colour and social class in sport: 'Football may favour red and blue above anything else, but Rugby Union with its links to public school has always been a little more adventurous.' He goes on to cite

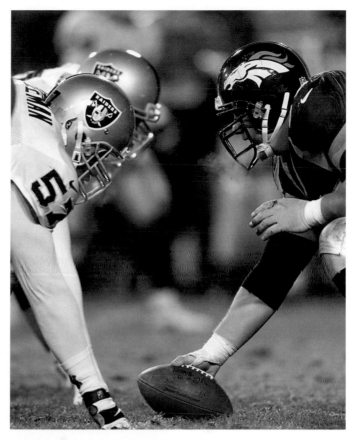

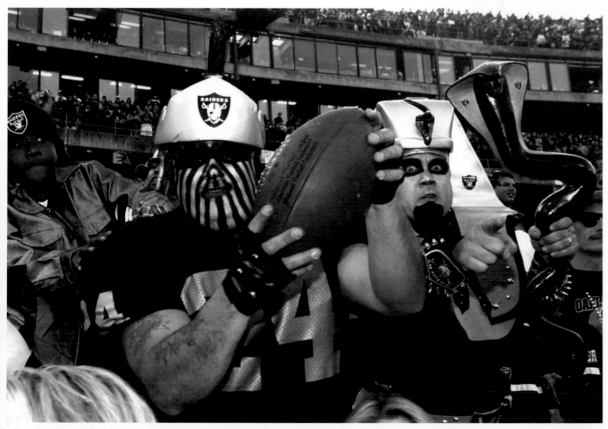

Sport is very big business and no aspect of the game is overlooked for its marketing potential, from the exuberant team names to the striking logos and use of colour and pattern. Parma supporters (opposite) show the impact of their team colours held high to form a sea of green, while the Denver Broncos and Oakland Raiders (above) demonstrate the importance of wearing distinctive colouring and intimidating logos. Enthusiastic Oakland raiders fans are shown (left) cheering a win against the Miami Dolphins during the AFC Divisional Playoffs at Network Associates Coliseum in Oakland, California.

Cyclists' shirts are emblazoned with sponsors' logos, but it is the stage and overall winner's shirts that have become more coveted than any trophy in the Tour de France. Erik Zabel of Germany is shown wearing the green jersey as the sprint winner in 1999, Lance Armstrong of USA is the overall stage-winner in the yellow jersey, while Richard Virenque of France wears the red spotted jersey as King of the Mountains.

Not all colour and pattern is used to intimidate. The relatively sedate game of golf has long sported its own distinctive use of harlequin colours and pattern which few sports have tried to rival. Set against a predominantly green background, the socks and sweaters create a colourful spectacle. This is particularly important for television viewers for what is one of the slower-moving sports to be televised.

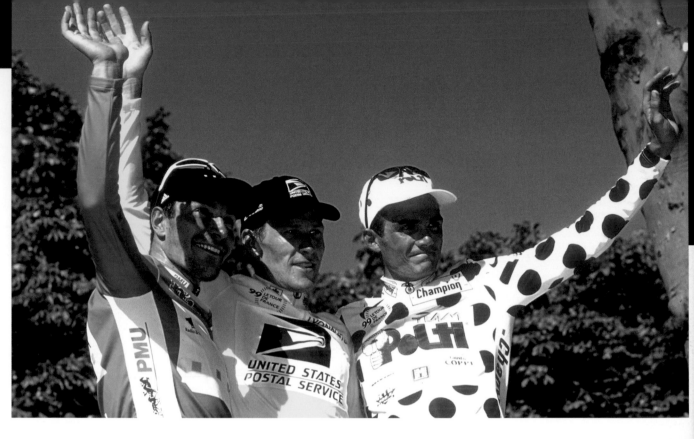

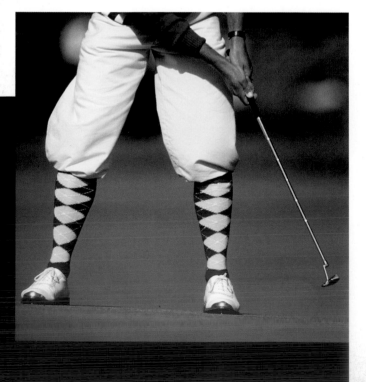

the example of London's Harlequin club who include pink and brown in their multi-coloured jerseys, a combination unlikely to be seen on many soccer pitches. Strong primary colours can dominate sports to the extent that teams are sometimes referred to by their colours. England's Manchester United fans refer to their team as 'reds', while in Rugby football New Zealand's All Blacks wear just that, an all-black Rugby strip. Both use colour to make them readily identifiable, but also as signifying power and strength to supporters and opponents. This use of colour has no role to play in the more sedate game of cricket; teams are dressed in clean whites with colour confined to cuff, neck and hat trims. When an attempt was made to introduce colour, it met with resistance from both players and supporters. The perception was that a move away from the purity of white would indicate a more aggressive approach to the game. The governing body, the players and the supporters had no wish to see cricket echo the more assertive nature of soccer.

While some colours allow for different interpretation, others have achieved a universal meaning. Gold is associated with success and usually an honour bestowed on the team or player rather than assumed. During the Tour de France, the Maillot Jaune (yellow jersey) is awarded to the leader of the race at the end of each stage. It may be held by several different riders during the course of the event, and is a temporary award until the final victorious cycle through the streets of Paris. Although yellow can sometimes border on gold, the Maillot Jaune is a bright lemon and can in no way be seen as gold. The most infamous breaking of this taboo against wearing the winner's gold was in the 1996 Olympic Games at Atlanta. The American athlete Michael Johnson wore a specially designed pair of Nike gold running shoes for his race. The audacity of wearing such shoes before winning the gold medal attracted more media coverage than the race itself. Imagine the embarrassment for Johnson and Nike if he had been placed second! The use of gold in this

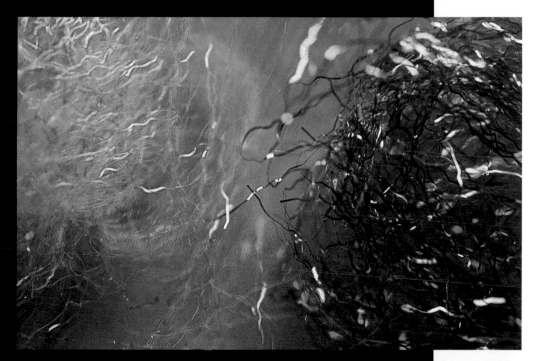

For non-competitive sports enthusiasts, being seen can be important for reasons of safety if training outside daylight hours. Day-glo and reflective fabrics are no longer purely functional, and manufacturers are finding ways of combining performance with aesthetic. Meadowbrook Inventions' holographic Angelina fibres (left) can be combined with other yarns to provide both reflectivity and colour, while Asia Sun uses its AAA reflective yarn in these woven fabrics (below).

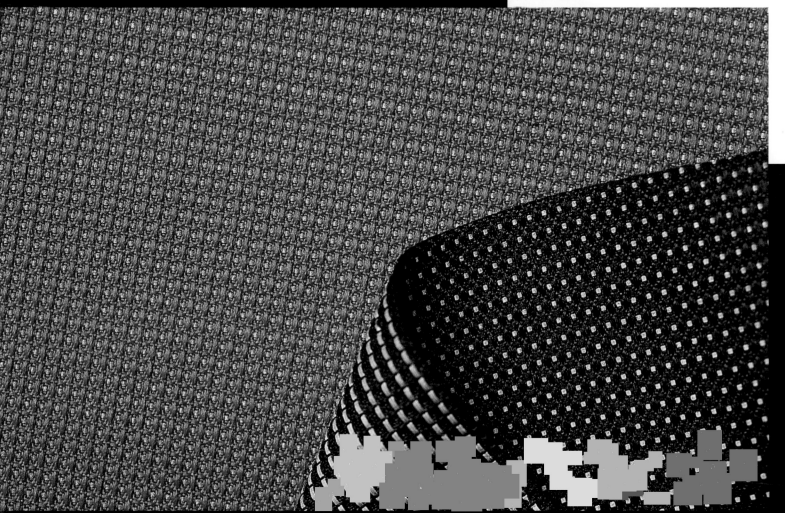

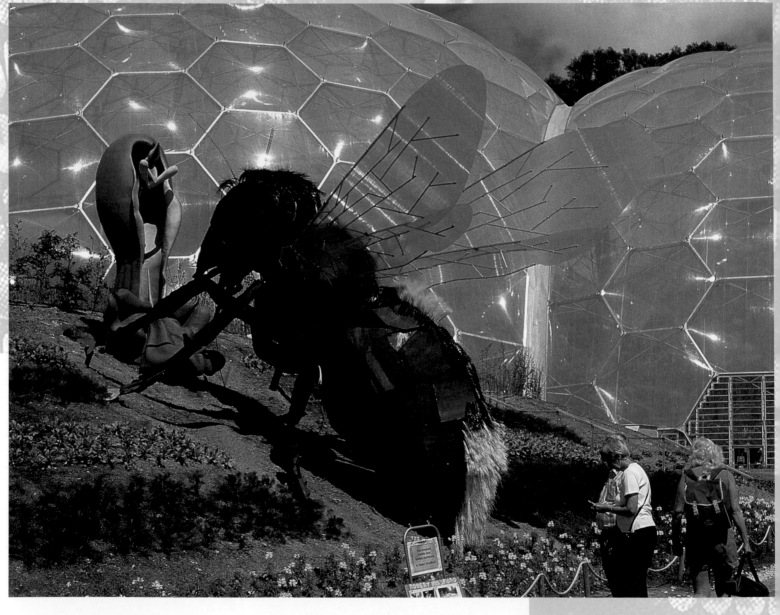

instance, however, had an undoubted psychological effect on competitors who were already aware that Johnson was the favourite to win the race. In the face of such supreme confidence it is difficult to see how he could have lost.

The use of colour and pattern in sports clothes mirrors nature where everything serves some purpose. Aesthetics can attract a partner or repel an opponent, and even the meaning can change depending on the way colour or pattern is utilized. The bright red of the poppy in a field, for example, attracts insects to pollinate it,

while the tiny shield bug uses an equally strong shade of red to quite different effect – it protects itself from predators by secreting repugnant odours from the top of its abdomen, and the brightness of the colour advertises this bad taste to birds who might otherwise be tempted to lunch on it. The colours found on the harder outer shell or exoskeleton of invertebrates can be used by the insect to create an optical illusion – a scattering, interference or diffraction of light. The colour can change in response to varying environmental conditions or to the threat of danger.

Colour and defined pattern combined make a stronger impact than either alone. The throat of the dragonfly is a combination of lime-green and black in a pattern that suggests the head of a larger and more intimidating insect, which has the desired effect of deterring attack from predators. The swirling pattern on the wings of the Peacock butterfly includes a circular design that to some predators looks like the eye of a larger creature, which again makes them less likely to attack. Some species of caterpillar have control over the use of their deterrent, choosing when and how to use their defensive pattern by puffing out their thorax

Nature provides numerous examples of the effective use of colour and pattern to attract or repel. Flowers rely on a combination of colour and scent to attract bees and other insects necessary for pollination. The model shown (opposite) is at the Eden Project in Cornwall.

to form a grotesque mask, and changing the tip of their tails to red.

Many sports adopt designs that combine aggression with attraction. Players need to intimidate their opponents while drawing the interest of supporters through spectacle as well as performance. Baseball stadiums attract some of the largest crowds in USA sports events, and there is also a huge television audience in sports bars and private homes. It is very much a team-spirited game where the culture is to participate, even as spectators, in groups. The game is the centre

of the experience, but the camaraderie, hamburgers, beer, cheerleaders and other entertainment combine to make it an experience. The players are part of this and dress appropriately. Protective shoulderpads and helmets communicate the aggressive tone of play, while colour, pattern and logos bring glamour and spectacle. Culturally the references are diverse, and include 1950s typography, comic-strip and motorcycle gang logo influences.

Motorcycling and luge also mix spectacle with performance, but with quite different results.

Wooda Corporation Ltd have laminated oval spots of holographic foil on to a lightweight synthetic jersey fabric to create this shimmering optical effect. While the base fabric provides some colour, the foil itself is without colour, and relies instead on its ability to pick up and reflect ambient colour from its surroundings.

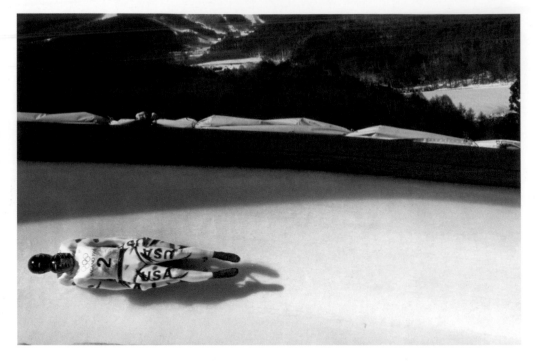

Two-man luge team Christopher Thorpe and Gordy Sheer of the USA make a dramatic spectacle in bright yellow with red and black trim, winning the silver medal at Nagano, Japan, in the 1998 Winter Olympics. The bright colours allow spectators and TV viewers to see them clearly against the snow .

The German company GKV have developed a range of Magic Mirror materials that are produced with and without a white PVC backing. They can appear as transparent as glass, or as reflective as a mirror. When artificial light hits them at a certain angle, a more dramatic rainbow effect is achieved. The technology is based on lenticular film.

There are common elements in these designs since some of the leading companies design for both sports. Pattern is selected and used to echo the contours of the body, emphasizing the fitness of the sportsman or woman and the ergonomics of their movement. The finished suits resemble exoskeletons in their performance and aesthetic, and the dynamic of the sport is communicated by the suit before it is even put on the body. Stripes and checkerboard motifs are used selectively rather than as the all-over patterns seen in football strips, or the garish horse-racing silks (where no design is too daring). This is an aesthetic choice made practical by the handmade element in the production of the motorcycle and luge suits. Vanson Leathers offer their customers customized motorcycle suits for professional road racing (see Chapter 3). The range of design possibilities is matched by the list of performance specifications that ensure maximum protection and comfort.

The use of dynamic motifs in sports design is often used to signify the high performance of the product, and, by association, the wearer. Converse and Hi-Tec sports shoes once enjoyed popularity for the simplicity of their pristine white designs. Colour and pattern, once shunned in sports shoes, came to signify their high technology. Patterns have moved away from the relatively 'static' all-over checkerboard black and white of the 1970s Vans to Puma's Cellerator Inhale which pays homage to the computer-games industry in its energetic design.

The movement of animals and insects is also reflected in the soles of many sports shoes. The speed of the cheetah and leopard have long been admired, but the gecko has come in for some recent attention. The gecko moves with great ease up walls, defying the laws of gravity. Scientists have analysed its feet to see how it manages this, and have found that the small reptile can turn parts of its feet into tiny suckers, which it can quickly activate then release, allowing it move with great speed while all the time remaining secure against falls. To develop a material that would behave like this would open many exciting new possibilities for the sports industry. In the meantime, the gecko footprints together with those from other animals have already inspired the myriad patterns to be found on the soles of running and training shoes.

THE LAST WORD

Organized sports began as a means of entertaining people, keeping them fit for work and war, and drawing society together. In the past century it has played an important role in each of these and other aspects of people's lives. The clothing worn and associated with sport has become an important signifier of this. Although not without its share of controversy, it is the positive aspect of sport that the clothes communicate, as sports style percolates into fashion, leisure, street and even office attire. The associations of youth, energy and enthusiasm remain transferable, despite the marketing men's attempts to quantify them. As with the question raised earlier about the nature of 'cool', what gives sport its universal appeal changes constantly in spite of the fact that it is such a global industry. It is this constant state of flux that ensures that sports design will never become tired. No designer or company can afford to become complacent or it will be overtaken by competitors in months rather than years. The result is constant innovation and refinement, a healthy basis for any design industry.

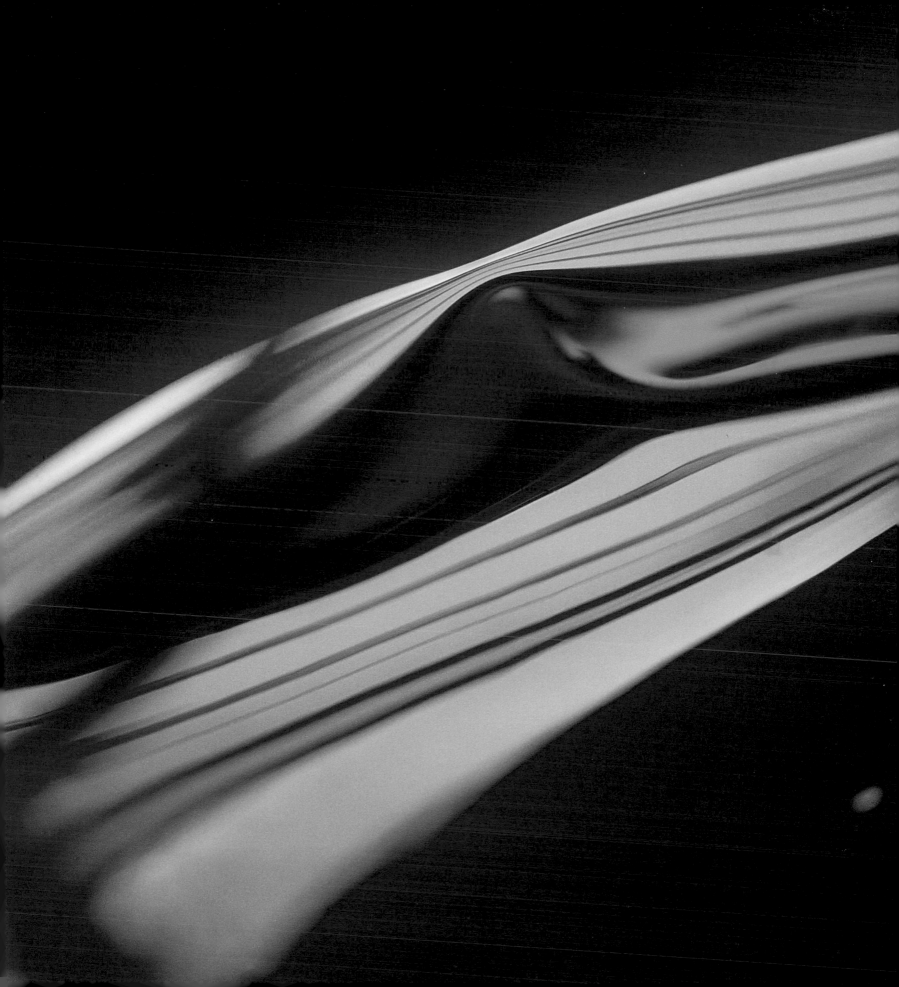

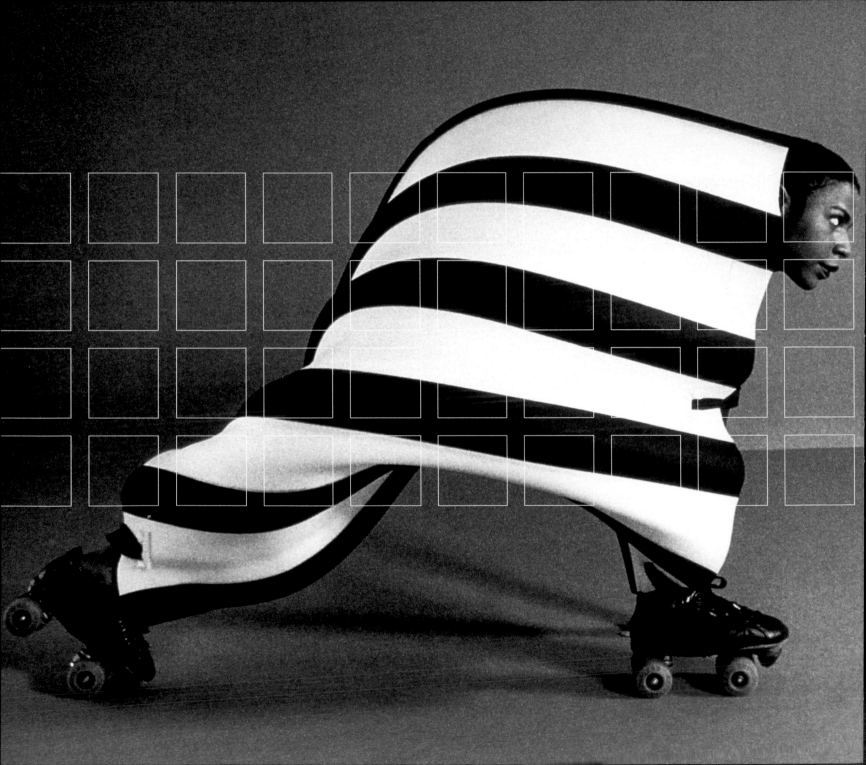

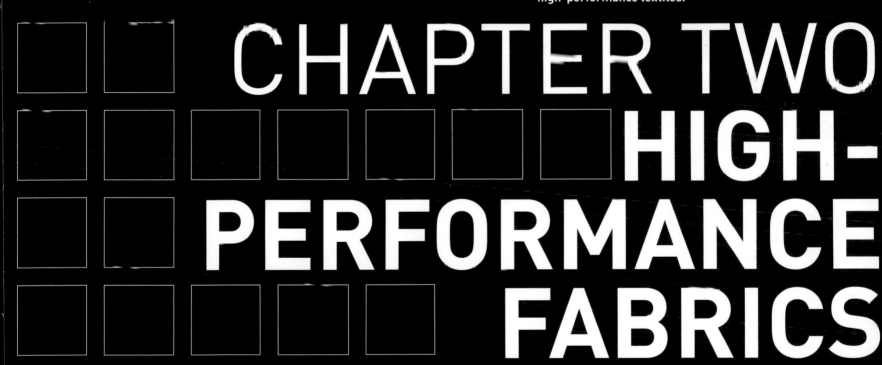

Since the 1990s there has been a great demand for out-of-the-ordinary sporting challenges. In growing numbers people are taking up seriously dangerous sports that push them to their physical and mental limits. There has also been more participation in 'street sports' such as kick-boxing, skateboarding and baseball. Yoga is the perfect non-competitive workout at any age, and older consumers, now known as the 'grey market', are undertaking more exercise – sports clothes for the more mature have to take account of physical changes. Sports clothing is a huge industry in the USA, and in the UK it accounts for almost half the sports goods market. International exhibitions devoted to sports are on the increase, and show the latest high-performance textiles.

CHAPTER TWO
HIGH-PERFORMANCE FABRICS

The textile industry invests heavily in research and development, and new processes and inventions are constantly being used for sports clothes. Many companies in this area work directly with textile researchers, designers and manufacturers to make functional materials in response to specific and sometimes extraordinary demands. Fibre and fabric engineering can produce very sophisticated materials that provide optimum function, efficiency and comfort as well as looking distinctive and handling well. Consumers expect technology to improve their personal best in their chosen sport, and have become very aware of what they are buying. Technical textile information is now given on garment tags, and these frequently list advanced performance characteristics.

Maria Blaisse, *Striped Square*, 1996–97. The dancer wears rollerblades and light, protective synthetic foam for Maria Blaisse's experimental dance project, *Kuma Guna*, as performed in Amsterdam. Strips of black and white industrial foam are laminated together, forming simple shapes.

Kombat 2000, the national Italian football team outfit, is made from Supplex and Lycra (both by DuPont). It wicks moisture away from the skin fast, making it efficient for high-energy sports. Supplex is polyamide-based but has a natural appearance and feel. Lycra is an elastane fibre, and its stretch property allows optimum movement.

FUNCTIONAL SPORTS CLOTHING

Extreme and dangerous activities require fully protective and durable clothing. Winter sports have had many highly functional textiles developed for them, and fabrics for summer sports are state-of-the-art textiles that are comfortable in hot weather because they can help control body temperature. Increase in demand has come at a time when sophisticated technological developments can produce textiles that answer these very specific requirements.

Clothes for team games, besides giving protection from the elements, must also be a defence against other players and their equipment. Climbers need protection in case of falls. In watersports, clothes help prevent drowning, and a one-piece wetsuit using the latest technical materials can keep the wearer warm for many hours, which could mean the difference between life and death. It is compulsory for Formula One motor-racing drivers to wear fire-resistant garments and helmets to protect the head from impact,

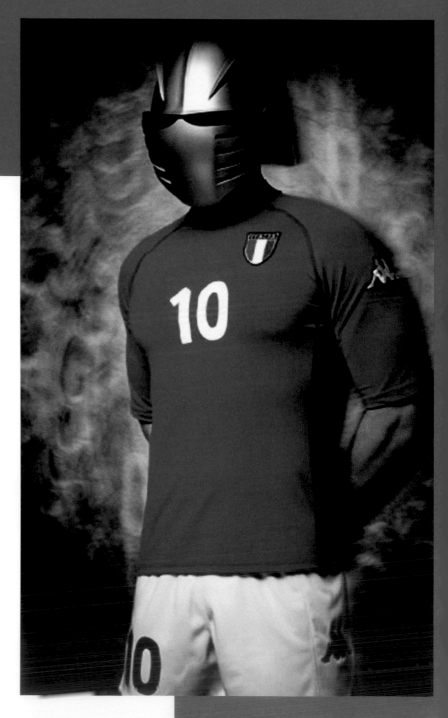

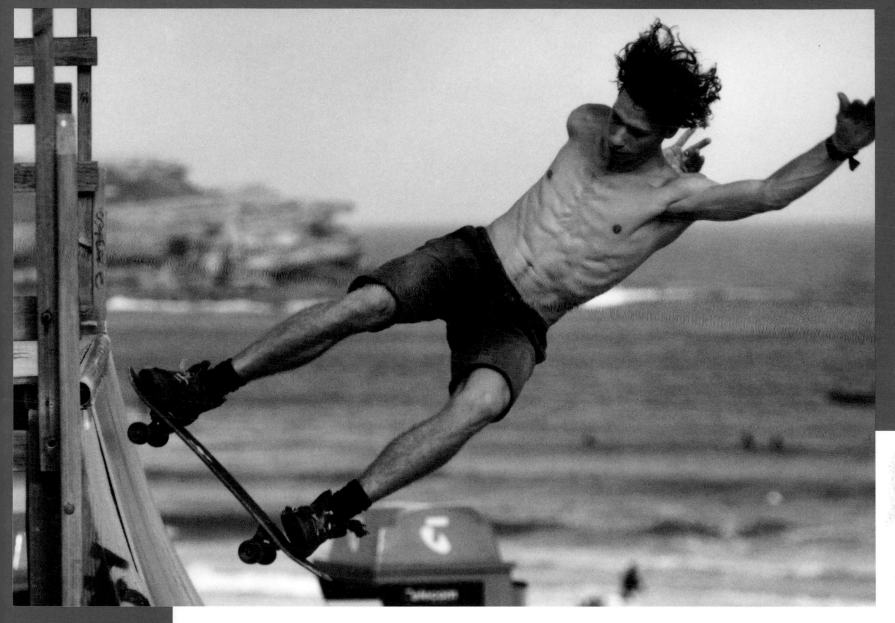

and this has led to a sharp decrease in fatalities. New textiles, lightweight, strong and durable, mean that there is no longer a need for bulk to protect the vulnerable areas of head, chest, arms, thighs, knees and genitals, and the materials chosen are rigorously tested to high levels.

Lightweight flexibles that offer superior protection were often first developed for space programmes or for the military, and the technologies have filtered down to sports. A case in point is Aerogel, invented in the 1930s, and used by NASA to insulate the probe Pathfinder on its mission to Mars. This ultra-lightweight material (only three times denser than air) is now being used for clothing, where it offers supreme insulation in conditions of extreme cold, but at a price – it is still very expensive. Velcro was originally designed for the US space programme in the 1950s, and is a very strong material as well as being flexible and lightweight. It is a fastening device that can be secured with one hand at places that are difficult to access, such as the wrists and ankles. It is sewn in strips to clothes or accessories, and is machine-washable.

A skateboarder pushes his performance to the limit on a half-pipe at Bondi Beach, Australia. He wears little but shorts and boots, nevertheless skateboarding fashion and protective wear now has its own strong cult following.

schoeller-keprotec, by the Swiss
company Schoeller, is a high-tech
fabric very resistant to wear
and tear. A textile incorporating
Cordura and Kevlar (both by
DuPont), rigorously tested, it is
used for motorcycle apparel
and trekking boots. schoeller-
keprotec-spirit is shown below
left, and technical schoeller-
keprotec materials below right.

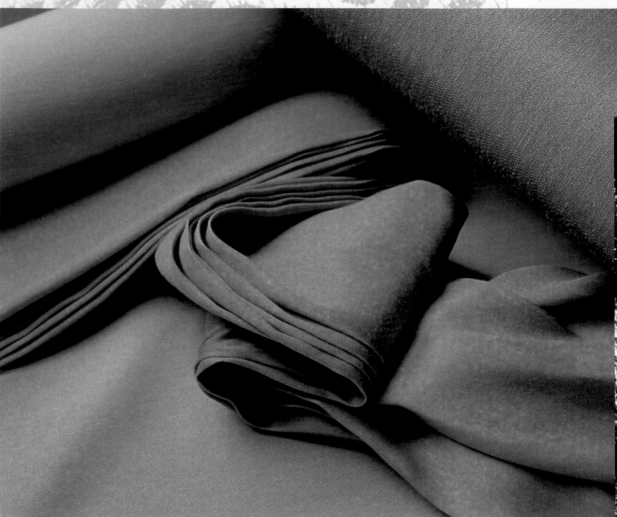

For ultimate protection, sophisticated textiles
are being produced that offer maximum
strength. These are rigorously tested, and
are designed for clothing and accessories
for extreme sports.

An important physiological function of the
human body is its ability to sweat. Activity
generates heat, and the body cools itself
down by the evaporation of sweat on the skin.

There are different types of perspiration – light
sweating (vapour-phase) to heavy sweating
(liquid-phase). Summer sports clothes need
to deal with liquid-phase perspiration. Sweat
has to be drawn quickly away from the skin
to the fabric surface to keep the wearer dry;
if moisture cools on the body there is an
unpleasant chilling effect. Effective clothing
must work with this system, and control both
the build-up of perspiration and heat loss.

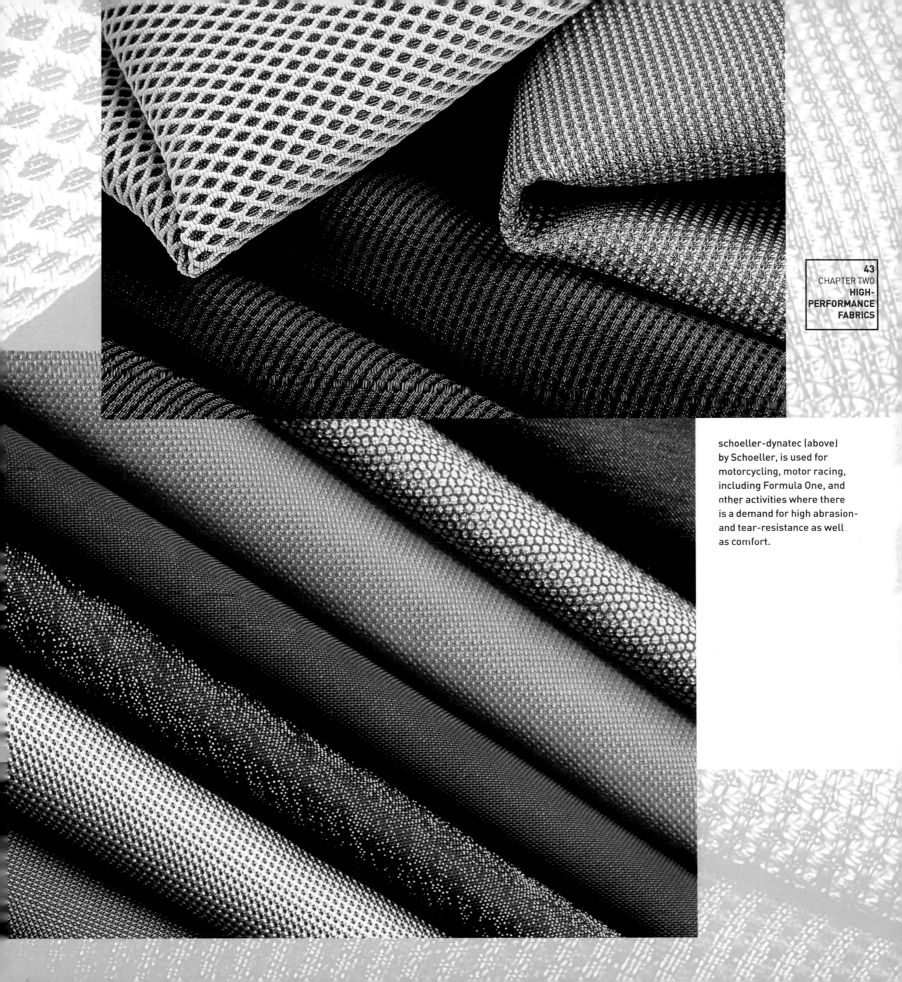

schoeller-dynatec (above)
by Schoeller, is used for
motorcycling, motor racing,
including Formula One, and
other activities where there
is a demand for high abrasion-
and tear-resistance as well
as comfort.

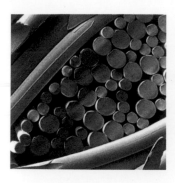
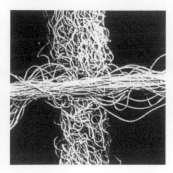
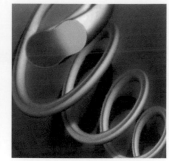

Tactel (DuPont) is made from a versatile nylon polymer derived from crude oil turned into Polyamide 6.6. Tactel HT (cross-section far left) uses technology developed for parachutes and hot-air balloons, and is very strong and abrasion-resistant. Tactel multisoft (centre left) is lightweight, strong and very soft. Tactel ispira (left) is elastic, strong and dries quickly.

HIGH-PERFORMANCE SYNTHETICS

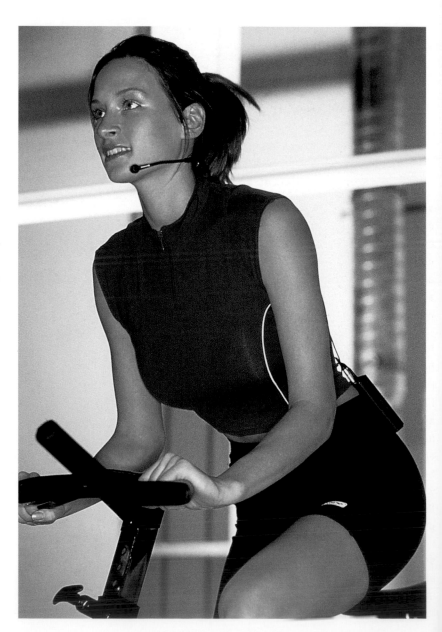

Advanced synthetics are now frequently chosen for outdoor winter sports because they are generally weatherproof while also being breathable, abrasion-resistant and durable. Most synthetics are thermoplastic (pliable when subjected to heat, taking on new surface effects and forms). Advanced industrial materials, including synthetic rubbers, closed-cell foams and nonwovens, can be laminated to achieve various effects, or vacuum-moulded to create surface relief or three-dimensional forms. Synthetic textiles, once thought inferior to naturals, are now increasingly appreciated by the general public.

Polyester

Polyester has been used for athletic wear since the 1950s, but really came into its own in the 1970s for leisure wear because of its easy-care characteristics. Polyester is used for many sophisticated synthetics, and most microfibres are either polyester or polyamide. Microfibres (defined as being a yarn of one denier or less) are ultra-lightweight and fine, soft yet very strong, making them both comfortable and highly functional. They can be engineered to be anti-static, anti-stress, UV-resistant, high-stretch and thermo-isolating (warm in winter, cool in summer).

Tactel aquator is a special type of Tactel (DuPont), which can be designed in 100% Tactel or blended with other fibres in the outer layer. Here it is blended with cotton, which absorbs moisture that the Tactel content then holds away from the skin, and 14% Lycra (DuPont) for stretch. Arena, have used this textile for its Instructor line – designed for professional fitness instructors.

The New Evolution workout collection by adidas uses DuPont fabrics. The high-performance polyamides Tactel and Supplex are blended with Lycra for an elastic textile that gives support while allowing maximum movement.

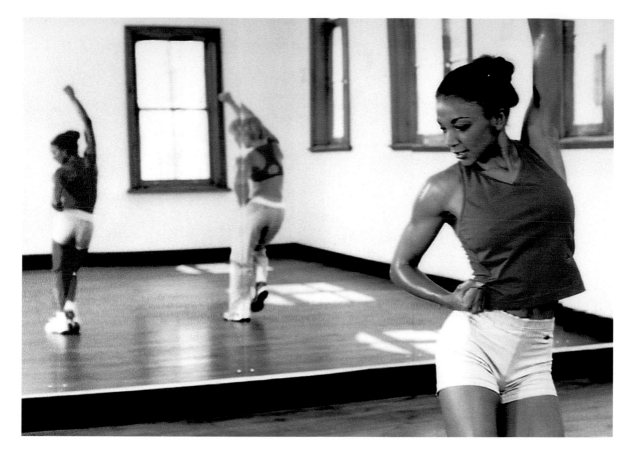

Various fleeces made of polyester were originally developed for mountaineering and exploring. Resembling a woollen fleece in appearance and texture, the new types are very lightweight and quick-drying (they are almost dry when removed from the washing-machine).

PCR (post-consumer recycled) polyester fleece derived from waste plastic bottles (from Malden Mills, USA, for example) offers high protection from harsh climates; minute air pockets insulate the wearer for a warm and very comfortable garment that is also environmentally sound. Different fabrics can be created for many different conditions, and variations include double-sided fleece, dense fleece with a smooth surface for extra weather protection and fleece that, it is claimed, blocks wind effectively in hostile conditions. First seen on the mountain slopes worn by skiers and climbers, polyester fleece is now also used for sailing as well as more general leisure and travel wear.

As polyester is a synthetic, it can be specially engineered to create a whole range of effects. The fibre can be given a grooved section to allow moisture to escape by capillary action so that it dries fast. The design of the fibre also enables it to act as a wick, drawing moisture rapidly away from the body to the outer surface where it evaporates. Other polyester fibres also work on the capillary principle, with a filament yarn used on the inside and a microfibre denier on the outside so that moisture is quickly taken from the wearer's skin, the inner face remaining dry even when the outer face is wet. Modifications to polyester can give it a high resistance to stretching, twisting and breaking, or to chlorine damage, or can impart a three-dimensional elasticity for increased comfort.

Polyamide-based

Nylon, or polyamide as it is also known, was originally created for technical and industrial use in the 1950s. Because it is a synthetic, it is easy to adapt – even its molecular structure can be altered – and it has many applications for sports textiles. Polyamide 6.6 is derived from crude oil and is used as the basis for many microfibres. High-tech fibre engineering allows polyamide to take on a variety of looks, handling qualities and performance properties, such as the rapid wicking of perspiration. Its inherent versatility from next-to-body-wear to specialist outdoor wear satisfies a wide and ever-changing market.

Polyamides can be treated, by air-texturing, for example, to give them a natural look and soft handle. Some even feel and look like cotton, but are abrasion-resistant, strong, lightweight, and, unlike cotton, quick-drying and easy-care. Polyamide blends well with many other fibres, including naturals, regenerated fibres and synthetics. A blend of polyamide with Lycra (DuPont) can result in a fabric that is comfortable and gives support, and a blend with Teflon (DuPont) one that is water-repellent and stain-resistant.

Neoprene/foam/nonwovens

Neoprene is a synthetic rubber-like polymer with perforations shaped like honeycomb cells, giving it good insulating properties. Since 1952, when Jack O'Neill invented the all-in-one neoprene wetsuit, neoprene has been the material of choice for surfing and diving wetsuits, as it is waterproof, lightweight, breathable, soft, warm, high-stretch, resilient and dries fast. Wetsuits were previously bulkier and less comfortable, but now there are special types of neoprene, including ultra-fine and super-lightweight. Carbon can be integrated into the fibre

Spartan Limited, 3D Dry Limited Edition. 3-DIS (Three-Dimensional Intelligent Skin) Carbon Cel neoprene by the Japanese manufacturer Yamamoto, is used for this wetsuit. It incorporates Spherical Carbon, which distributes stress, and an FE polymer, which prevents 'self-curing'. On the outside of the inner layer and on the inside of the outer layer is a titanium coating finished with polytetrafluoroethylene (PTFE). The two layers trap air for better insulation, and the seams are chemically bonded.

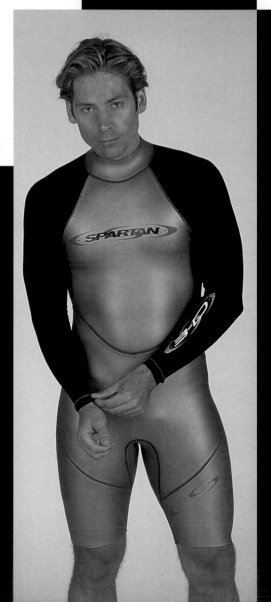
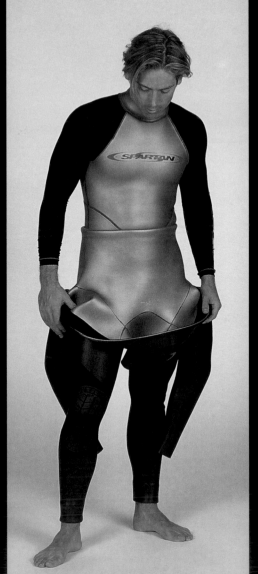
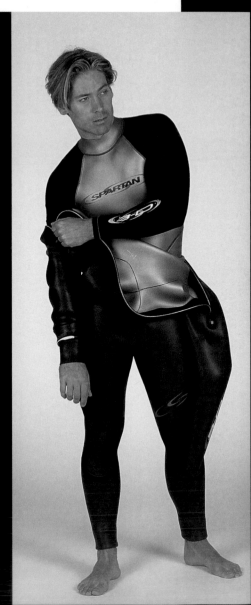

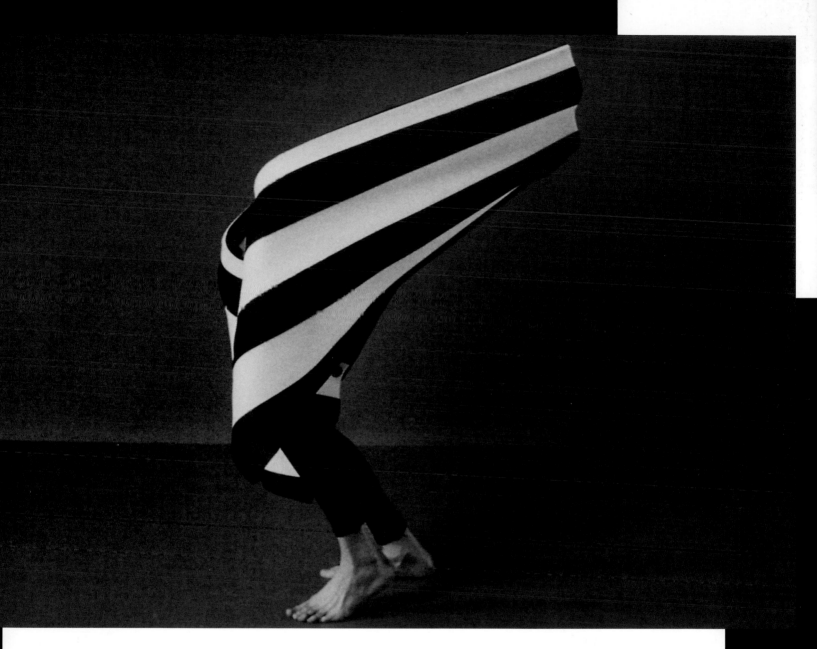

Maria Blaisse, *Striped Square*, 1996–97, from the dance production *Kuma Guna*, Amsterdam, choreographed by Susan Rethorst. The Dutch designer Maria Blaisse researches the essence of form to create powerful performance works. This dynamic image emphasizes movement and speed. Soft, flexible synthetic foam is an ideal material for performance, as it springs quickly back to its original shape when crushed.

to distribute stretch and compression properties evenly, which prevents stress build-up; any shock or load is taken across the entire wetsuit – localized, this would cause a weak area. Stretch occurs without loss of density to the neoprene so the wearer keeps as warm as possible. Neoprene can be bonded, which makes it extremely durable, and the introduction of certain types of polymer can prevent 'self-curing' and maintain flexibility.

A wetsuit made from these new-generation neoprenes is totally protective and feels like

a second skin. This material is now being used for many sports, and research and development has produced new combinations, including bonded neoprene and jersey, and neoprene with polyester fleece that out-performs other polyester fleeces. These thermoplastic textiles can be machine-moulded to create very lightweight and flexible waterproof garments.

Synthetic foams are often used in sports clothes because they are ultra-lightweight, soft and flexible, giving both ease of movement and protective volume. Foam

Rhovyl Sport fleece top. The French company Rhovyl has used the PVC-based chlorofibre Rhovyl'Up. Developed specifically for such sports as skiing and mountain climbing, this antibacterial textile has high-performance properties and extreme comfort. Its capillary action wicks sweat away fast, helping to maintain a constant body temperature. It insulates and is flame-retardant.

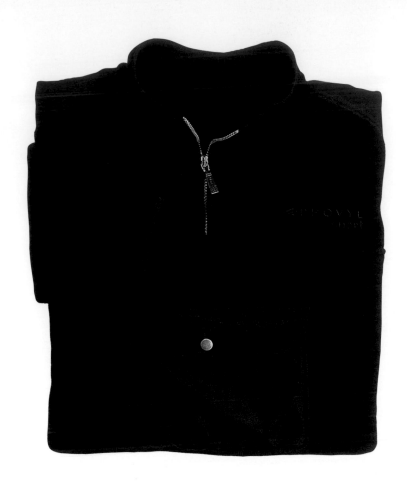

Lucy Orta, *Refuge Wear, Double Cocoon*, commissioned by Expofil 2000. This artwork comments on the nature of survival. Its multi-functional sleeping bag/shelter for the new urban nomads utilizes the latest high-performance materials. Double Cocoon is made of a velvet Rhovyl AS antibacterial chlorofibre knitted textile, with Meryl Nexten (Nylstar) coated with Teflon (DuPont) between a microporous polyurethane and Trevira fleece, which is laminated with Isofilm (Eschler) and silk-screen-printed. The hollow construction of the Meryl Nexten fibre reduces weight and provides insulation. The print communicates a message using universally understood imagery – here a compass and a rope.

naturally absorbs stress and energy from an impact and spreads the force. Closed-cell foam is very versatile: it can be rigid and unyielding or fluid and soft. Helmets with their rigid outer shells often have linings of compressible foam. When the energy is absorbed the foam is crushed and protects the wearer's head (once this has occurred, the foam holds no more energy and the helmet must be replaced).

Nonwovens were first developed for medical or protective purposes, and are now seen in the manufacture of clothes both for sports and fashion. A nonwoven is made of a web of fibres, and these fibres are bonded using a variety of techniques, such as heat treatments and water jets, friction, interlacing, glueing, needle-punching, or combinations of any of these. The cloth once bonded can then be dyed and coated.

Nonwoven fabrics are not generally as stable as a woven or knitted construction, but they can be given greater tensile strength by bonding them with a membrane. New nonwovens can be ultra-lightweight, and some have a high percentage of Lycra for elasticity. Others can be micro-perforated to give them an insulating property, and very fine sheets of nonwovens can be fused to other fabrics to make them multifunctional.

Aramids and chlorofibres

An aramid is a particular type of nylon (polyamide) that has been engineered to include six-membered carbon rings in its molecular structure. Aramids are generally very strong and also capable of withstanding extremely cold temperatures. Kevlar (made by DuPont) is an example of an aramid fabric which can offer a tough, dense surface which absorbs energy and can even prevent the passage of bullets. Kevlar was originally developed for spacesuits and space vehicles in the 1950s, but is now used in sports clothes and equipment. This high-performance textile resists abrasion, and is one of the strongest

and most durable materials available. Aramid microfilaments are being developed in Japan where research has produced very strong and lightweight aramid microfibres that are used for their protective and performance capabilities.

Chlorofibre is a generic name indicating that more than 50 per cent of the textile's make-up is polyvinyl chloride (PVC). Chlorofibres are generally mixed with other yarns, such as cotton, silk, wool or acrylic, to produce a functional textile. The chlorofibre content helps the textile retain its shape and enables it when crushed to return quickly to its original state. These chlorofibre-based fabrics have significant advantages for those who take part in highly active and energetic sports. Textiles can be produced with a variety of useful performance characteristics – they can be insulating or flame-retardant, for example, and the synthetic content of the textiles gives the clothes made from them easy-care characteristics.

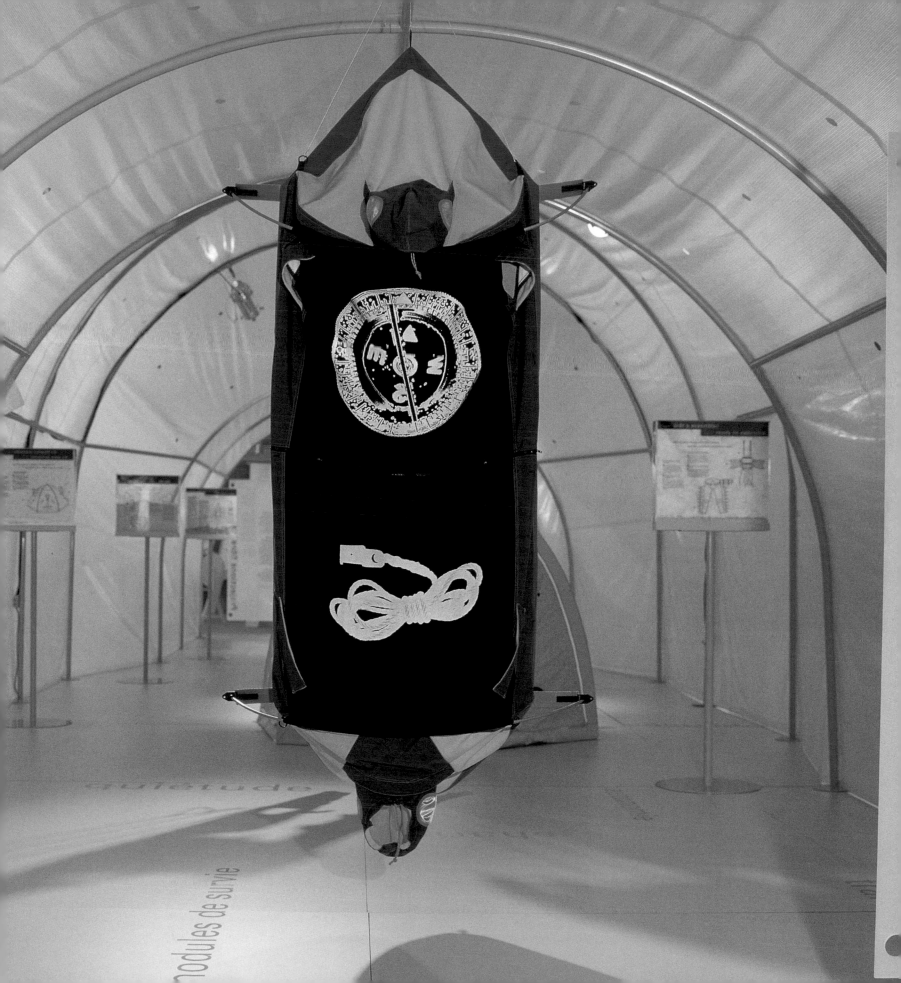

A blend of Amicor and cotton is used for tennis wear by the German company Essence. Amicor is the trade name for specially engineered antimicrobial fibres by Acordis. They keep clothes smelling fresh for longer by preventing the growth of bacteria when the body sweats. The special acrylic fibre is constructed with a core that emits the antibacterial agent (Triclosan by Ciba) only when required so that the property will last – usually around 200 washes.

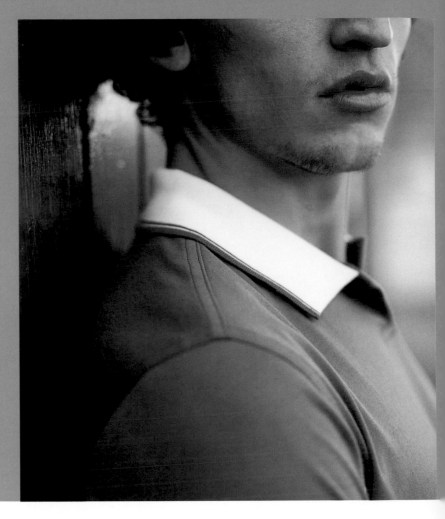

MICROTECHNOLOGY

Microtechnology has produced extremely sophisticated materials that have revolutionized the sports market, such as fabrics made from microfibres. Innovations in technically advanced textiles for performance wear has led to very fine deniers, including high-performance microfibres and ultra-microfibres for 'second-skins'. Most are made from either polyester or polyamide filament. The old attitude to synthetics was that they were uncomfortable during activity, but these new synthetics have transformed their reputation.

Microfibres usually blend well with other fibres to extend the range of their performance qualities. A cloth with a micro denier can be totally designed and engineered – from the internal core to the outer surface – to answer specific needs; microcrimped loops, for example, create flexible and durable fabrics. Texture and look is an important feature of today's fabrics, and these fine fibres can be air-textured (blasted with air to roughen the surface) or given a lively surface interest with various yarn twists.

The Japanese word for a new synthetic fibre is 'shingosen'. Researched and developed in Japan since the 1960s, many are polyester-derived. The aim is to improve on, not to imitate, natural fibres. Shingosen are distinct from other polyester fibres in their utilization of the latest in technology, including microtechnology.

Microencapsulation technology has developed fabrics with a variety of 'health-giving' and 'well-being' substances contained in minute bubbles suspended along their fibres. As the textile creases when worn, the bubbles break and gradually release their contents into the skin of the wearer. Originally developed for astronauts, for survival wear, for protective wear and for reusable surgical gowns, these fibres are now being used for sports clothes and both ready-to-wear and high fashion. Microfibres can be impregnated with vitamins, healing substances and fragrances, including essential oils that reduce stress or prevent insomnia, or aloe vera moisturizer with its antibacterial properties. Sensors built into the fibres can enable the textile to respond to certain stimuli. A fabric of the future could well contain many small polystyrene balls to massage the wearer and relieve tension.

Antimicrobial fabrics guard against disease by repelling and fighting bacteria, though not destroying them totally, since they play an important role in the ecosystem of our bodies. By monitoring a wide range of microbes, these fibres can inhibit bacteria and such unwelcome fungi growth as athlete's foot, which tends to thrive in the hot, damp environments on an active person's body. Antimicrobials can also prevent body odours. There are some materials that are naturally antimicrobial – both copper and ceramic are used to prevent the growth of bacteria.

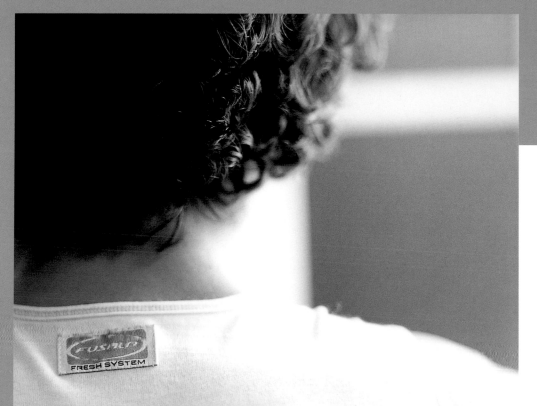

Base layer of Amicor blended with polyester by the French company Fusalp which produces specialist wear for activities such as mountaineering and skiing. Amicor (by Acordis) blends well with most fibres, both natural and synthetic – only low percentages (around 20%) are needed for the textile to be effective.

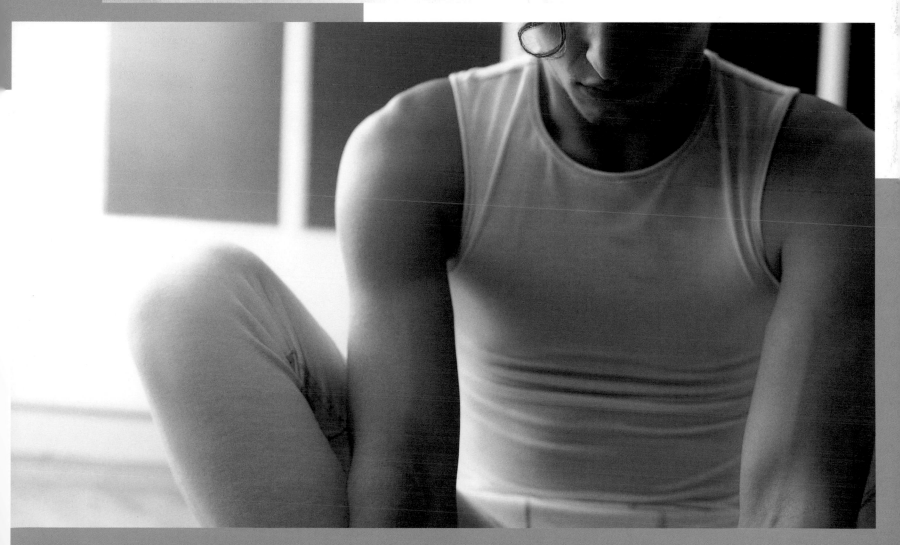

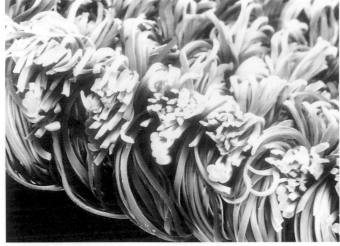

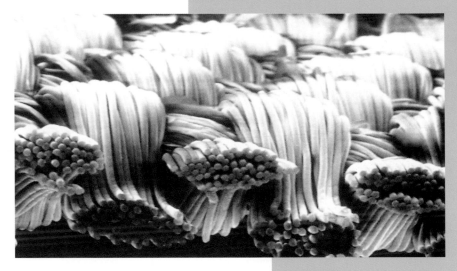

Meryl Nexten (Registered trademark by Nylstar – polyamide fibre). This hollow fibre (opposite) from the Meryl range offers high insulation – air is trapped in the fibre core. Blended with other fibres such as cotton, linen, wool and viscose, it is used for both base-layer and outer-layer sports clothing, especially skiwear. It is ultra-lightweight but its bulk ensures that it drapes well, which also makes it popular for ready-to-wear tailoring.

Meryl Satiné (Registered trademark by Nylstar – polyamide fibre). Meryl is a range of speciality yarns made from ultra-fine polyamide that offer superior properties, and are used for clothes from extreme sports to casual wear. Meryl Satiné has a fibre with a lengthened rectangular cross-section that gives it a sophisticated sheen. It also has an attractive soft handle, good abrasion-resistance and resists pilling. The subtle sparkle of this fibre has many applications, including next-to-skin bodywear.

Meryl Microfibre (Registered trademark by Nylstar – polyamide fibre). Microfibre specialities by Nylstar's Meryl can be used for very fine, closely woven or knitted fabrics (a woven cloth is shown above). Meryl textiles are ultra-soft, weatherproof, comfortable and breathable. They are suitable for lightweight garments next to the skin, especially for sports base layers.

Using microtechnology, an antibacterial or antifungal agent is added either at the yarn-construction stage or as a finishing treatment. A commonly used antibacterial agent is Triclosan (manufactured by Ciba) which is found in toothpastes and mouthwashes. Benzyl benzoate is the agent in textiles that protect against dust-mite allergy because it removes the fungi and bacteria on which dust-mites feed. These fibres blend well with natural, regenerated and synthetic fibres, often at low percentages, which enables the main fibre to retain its look and texture. When the active agent is an integral part of the fibre, the effect tends to last the life of the garment (or up to around two hundred washes) since it emits the substance slowly, and only when needed. Sometimes the agent works by penetrating the fibre itself as well as coating the surface. Clothing made with these speciality fibres smells fresh for longer, and will need washing less often than conventional fibres; it also tends to be non-irritant and therefore appropriate for asthmatics and those with skin allergies.

Cotton is popular in sports attire for its soft handling qualities, but, being naturally very absorbent, without an antimicrobial agent it provides a breeding-ground for bacteria. Antibacterial textiles are used in next-to-skin active sportswear, jacket linings, fillings (wadded fabrics), for multifunctional clothing – in particular adventure and travel wear, and for underwear-as-outerwear in the fashion world. Antibacterial and antifungal textiles also tend to be used for socks and for liners for athletic footwear.

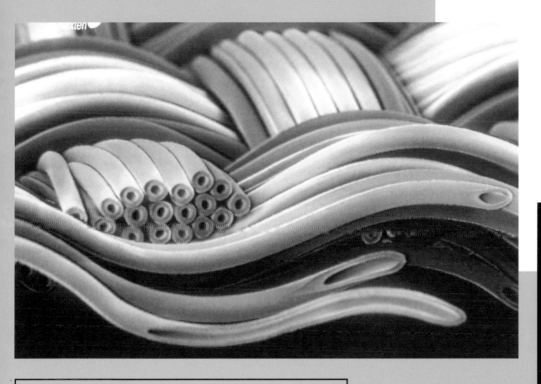

CoolMax (DuPont) is made of a very high-density Dacron polyester which is a hydrophilic polymer. This fibre has a grooved section to allow moisture to escape by capillary action and it therefore dries fast. It is shown here in combination with Tactel aquator (by DuPont), and with Lycra (also DuPont) for a sports bra by Triumph.

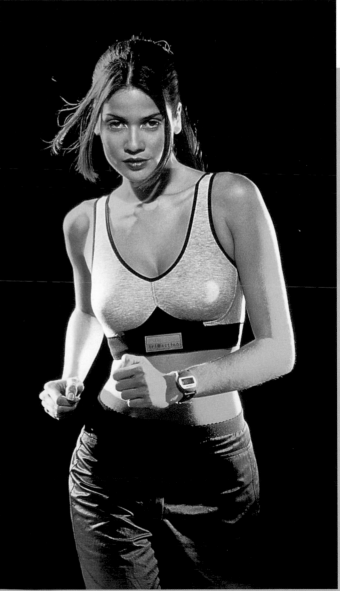

THERMOREGULATORS

Thermoregulating textiles are a development of the new technology. They work well in both hot and cold conditions, so clothes do not need to be removed during activity or added when cooling down. Conventional fabrics allow more heat loss which may prevent the wearer from performing to the best of his or her ability. Thermoregulating fabrics are very suitable for such sports as mountaineering and tennis, and also for beach and travel wear.

There are advanced technical fabrics that have specialist finishes in the form of water-resistant and breathable thermal-control membranes made of polyurethane resin. The molecular structure of the membrane varies according to temperature – when it is low, heat retention is efficient as the polymer molecules tighten up and insulate the wearer, and when high, the molecules move freely and away from each other to allow the fabric to breathe.

Hollow fibres

Some textiles use hollow fibres that trap air and insulate the wearer efficiently. This is a relatively new field, and is very successful owing to advances in fibre-engineering. Fibres can be made ultra-lightweight (up to 130 per cent lighter) with a hollow core construction that provides insulation by trapping air both inside and in between the fibres for maximum effect. Hollow fibres are generally blended with other fibres. Depending on the fabric structure, the textiles can be very fine, breathable, waterproof, quick-drying, provide good warmth-to-weight ratio and possess a volume. They are used for both underwear and outerwear in a range of sports activities.

Phase-change materials

Textiles for active wear should be capable of assisting the wearer to maintain a constant body temperature. This makes for comfort at most levels of sports, and possibly survival in dangerous and extreme sports. Sports clothes generally follow the body's contours, and, ideally, moisture from the perspiration should travel through the fabric to the outside surface as quickly as possible for the wearer to feel dry and comfortable. A fabric is required that removes the heat and stores it, to release it gradually when needed to keep the wearer at a constant temperature for longer. This is exactly the science behind the latest phase-change materials (PCMs), which absorb body heat and store it to release it later.

Phase-change technology, originally developed by NASA, enables a textile to adapt to changes in the weather and to environments from the Arctic to the Sahara.

In all sports, the muscles need to be kept at an optimum temperature to operate to their full potential. PCMs can help prevent the muscles from seizing up, and are useful for both warm-up and cool-down clothing (significantly reducing the risk of chilling). Phase-change technology uses materials that respond to both body and environmental temperatures, for example, paraffin wax. This can be added in the form of a microthermal membrane, which, making use of microencapsulating technology, contains the phase-change material within an acrylic shell. This membrane is incorporated into the actual fabric, between an inner and an outer layer. Alternatively, a garment lining can be given a PCM film with a plastic coating. Excess temperature is absorbed by the PCM which liquefies and distributes the heat evenly before storing it. As the temperature drops, the material becomes solid, and gradually releases the stored heat. In this way, overheating is prevented, and warmth will be generated after energy is expended.

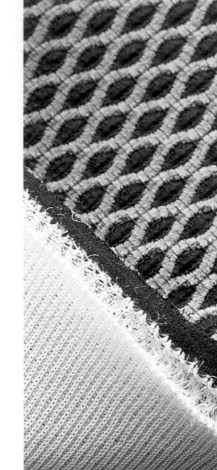

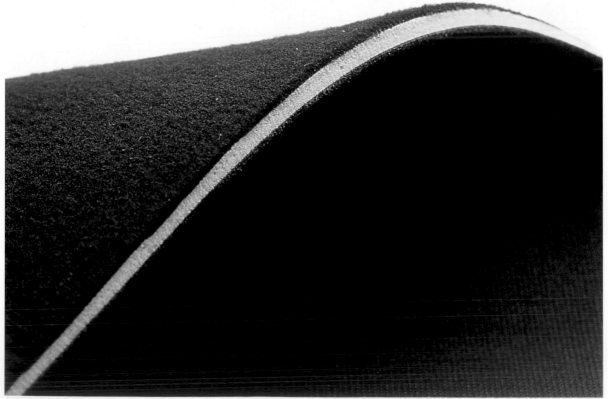

schoeller-ComforTemp (left and above) is produced by Schoeller, and ComforTemp is a registered trademark of Frisby Technologies, USA. The textile actively balances out temperature extremes and is based on phase-change technology. This high-tech textile has microcapsules that trap paraffin wax to regulate body temperature. The three-layer structure of the textile can clearly be seen.

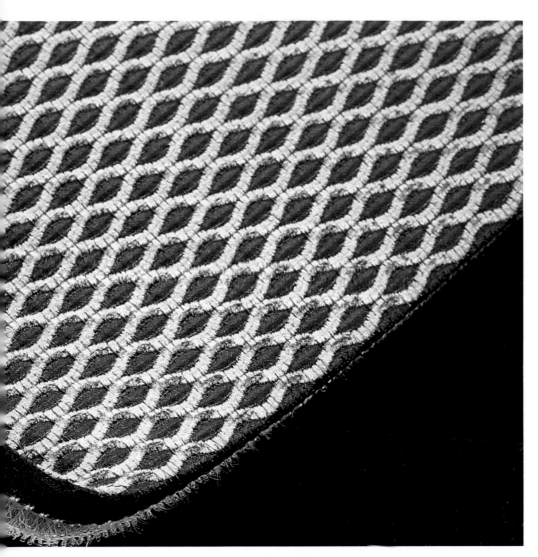

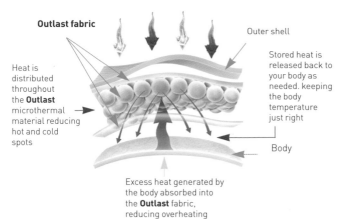

FABRIC
Harsh outside environment

Outlast fabric

Outer shell

Heat is distributed throughout the **Outlast** microthermal material reducing hot and cold spots

Stored heat is released back to your body as needed. keeping the body temperature just right

Body

Excess heat generated by the body absorbed into the **Outlast** fabric, reducing overheating

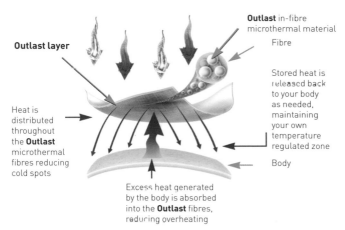

FIBRE
Harsh outside environment

Outlast in-fibre microthermal material

Outlast layer

Fibre

Heat is distributed throughout the **Outlast** microthermal fibres reducing cold spots

Stored heat is released back to your body as needed, maintaining your own temperature regulated zone

Body

Excess heat generated by the body is absorbed into the **Outlast** fibres, reducing overheating

Outlast Technologies, Inc, uses phase-change technology (right) for a microthermal material that absorbs excess heat, evenly distributes it over its surface and stores it in order to release it gradually as the body cools after activity. This technology can be used as a fibre, fabric or foam, and a material such as paraffin wax is microencapsulated in an acrylic shell. As it absorbs heat the substance liquefies, and when cool it solidifies.

Some PCMs are even capable of absorbing light and storing it to release it later in dark conditions. These highly functional fibres that create their own microclimate between the fabric and the skin are generally unaffected by water, and add minimum bulk. They provide efficient protection, and are particularly popular for motorcycling and skiing, though they are also used for clothes and footwear in many other sports.

Thermochromic textiles also have their place in sports clothing. These change colour with variations in body temperature – from green to purple to yellow, for instance. This decorative flourish could also have a functional use, such as signalling to the wearer when to stop physical exertion.

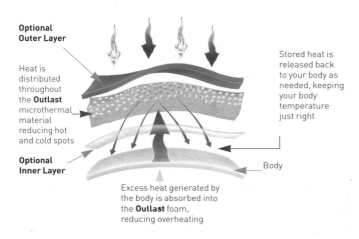

FOAM
Harsh outside environment

Optional Outer Layer

Heat is distributed throughout the **Outlast** microthermal material reducing hot and cold spots

Stored heat is released back to your body as needed, keeping your body temperature just right

Optional Inner Layer

Body

Excess heat generated by the body is absorbed into the **Outlast** foam, reducing overheating

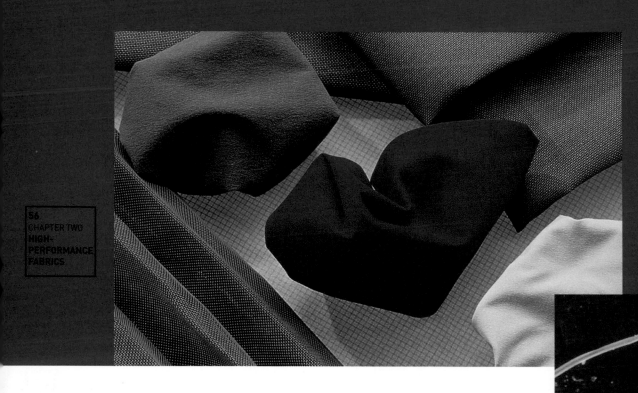

schoeller-adventure. Different stretch materials by Schoeller are shown (left). Elasticity is very important for sports attire, as it allows extreme movement and efficient recovery. These fabrics are also comfortable for the wearer while still looking good.

STRETCH TECHNOLOGY

A stretch property is vital in all sports clothing, and many of the latest fabrics are ultra-fine, lightweight and capable of extreme stretch in every direction. Natural bi-stretch textiles were initially designed for activities like swimming which need garments that are flexible and responsive to every movement. Elastane fibres can totally transform sports clothing – even bulky clothing can have elasticized cuffs and trouser hems to prevent water and wind penetration.

Wool jersey is the original stretch fabric with its natural crimp giving it elasticity. Many versions of fibres (generally synthetics as these can be engineered throughout their entire manufacture) offer stretch capabilities. Elasticity has now become a requirement in all forms of clothing. Clothes fit better and are more comfortable, and allowance can be given for bending, stretching and vigorous activity if necessary. A degree of stretch also means that the textile will naturally bounce back into shape. The 1980s skin-tight, clingy clothing allowed maximum movement, showing off an athletic physique, and was used for all kinds of sports, such as roller-blading, jogging and aerobics. Using the new stretch textiles, seaming and tailoring can be kept to a minimum while still achieving a flattering fitted aesthetic.

Stretch synthetic fibres (in particular DuPont's Lycra) have transformed the look of clothing in the last two decades. Some super-elastics can stretch up to 500 per cent and possess very good shape-retention. Most are also crease-

Elité (Registered trademark by Nylstar) shown before and after dyeing, is made from modified polyester. It has a three-dimensional elasticity and high resistance to breaking. Speedo, Arena and Aquarapid have all used it for swimwear, as it is lightweight, chlorine-resistant and comfortable next to the skin. It takes a range of dyes well, and its production is not harmful to the environment.

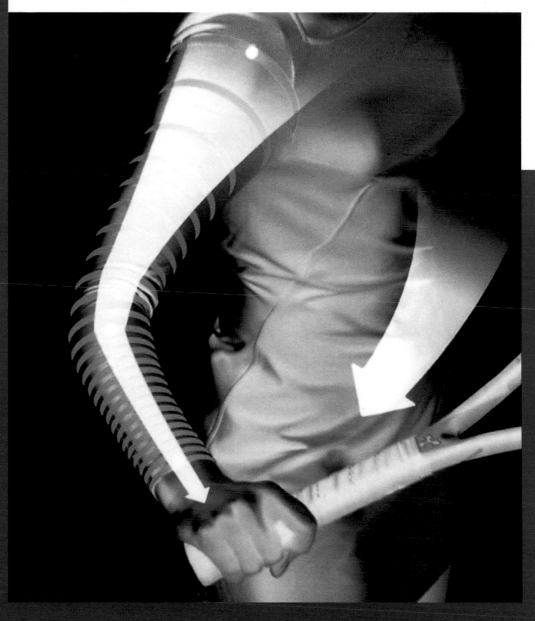

The One-Armed APPrecision Polo is made from DuPont's Lycra power with adidas ClimaLite fabric technology (below). Lycra power was first used by adidas for the athletes in the 1996 Olympics in Atlanta, USA. Lycra power reduces muscle vibration to allow for a more accurate tennis stroke; and Anatomically Placed Protection (APP) offers sports-specific protection from the environment and from injury. The ClimaLite fabric developed by adidas manages moisture effectively, as sweat is wicked away from the skin to evaporate in the air outside the garment.

resistant, durable, fast-drying and can be mixed with a variety of fibres (to give either a natural or a high-tech appearance and handle). The unique properties of leather can be improved by incorporating a degree of stretch. Here, nature and technology are fused to produce an elastic material with wider applications in clothing and accessories, including footwear. Laminating techniques are used, and subsequent stretch-and-recovery capabilities can be excellent. This takes stretch into a new area, as working with skins is very different from working with knitted or woven textiles.

New-generation stretch nonwovens have wide-reaching applications for active wear. Techno-stretch fibres can offer support by providing muscle compression to combat fatigue, and help sports people, dancers and those who exercise to reach their optimum physical performance. Generally, the higher the percentage of elastane the more beneficial the effect. Although stretch fibres can be used to create body-conscious shapes, they are also being used for a relaxed, less clinging fit and ease of movement. Well-being, mobility and speed are emphasized – all considered essential for today's active lifestyle. Superior stretch fibres have been used for all sorts of garments, including sports bras and other close-to-skin bodywear, swimwear and outerwear for athletics and exercise. Lightweight layers and linings with maximum stretch make for multifunctional clothing.

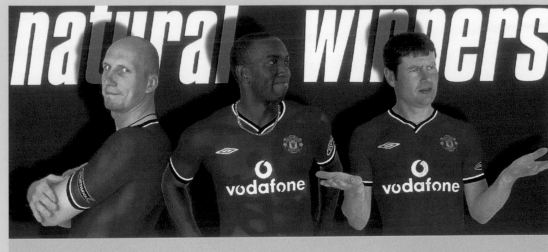

The Woolmark Company, Sportwool. This high-performance textile is made of Australian merino wool with polyester. The fabric accelerates the wicking of moisture-vapour molecules from the skin to the air outside the clothes. The Woolmark Company, Umbro and Manchester United worked together to develop the home soccer shirt for Manchester United, launched August 2000 (right).

TECHNO-NATURALS

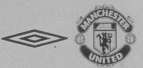

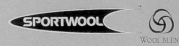

Discover for yourself why Manchester United think their new Sportwool™ shirts are so cool it is like having nothing on…

Innovative in design and production, today's new sports textiles use both synthetic and natural yarns. Natural fibres were previously considered unsuitable for high performance – synthetics, which can be controlled at every stage of their manufacture, were the top choice. Natural fibres, however, are now being combined with synthetics and are given sophisticated treatments to improve their performance. Customers like this new group of 'techno-naturals' or 'super-naturals' because of their familiar look and handle.

Advanced synthetics are frequently combined with such fine quality natural fibres as pure wool, silk, cotton and linen. Some techno-naturals are made from totally natural materials but are manufactured using new techniques. Most, however, are blended with technical synthetics or given sophisticated finishing treatments (coating, laminating and bonding). A softer look is often achieved by blending thicker natural yarns with synthetic. Their volume can be reduced by up to 50 per cent with the latest super-light, thin materials, and in this way traditional heavier wools can be streamlined. Synthetics are now often given finishing treatments to imitate natural fibres, and these are very

popular in sports clothes and also appeal to a wider market. Synthetic yarns can be given a crimp or texture using air-jet technology to create lively surfaces. Balancing natural and synthetic can often combine the best qualities of each. Now wool, silk, cotton and linen can all be easy-care – they can be washed with other fibres without risk of shrinking or going out of shape.

People tend to believe that all things natural are good and all synthetics harmful, but this is not necessarily the case. Natural cotton may need bleaching, dyeing and finishing, all of which can harm the environment, while synthetics, because they can be specifically engineered, do not always require these processes. The new techno-naturals are usually eco-friendly fabrics, and the development of organic materials means an increasing number of environmentally sound products.

Wool

Wool has an advanced and complex structure made of a protein similar to the protective outer layer of human skin. Layers of dense wool give increased protection from the elements in winter, while a good choice for summer sports is the long, fine wool of

the merino sheep – comfortable to wear. Wool's crimp gives it natural stretch, resiliency and recovery, and it is also absorbent, soft and light. It manages moisture efficiently, moving it rapidly away from the skin, thereby helping to regulate body temperature. Woollen garments drape well and are crease-resistant. Techno-wool, with technical improvements in addition to its natural properties, is now popular for sports.

Cool Wool by The Woolmark Company is a very lightweight fabric, with all-year-round applications, including next-to-skin sports clothes. Woollen fleeces rival polyester fleeces. Wool and hair textiles can possess many looks and textures in various weights, from natural luxury with mohair, angora and cashmere to alpaca and camel hair and the new lightweight felts. Cashmere is used for after-exercise when the wearer wishes to avoid chilling. It is also popular with those embarking on less physical activities, such as yoga and meditation where it offers both style and comfort.

For active wear, wool is best blended with such synthetics as polyamide, polyester or elastane. A combination of 30 per cent wool

The Australian cyclist Jay Sweet won gold at the Commonwealth Games in 1998 wearing the revolutionary new Sportwool (The Woolmark Company) made from merino wool blended with polyester. The textile proved very suitable for close-fitting cycling clothing as it keeps the skin dry and comfortable.

and 70 per cent polyester offers moisture control as well as insulation to keep the wearer warm in winter and cool in summer. When combined with a stretch yarn, such as Lycra, wool's natural elasticity is enhanced. Wool, traditionally a winter yarn, can be blended with cotton for summer trans-seasonal garments. Merino wool, a high-quality yarn, can be blended successfully with a range of other fibres, including silk, cashmere, linen, viscose, TENCEL (Tencel Ltd), polyester, polyamide and Lycra. In addition, a very fine merino wool can be used as an inner face to a fabric with an outer face of polyamide. The resulting textile is soft and absorbent next to the skin, but has a hard, weatherproof exterior to protect from the elements.

Pure lambswool can be blended with unusual fibres, such as steel, for a combination of softness with strength. DuPont have been looking into blending its synthetics with natural yarns – mixes of polyester and wool, for example, to give softer and more durable cloth. Some companies are investigating organic wool, and others are trying wool mixes for crease-resistance and to prevent pilling. The names of The Woolmark Company's Easy

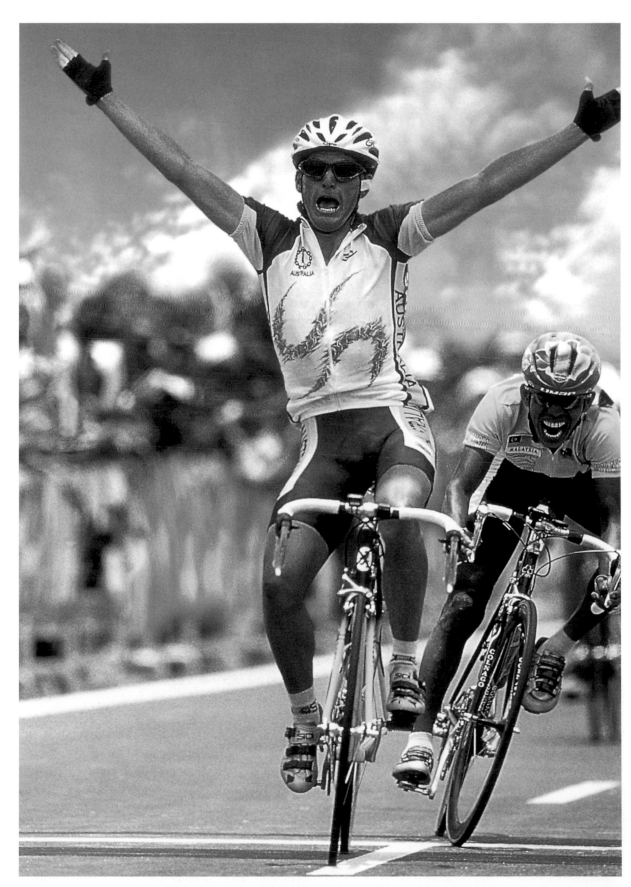

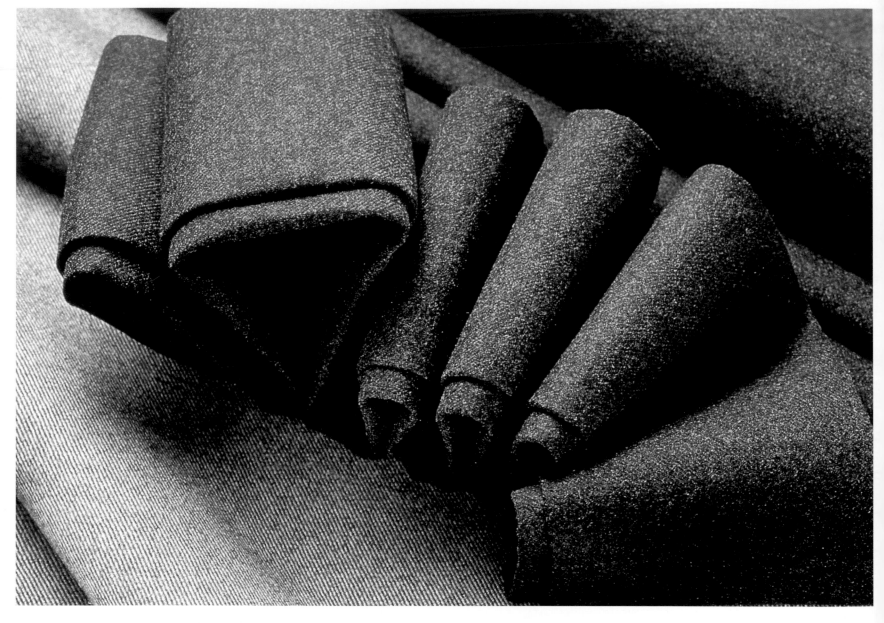

Care and Wear Wool programmes indicate which of its products are non-crease and more durable. Some of the latest blends have a 'Total Easy Care Wool' tag, indicating that garments can be machine-washed and even tumble-dried without shrinkage or loss of elasticity or recovery.

Bonding as well as blending can be used to create new techno-wools in which wool or its blends are heat-fused to other fabrics (usually synthetics). Wool bonded to a waterproof, breathable membrane looks natural but is extremely functional.

Today's finishes can vary from simple brushing of the surface to create volume and trap insulating air to invisible treatments for ultra-violet protection and thermoregulation. Wool with Teflon gives an easy-care textile that repels water and is stain-resistant.

Resin coatings can be synthetic or natural (perhaps from renewable sources), and polyurethane resin can be used to ensure a waterproof textile. Microporous membranes can be fused to wool, and wool can also be laminated to polyester

schoeller-techno-Loden by Schoeller. Loden is a dense woollen textile which keeps the wearer warm and dry when used for outdoor wear. When combined with new developments in textiles, its performance is further enhanced.

microfleece. The Envirowool process results in an absorbent textile with antibacterial properties that will not shrink or felt; this treatment is environmentally friendly as no chlorine is required.

Linen

Linen is a fibre usually thought to be suitable only for summer clothes, but multifunctional techno-linen can suit all seasons, even winter. Linen, like wool, is a naturally high performance textile, and it can be either woven or knitted. Ideal for hot days, it has an instantly recognizable look and texture. It is very absorbent and crisp, and is naturally antimicrobial, but one slight disadvantage is that it creases readily, especially when woven, though some like this characteristic.

Linen as a 'techno-natural', however, has been blended with other fibres, both natural and synthetic, to give high-performance qualities yet retaining its individual character. Popular mixes include wool and linen to give a hairy, felted quality; cashmere, or silk, with linen for a soft, smooth look and texture; and CoolMax (DuPont) with linen for outdoor wear. Finishing treatments can also transform linen – brushing for an ultra-soft surface; glazing; printing; quilting; coating with oil, wax or metal.

Cotton

The super-absorbency of cotton, with its naturally soft yet crisp handle and excellent recovery, makes it a very good choice for summer sportswear – especially for tennis and golf.

Mercerized sea-island cotton (cotton with long, fine fibres from islands off the USA) is high quality and has a surface sheen. When cotton is wet, it quickly becomes saturated and uncomfortable, but the new techno-naturals can improve on this. Densely woven cotton is weatherproof; it has been worn by sailors and aircrews, mountaineers and explorers in the most extreme conditions.

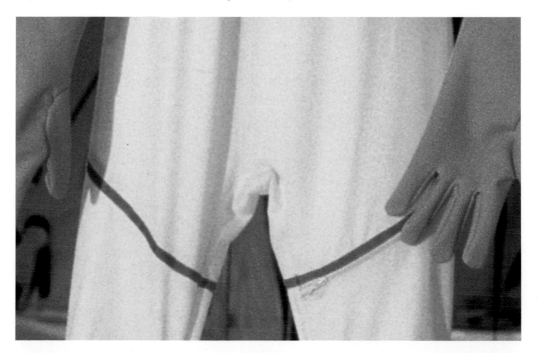

Lucy Orta, *Oxygenation Kit* (detail), commissioned by Expofil 2000. Part of the *Urban Life Guards* series, this suit is made from pure wool treated by the Envirowool process by De Martini-Bayart. This process uses no chlorine and is therefore environmentally friendly.

Prada Sport Menswear, Spring/Summer 2001. Trousers are made of a twisted cotton gabardine with one-way stretch that has been given a Teflon (DuPont) finish to make the textile showerproof and stain-resistant. The towel is made of a bacteria-resistant cotton.

TENCEL, Jersey Textures, Autumn/Winter 1999/2000 (opposite). TENCEL is the registered trademark of Tencel Ltd. Its name comes from 'tensile strength' and 'cellulose'. Made from wood pulp, it is soft and absorbent. TENCEL jersey is very comfortable, and its efficient wicking properties make it a good choice for sports. From right to left: TENCEL and polyester by Rueff (Austria); TENCEL, wool and Lycra (DuPont) by Albaud (France); and TENCEL A100, cotton and Lycra (DuPont) by Calamai (Italy).

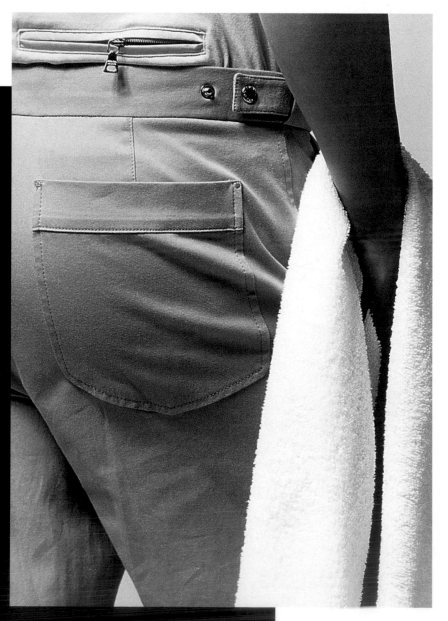

Cotton now has many applications for a wide range of sports.

Very fine cotton corduroys suit the relaxed informality of casual clothes. Cotton and polyamide mixes have been widely used in sports clothing because they perform better than pure cotton. Cotton stretch (with Lycra) is also appreciated for its absorbency and ease of movement. Research and development into cotton fibre has produced cottons that absorb less water and therefore dry faster while still keeping the look and feel of traditional cotton. This new-generation cotton is a much more versatile option for sportswear; it performs well in both hot and cold climates. In some fabrics the cotton fibres are oriented in parallel lines to ensure a very soft, silky cloth that is strong and resistant to abrasion and creasing.

Denim has come a long way from the image of traditional workwear or weekend wear. The classic cotton indigo in all its variations is still a significant seller, but various finishing processes have produced a whole new range. Now there is coloured denim with subtler colours and over-dyeing; aged denim; raw and unfinished denim; 'dirty' denim; denim with such fibres as Lycra; and denim woven with irregular yarns for a unique, 'imperfect' and deconstructed surface. This raw look is very much in demand, and, although the fabric appears damaged, it is in fact very strong. Pigment coatings on the reverse

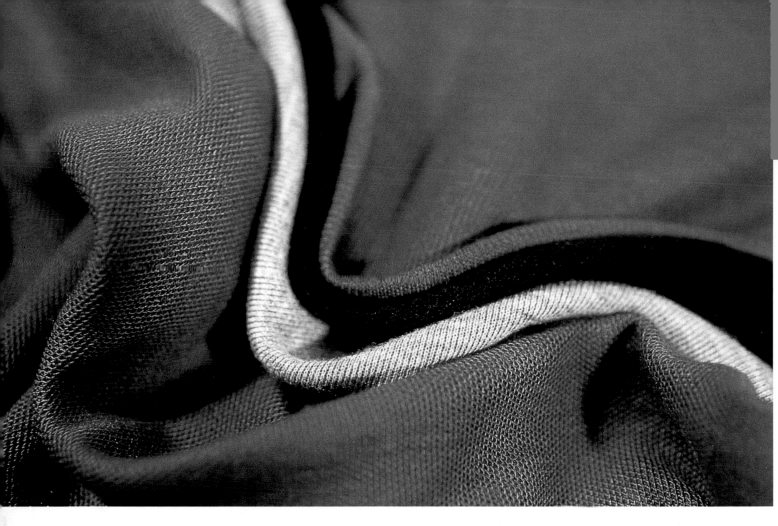

of denim can give an unusual look, while water-splash effects and shiny glitter surfaces are also popular.

Denim was rarely chosen for sports clothes because it becomes heavy when wet and takes a long time to dry. Its natural strength and durability, however, can be enhanced when blended with other fibres, both synthetic and natural. Often these blends provide a particular function, such as moisture-control and management, antimicrobial qualities for active clothing, or increased abrasion-resistance and anti-static properties. Cotton can be mixed with synthetics – Lycra for stretch denim, Tactel (DuPont), Amicor (antimicrobial fibres by Acordis) – and with regenerated fibres – TENCEL A100 (a new version of TENCEL by Tencel Ltd) for performance wear and sports.

Many designers blend TENCEL and denim to give a softer, less absorbent textile, which looks and feels good, and will dry faster when wet. Cotton can also be blended with naturals – linen, wool, silk, cashmere – giving a new look, handle and performance. There are also combinations of denim and stainless steel, copper and carbon fibre.

Denim with the synthetic polyolefin has been engineered to give it a refined wicking system which transports body moisture very quickly to the surface of the fabric where it evaporates. The new denim can therefore be worn for competitive sports, keeping the wearer dry and comfortable. Denim can also be bonded with polyamide net which is aimed in particular at the sports market. In the future, we are promised denim finishes that will

make the textile totally water-repellent and even bulletproof.

With biotechnology, a plastic polymer-infused cotton can be produced that eliminates the need for dyeing. An electrical discharge of metal particles coated with DNA can be introduced into the cell of the cotton to modify permanently the cellulosic fibre core. This genetically modified fibre still looks and feels like pure cotton, but performs better, is crease- and shrink-resistant, less absorbent and comes in various permanent colours.

Organic cotton used to be a niche market, but is now widely available. No pesticides or chemical treatments (dyes, finishes, etc.) are used in its production. Now new developments have improved its feel as

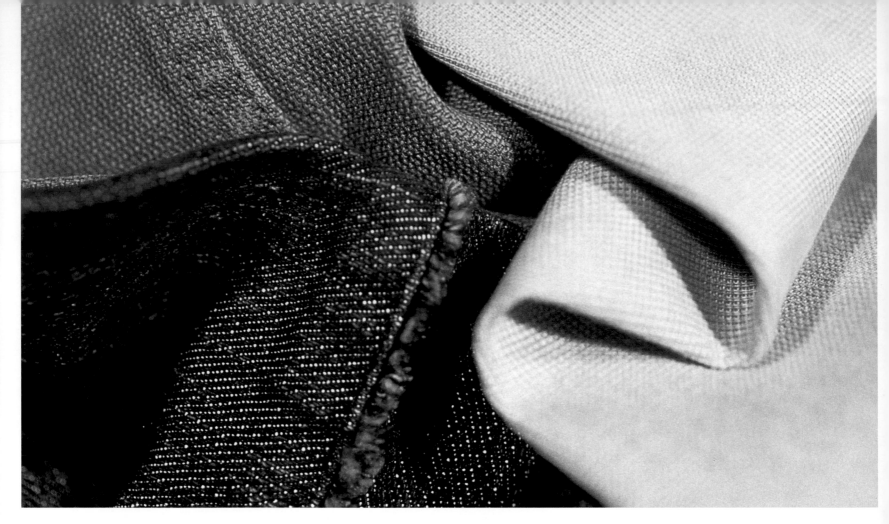

well as its look. Nike and Patagonia in the USA have used organic cotton, as have Esprit in their 1990s E Collection – promoting its use both for sports and for fashion. More companies now produce organic cotton, and the yarn is available in many weights and types, especially fine yarns which are then densely woven for protective textiles. Organic cotton is also being blended with technical fibres for high-performance sportswear.

Regenerated fibres/natural chemicals

Regenerated fibres, or natural chemicals as they are sometimes referred to, are derived from natural sources, which are chemically treated to extrude the fibre. Examples include viscose rayon whose raw material comes from replenishable sources of wood pulp (eucalyptus or American pine), which is then treated and made into an attractive, soft fabric with distinctive performance properties, and which is also environmentally sound.

These cellulosic fibres tend to be absorbent and comfortable. They look and feel natural and also drape well. They can facilitate the rapid movement of moisture from the skin, protecting the wearer from temperature fluctuation both on the body and from the external environment. As the manufacture of the fibre is partly synthesized, it can be controlled and modified to create a wide range of appearance, texture and performance capabilities. Invisible care properties can also be built in for many end uses for clothes used in both professional high-performance sports and for leisure activities. For a silky, smooth appearance and handle as well as increased strength, the fibres can be made to lie parallel with the fibre axis. The fibre can be crimped to provide elasticity and also to trap air between them for insulation. Regenerated fibres blend well with other fibres, both natural and synthetic. They are very soft and comfortable, making them a good choice for base layers in active wear. Knitted regenerated fibres tend to offer both comfort and function, and have

TENCEL, Urban Sportswear, Autumn/Winter 1999/2000. TENCEL is the registered trademark of Tencel Ltd. TENCEL blends well with other natural, regenerated and synthetic fibres without overpowering their specific characteristics. The fabrics shown here are a blend of TENCEL and cotton by Cotonificio Veneto (Italy) and TENCEL, cotton and rayon by Nien Foun (Taiwan).

efficient wicking properties, making them suitable for sports clothes at all levels. When densely woven, these cellulose-based fibres are very suitable for active outerwear.

Leather

Leather is a very good protective material, but its main disadvantage is that it is not totally waterproof. There are now improved ways of processing and tanning leather to make it very lightweight and supple enough to be used even for next-to-skin bodywear. Leather mesh can be made using sophisticated laser-cutting, while stretch leather combining leather with Lycra can be made into body-sleek clothing. This has great potential for protective sports attire where increased body movement and stretch recovery are required. The new stretch leathers are also being incorporated into footwear because they provide better shape-retention and are very comfortable to wear on the feet.

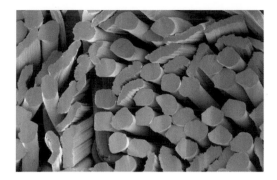

Viloft is an engineered viscose thermal fibre by Acordis. Most Viloft is spun in a fifty-fifty blend with polyester, and the magnified cross-section (above) shows how the flat Viloft and more rounded polyester create pockets of air for insulation. There is Viloft active, Viloft thermal, Viloft micro and Viloft spirit; the fabrics have a natural look and soft feel, and they manage moisture and temperature well. The diagram (right) shows how a Viloft fabric wicks sweat away to the air outside the clothes.

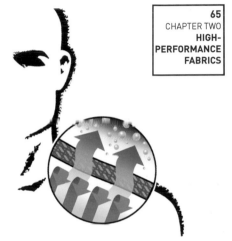

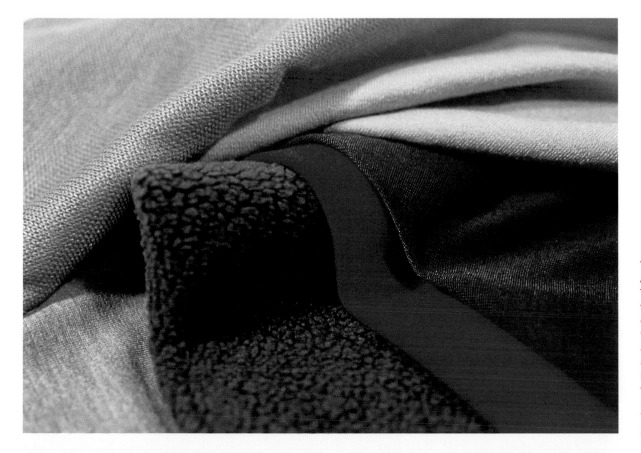

TENCEL, Comfort Cocoon, Autumn/Winter 1999/2000. TENCEL is the registered trademark of Tencel Ltd. TENCEL can be blended with other yarns for fluid and lustrous fabrics that are extremely comfortable as well as functional. Examples shown here include TENCEL with fine wool, cashmere, angora, silk, polyester, polyamide and viscose. Textiles by Luigi Botto, Albaud, Jackytex, Becagli and Otten.

TECHNOLOGY TRANSFER

Textiles are being combined with non-textiles using technology transfer – that is, the adoption of many advanced developments in textiles originally intended for industrial or medical use. Fluid and stiff materials, wool and plastic, for example, are combined to give diversity of shape, protection and enhanced performance capabilities. Paper is cellulosic which makes it very compatible with textiles, and there are blends of paper with cashmere. Wood has even been combined with high-tech 'sports' textiles to create new flexibles. Metals and ceramics can be mixed with synthetic or natural fibres. These new composites, it is claimed, take the best qualities from each material. Fibre optics can be woven into cloth to send and receive information for potential applications in sports clothes. Latex blends give an attractive rubbery feel with improved grip, and it is predicted that these new flexibles will be a large area of growth – they can offer multifunctional and versatile characteristics for many different applications in everyday wear as well as in specialist sportswear.

Metal

When combined with a textile, metal can lend a whole new dimension – cashmere mixed with steel contrasts a sense of luxury with the strength of metal. When the cloth is deformed it is capable of returning quickly to its original state, it is malleable, and it has a new handling quality and appearance.

Silver has long been known for its inherent medicinal and therapeutic properties and was originally used in the medical world for bandages. Microfibres can be coated in silver which can withstand up to a hundred washes. The silver reflects body heat to keep the wearer warm, and additional benefits include antimicrobial, anti-odour, thermal-conductive and anti-static properties. A whole range of textiles can be silver-coated – knitted, woven and nonwoven. This technology was originally developed as a medical or an industrial fibre, but is now being utilized as a high-performance textile for sports and even general clothing.

Titanium and aluminium are often used for linings, and will provide thermal insulation by reflecting body heat; titanium-lined neoprene is used for wetsuits (see p. 46). Copper-plated fabrics are often given a very fine coating of polyurethane to prevent the copper turning blue/green through atmospheric oxidization. One major disadvantage of using metals in textiles is that they will only flex for a certain number of times before succumbing to metal fatigue, and the position of these materials has to be confined to non-flex areas. Then there are the micro-metal fibres whose yarns retain heat for use in winter sportswear.

Many companies are developing UVA and UVB screening technology, since ultra-violet rays cause premature ageing, long-term damage to the skin and cancer, and exposure is

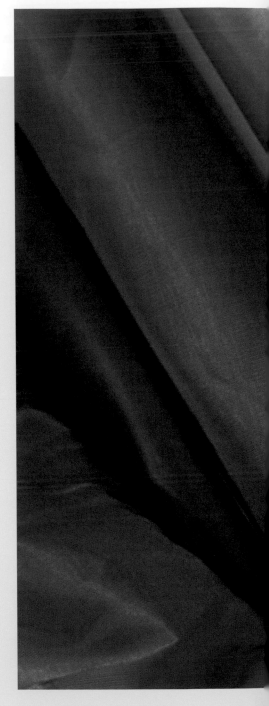

increasing with the depletion of the ozone layer. To combat this, titanium dioxide, for example, can be added to sun lotions. This pigment absorbs ultra-violet rays and reflects light, and can also be incorporated with synthetics to create a permanent effect. Darkly dyed clothes tend to be better at absorbing light and ultra-violet rays – black is often worn in hot countries.

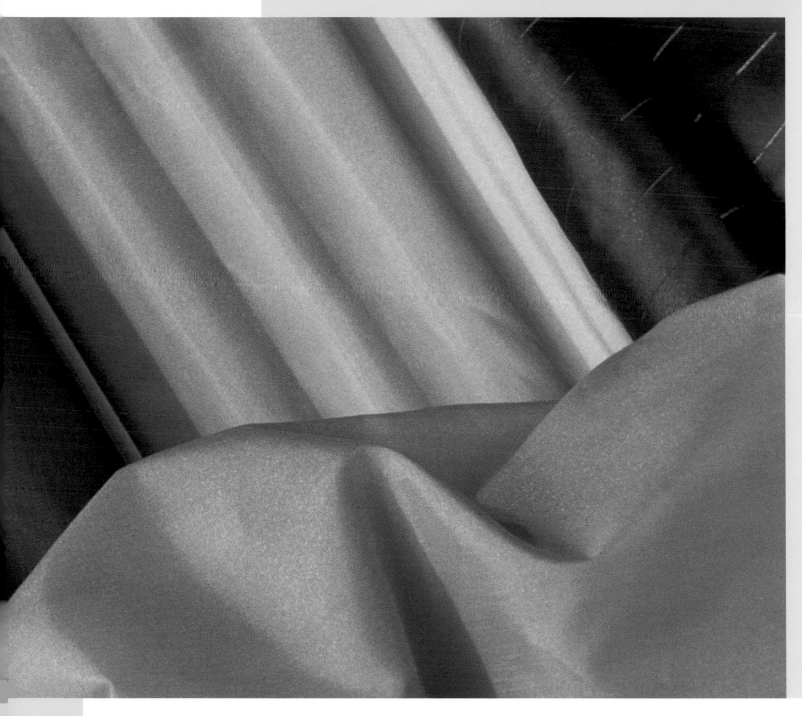

UV-blockers reduce ultra-violet ray absorption by the skin, and are similar to dark dye in the way that they operate. A denser textile also gives better protection, and the disadvantage of added weight with increased density can be avoided by choosing a microfibre fabric. These UV-protective textiles are generally used for such outdoor summer activities as cycling, golfing, tennis and sailing.

Carbon

Originally developed by NASA, high-tech materials that incorporate carbon fibre have distinct advantages because the carbon content makes them incredibly strong, durable and lightweight. Carbon is also capable of resisting extremely high temperatures while remaining flexible. It imparts anti-static properties and protects schoeller-spirit with silk and metal. Schoeller combines these materials to produce a textile that is lustrous and malleable, with good shape-retention and a new handling quality. Schoeller's combinations of materials frequently offer high-performance qualities as well as looking good.

Lucy Orta, *Body Architecture – Vêtement Collective x 6,* commissioned by Expofil 2000. This tented piece on an aluminium telescopic framework consists of hoods and sleeves which can be transformed into six detachable ponchos, one of which is shown converted. The tent walls/ponchos are made from a nonwoven Rhovyl chlorofibre laminated with a waterproof and fireproof PVC membrane. The sleeves are made of Corterra by Setila, and the hoods of a polyester and viscose fabric with a ceramic coating by Avelana to protect from ultra-violet rays.

from electro-magnetic waves and electro-static radiation. Carbon, however, cannot be spun like most yarns because it does not easily melt or dissolve. Instead, carbon fibre is frequently incorporated with resin as a laminate, and in this way has revolutionized sporting accessories and equipment. Textiles can be impregnated with carbon so that they absorb odour, making them highly suitable for active sports footwear. Hyper-carbon is extremely tough, and carbon textiles have been used in bulletproofing, and by Formula One racing teams for their high-performance and protective qualities.

Glass and ceramic

Glass and ceramics are both silicates. Fibres made from these materials are good insulators, and are also fire-resistant and durable.

It is claimed that fabrics incorporating glass can filter both X-rays and gamma rays. Recycled glass blends well with other fibres, and textiles can even be spun from glass microfilaments.

Fibres can be combined with ultra-fine ceramic powder to absorb heat and give protection from both electro-magnetic waves and ultra-violet radiation. The ceramic powder is incorporated in the core of the yarn, and gives a high sun-protection factor by both absorbing and reflecting the sun's rays. When sealed into microfibres, the ceramic powder makes a particularly high-performance textile. With other fabrics, some of the radiation passes

through the fabric and some, though still reflected, passes through to the body.

Woven and knitted with other yarns (such as cotton or polyester) these ceramic-based textiles have high-function characteristics that make them very useful for all kinds of sport. They can help maintain an even body temperature in extreme heat or cold, and certain cotton and ceramic mixes are capable of keeping the wearer's body temperature several degrees below outside temperatures. Some thermochromic ceramic fabrics change colour when the wearer has been exposed to too much sun. Others can store solar energy to keep the wearer warm, which could be very useful for preventing swimmers chilling when out of the water.

Silicone

Silicone, a polymer, has properties that are very useful for sports clothes and sports footwear. It prevents friction, repels moisture, is flexible, elastic and strong. Most types of silicone are resistant to chemicals and insensitive to temperature change. In the construction of a garment, silicone can improve waterproofing – it is either used in conjunction with sewing for a very strong bond, or to 'seam' the fabric directly where no sewing is required. This reduces bulk and the possibility of friction to give a close and comfortable fit. The application of silicone prevents a woven cloth from fraying and a knitted fabric from laddering, and is used to impregnate carpet to make dry ski slopes and ski-simulator machines.

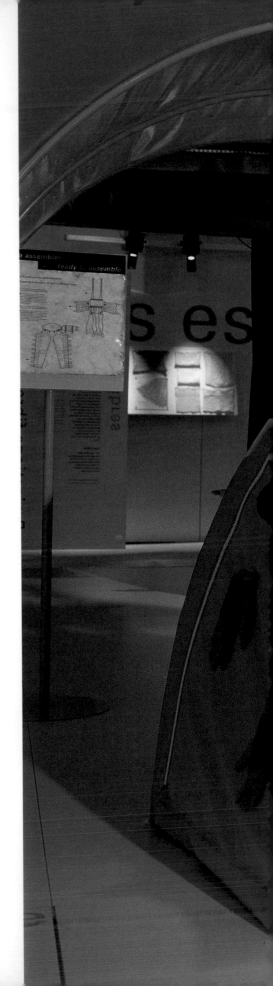

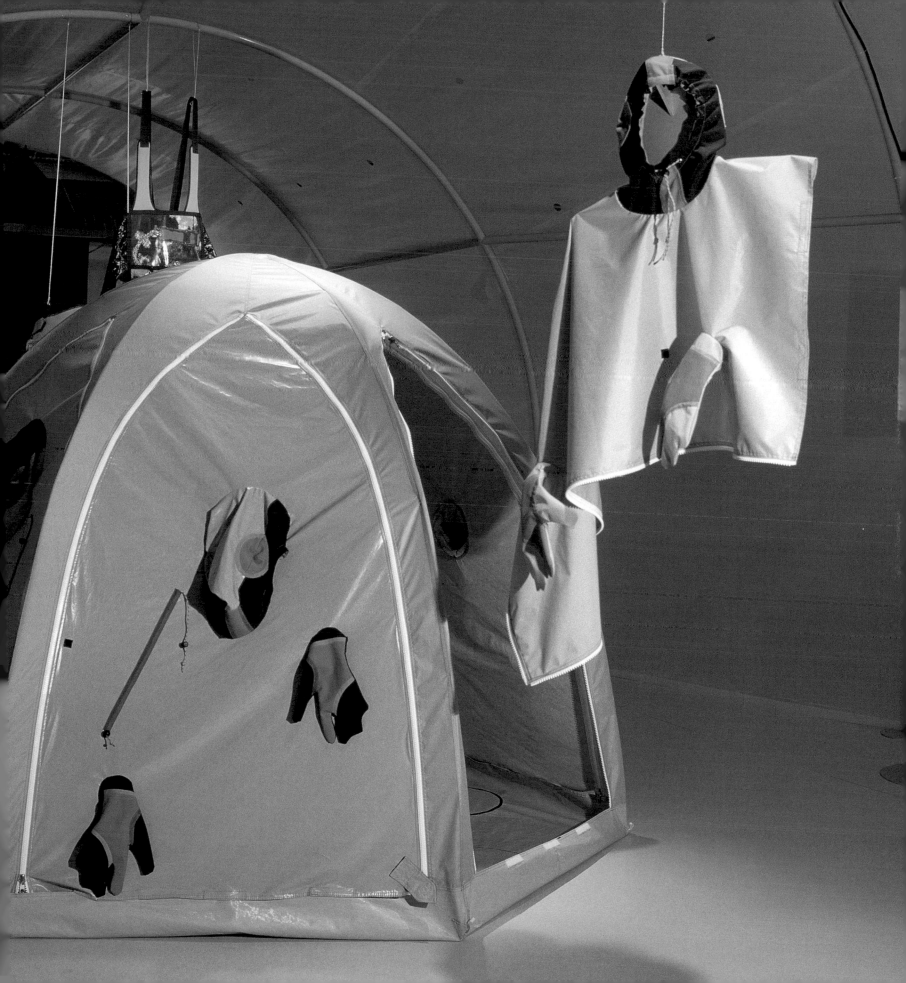

Reflec Technology, reflective print. A reflective water-based printing ink allows the cyclist to be seen at night or in conditions of poor visibility from up to 200 metres (almost 220 yards) away. Reflec Technology make reflective screen inks for fabrics or tape for high-visibility garments and accessories.

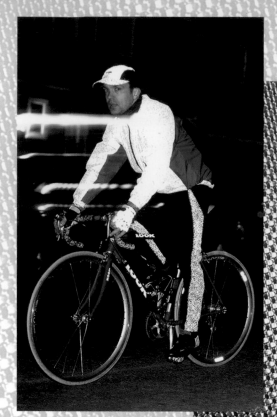

REFLECT-OPTIC TECHNOLOGY

The creation of reflective textiles uses the concept of the 'cat's eye' (the reflective devices set in the centre of roads) and state-of-the-art microtechnology. Originally this technology was developed for safety workwear and high-performance sports gear for conditions of poor visibility – night-time cycling, running and motorcycling. It is now used in sports clothes at all levels, and also for fashion, both prêt-à-porter and haute couture. It produces a highly reflective surface when low-lit (from light up to 200 metres, 220 yards, away) and many companies are increasingly using it for both sports footwear and garment detailing. Reflect-optic technology can be used in printed textiles where microscopic glass spheres, half-coated in aluminium, are suspended in textile ink and applied to the fabric using rotary printing techniques. Printed on a textile, or a reflective prism on tape, or patches positioned on the body, they shine in safety yellow at night and in conditions of poor visibility.

Even a dark-coloured print will throw back a bright white light and the reflection of coloured light is being researched. The reflective print is invisible in natural daylight when printed in the same colour as the substrate, which leads to interesting effects – patterns suddenly appear as bold imagery after dark. The printed cloth can be washed many times without substantial loss of the reflective property. The minute glass spheres can also be incorporated directly into a textile, which gives it the additional advantages of being very fine, soft and flexible.

schoeller-reflex materials. Reflective textiles by Schoeller. These are interesting visually, but they are also abrasion- and tear-resistant, and the wearer is visible from a distance of up to 100 metres (110 yards). These fabrics use Cordura (DuPont) and retroreflective Scotchlite (3M). The weave used protects the many tiny glass balls which reflect light.

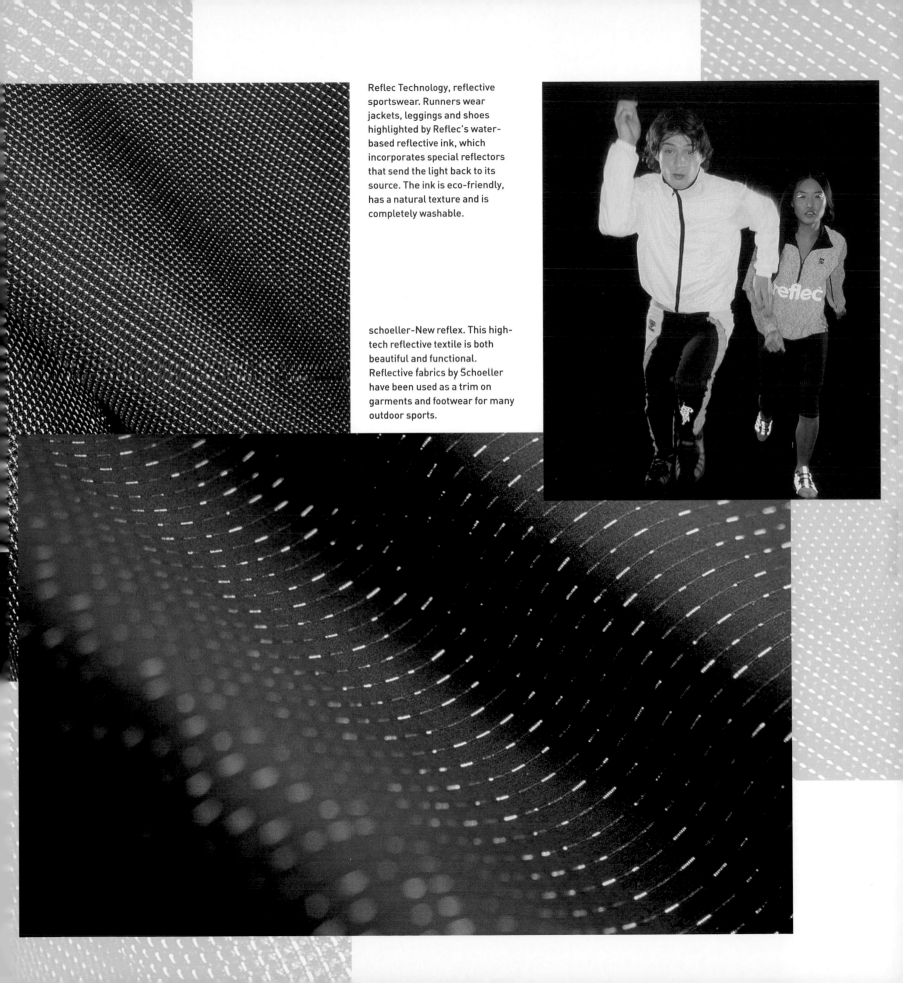

Reflec Technology, reflective sportswear. Runners wear jackets, leggings and shoes highlighted by Reflec's water-based reflective ink, which incorporates special reflectors that send the light back to its source. The ink is eco-friendly, has a natural texture and is completely washable.

schoeller-New reflex. This high-tech reflective textile is both beautiful and functional. Reflective fabrics by Schoeller have been used as a trim on garments and footwear for many outdoor sports.

Toray Industries, Inc. Entrant Dermizax-EV (top right). The Entrant fabrics series is intended for active wear, and there are many variations that use advanced finishes. This textile has a water-repellent membrane with improved moisture permeability (MR stands for Moisture Release). making it especially suitable for snowsports and climbing.

Toray Industries, Inc. Entrant-DT (below right). This microporous coated fabric is lightweight, waterproof and breathable. Soft, with a dry smooth texture (DT stands for Dry Tech), it is intended for cycling, running and hiking.

Toray Industries, Inc. Entrant GII-XT (far right). This microporous coated fabric is made of two polyurethane resin components which produce a 'pumped-up' effect and rapidly wick away sweat. Wind- rain- and snowproof, it is suitable for many outdoor winter sports.

Lucy Orta, *Life Raft keep afloat and surf the urban wave,* and *Life Line rescue aid for disorientated persons* (details opposite), both part of the *Urban Life Guards* series commissioned by Expofil 2000. The wader suit with heat-moulded pockets is made of Trevira coated with Teflon (DuPont), and the boots of 3D Meryl (Nylstar) jersey. The life-saving ring and jacket are made of Tactel HT (DuPont).

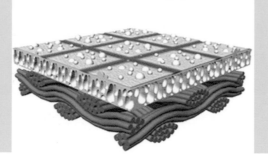

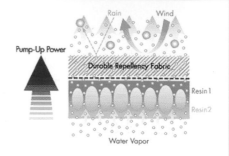

FINISHING TREATMENTS

Finishes can totally transform textiles and give them a whole array of sports applications. A finishing treatment on a lining increases high performance but does not alter the face fabric. Textiles can be enzyme-dyed, which is less harmful for the environment, while simple brushing of the surface gives volume, softness and warmth. The latest finishes give textiles a new aesthetic, a 'good-to-wear' experience and superior performance, with most offering a degree of protection from the elements. Finishes can make fabrics trans-seasonal, multifunctional and reversible, and are used on both naturals and synthetics with great success.

Traditional outdoor wear uses waxed cottons and linens, cottons and wools treated with resin, felts backed with jersey and oiled yarns for knitted garments, all of which give excellent warmth and protection from the weather. The latest finishes, however, are new versions of oiling and waxing – oils can be exuded to give practical water-repellent surfaces. Barbour, the outdoor-clothing company, have even developed a wax coating that has no odour or oily feel. A waterproof textile with high breathability will be efficient and comfortable for such watersports as white-water canoeing and kayaking, and will also shield from rain

in the city. New treatments make leather windproof and waterproof, and therefore ideal for sports footwear.

Not so very long ago a fabric could not be both weatherproof and breathable, but sophisticated membrane technology in the form of new coatings and laminates have altered this. Both visible and invisible coatings now make it possible for a fabric to carry sweat away and for air to circulate around the body. Ultra-fine and super-light treatments can give improved function to traditional cloth without much increased weight, and textiles can be made rain-, wind- and fireproof, and flame-resistant while also being breathable. Specialist coatings with carbon fibre can protect the wearer against pollution, which could be useful for motor racing.

Some of the new finishes provide a barrier to dirt and staining; a polyurethane resin coating, for example, can give stain-release properties. Such resin finishes on synthetic substrates can also provide a protective barrier for jackets and tracksuits for wet-weather and winter sports. Another material used for coating is Teflon

(polytetrafluoroethylene, PTFE, made by polymerizing tetrafluoroethylene). It was developed for the US space programme, and functions through molecules building up around the fibre as a protective layer. It has a very low surface friction which is useful in sports clothing. Treating a textile with Teflon gives it a technical look and tactile quality while providing protection from showers and stains. Liquid simply rolls off its surface – a particularly useful property for wet-weather sports. Like silicone, Teflon can reduce water drag, and is ideal for clothes for swimming, skiing and snowboarding. On clothing for round-the-world sailing, Teflon coatings on the shoulders shield where protection is most needed. On the inside legs of tracksuit bottoms or leggings such a coating increases durability by reducing friction, and on trouser bottoms is practical for outdoor sports.

Invisible finishes can defend against the extreme conditions encountered in snowsports, mountaineering and exploring, and can also be used for survival wear. Very fine films can be laminated between a lining and a face fabric. On a face fabric an ultra-fine treatment does not hide the underlying textile, and appearance, texture and drape are less affected. In clothing for most outdoor winter sports it is important for a fabric to transport perspiration from the skin to the air outside the garment and remain water- and windproof. There are generally two methods of creating breathable, weatherproof textiles, using either microporous or hydrophilic technologies. The first works by means of very fine holes in the membrane that allow perspiration to escape as water vapour and move quickly from inside to outside, but prevent water in the form of rain, mist or snow from penetrating. The second attracts water molecules and allows warmer water vapour to move through the membrane to the cooler temperature outside the garment (water molecules always move from high to low temperatures). Seaming generally involves special adhesives, taping and lining to make clothes totally windproof and waterproof, all very desirable properties in protective sports clothes.

Microfibre fabrics are also given advanced finishing treatments to create waterproof, breathable textiles. In addition, when combined with other technologies, coatings can offer, for example, ultra-absorbency from finishes with a foam construction. Some work by utilizing two membranes, such as a very lightweight, breathable polyurethane membrane with ultra-fine pores together with a water-repellent membrane to provide supreme comfort and protection.

An invisible finish can be virtually undetectable and therefore the look and feel of a traditional cloth can be retained. With the new finishing treatments, a workaday cloth like denim can be transformed into a fabric suitable for professional sports. Raw textured cotton, linen and silk can all be given high-tech finishes that are not readily apparent. Chemically laminated cotton dries fast because the molecular structure of the cotton fibres has been changed. The fibres are aligned so that they are parallel to the axis, which gives the fabric a softer handle and a smoother appearance. It is also resistant to creasing or wrinkling, and only has to be wiped clean.

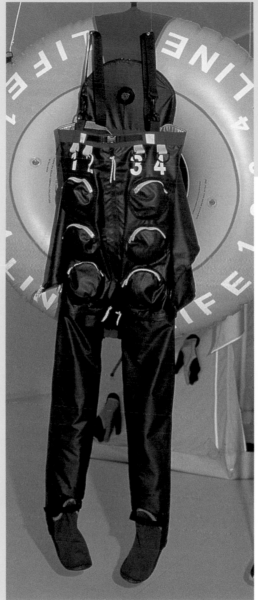

A typical summer fabric, cotton or linen for instance, or a fabric such as wool which is usually considered a winter textile, can be made trans-seasonal by giving it one of the new finishing treatments. Coated hessian with a felt backing retains its natural look but the finish gives it sophisticated performance qualities. Antibacterial finishes, invisible to the naked eye, have now been used on both natural and synthetic textiles for sports and leisure clothes. And some fleeces are laminated to windproof membranes to give them additional high-performance characteristics.

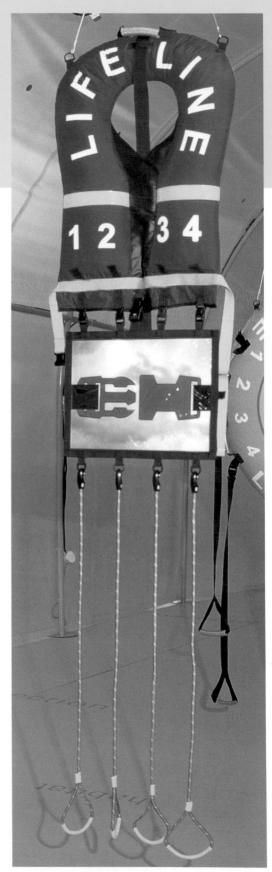

schoeller-WB-400 by Schoeller. This is a high-stretch textile, with a three-layer structure, which is comfortable and gives all-weather protection. Performance fibres are blended with Lycra (DuPont) on the outside, and the WB-400 membrane is a built-in acrylate laminate which prevents penetration from rain, wind and snow. The fabric has a warm, soft fleece lining and good shape-retention, and is durable, breathable and easy-care. Shown here are different qualities of textile with the WB-400 membrane.

The fact that many coatings are invisible can be a disadvantage, however, because customers generally like to see what they are getting for their money. As a result, some companies are working on the aesthetics of textile finishing, recognizing that style and performance in sports clothes need to be intrinsically linked. Visible treatments can create a new look and often a futuristic appearance. The enhanced functional properties are part of the new textile's attraction, and can play a large part in its marketing. Active wear tends to concentrate on finishes, such as coating and laminating, rather than traditional prints, preferring all-over effects. Conjuring up images of city steel and asphalt, metallized finishes use a variety of techniques including oxidizing, burnishing and bronzing. Light-reflecting, pearlescent, iridescent and moiré (water-like) finishes are also widely used.

Stained, smudged and discoloured looks are popular for many sports, and this aesthetic has come from the fashion world. Stone- and sun-washed finishes are intended for both sports and travel wear and give a functional look. A textile can simply be washed and given whitening treatments for a slightly faded, aged appearance, while bleaching makes a fabric softer and less obviously 'technical'.

Prints in favour tend either to have a technical feel with computerized and pixelated imagery, or are based on micro patterns found in nature. Over-printing can create a kinetic or optical look, and diagonal prints can give a dynamic feel, emphasizing speed. Further surface interest can be achieved through the use of heat-reactive chemicals to create contoured and embossed effects. Thermoprinting gives irregular textures and uneven 'destroyed' surfaces, and is typically used on bonded neoprene with a polyurethane coating for a high-tech, street-inspired, sporty look. Transfer prints are used with flocking and embossing techniques on sports clothes purely for their visual appeal.

Other visible finishing treatments include holographic and *changeant* effects (fabrics that can change colour in response to temperature fluctuations have many potential uses), and a finish that is sensitive to ultra-violet light.

Spattering describes a range of fine metal coatings that can alter the look, touch and performance. Woven polyester tends to work the best, and various metals can be employed. An aluminium coating is capable of retaining the wearer's body heat and of reflecting the sun's rays to keep the body cool – properties that could prove crucial in extreme conditions.

Tactile coatings can give a subtle, non-slip touch – a talc-like handle and a fine latex feel, either matt or lustrous. Such finishes are often achieved using microporous membranes on ultra-fine synthetic or nonwoven substrates. A non-slip property is obviously useful in many sports, as it is also for micro mobiles and hand-held information/ communication systems, but was originally intended for medical hygiene materials. Interesting textures can be created by lacquering the surface for a crisp, papery or crackly handle. Specialist finishes can mimic the skin of a reptile or fish, or employ polyethylene to imitate the skin's pores for a skin-grain finish. A very fine coating of polyvinyl chloride on a knitted textile can impart various textures, ultra-smooth or piqué, for example.

The thinnest of transparent coatings can give beautiful shot-silk effects, while microjersey textures can closely resemble a woven cloth.

Silicone coating and printing offer low resistance, and are water-repellent and flexible. These are useful qualities for clothes and shoes for time-based sporting activities, such as speed-skating and sprinting, where shaving off fractions of a second is often what is needed to win. Since silicone repels water, silicone printed in stripes on swimwear, and in particular on headgear, can reduce drag and help speed a swimmer through the water, as well as reducing the chill factor after swimming. Lightweight swimwear made from a synthetic and Lycra, with alternating rough and smooth stripes of silicone is very efficient.

Silicone can be used either on the fibre or on the fabric, and either on a natural or on a synthetic, making it a versatile finish with many applications. When silicone is used in concentrated form, coatings are abrasion-resistant and water-repellent, and very useful for outdoor activities and watersports. When dilute, silicone gives a flexible and easy-care finish. A very fine coating creates a fabric which can be washed or dry-cleaned and the coating is often permanent. Fabrics with a silicone finish tend to keep their shape after repeated washing; they are also non-shrink as well as being crease-resistant. A silicone coating can also prevent a wool from pilling (forming little bobbles all over the surface of the garment) which can be unsightly.

Schoeller fabrics with several different coatings (below). The finishing treatments can alter the underlying textile's look, and give it smooth or textured surfaces, as well as high-performance qualities.

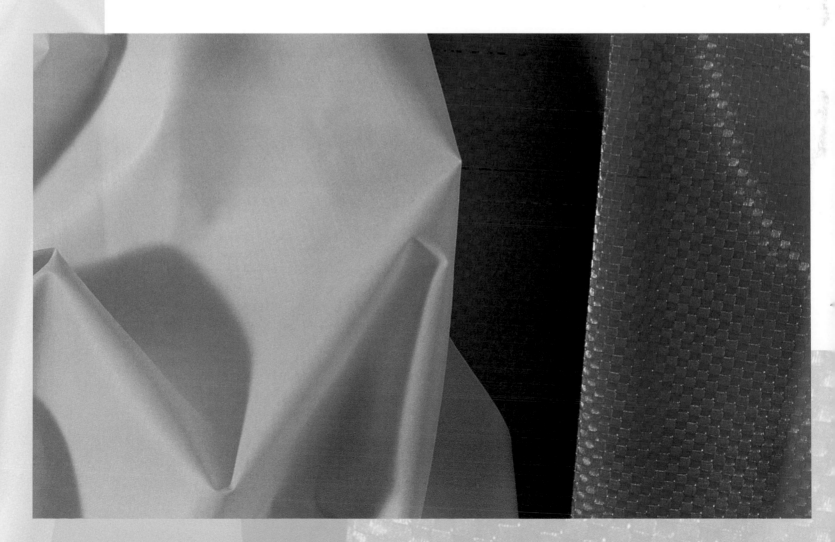

Lucy Orta, *Habit Kit easy to assemble* (foreground), commissioned by Expofil 2000, part of the *Urban Life Guards* series. The back of the harness is made of a ripstop fabric, Meryl by Nylstar. This is ultrasound-quilted to an absorbent mesh knit of Rhovyl chlorofibre. The front of the harness is CoolMax and Lycra, both by DuPont. The reversible leggings are in Nylstar's Meryl Nexten bonded to a micropolar Filifine jersey by Tergal Fibres.

FABRIC CONSTRUCTION

The actual construction of a textile plays a part in its suitability for sports attire. The linked construction of knitted fabrics gives elasticity, and the latest jerseys are super-light and ultra-fine. For warmth and comfort in adverse conditions, textiles may be brushed, bonded, padded (with goose feathers and down or synthetic foams), quilted or wadded to give a lightweight volume with little excess bulk. They can also be multi-layered and reversible.

Technical knits that are moisture-wicking tend to be more open in structure on the back than on the face, and airy weaves with cellular construction let air through. In such openly structured weaves, moisture from perspiration passes more quickly through. Examples of this include Aertex, a traditional sports fabric, which is widely used. Technical leno weaves (with a twisted warp to create an open lace-like effect) are effective at trapping air and can therefore assist in keeping the wearer at a constant temperature. Nonwovens and coarse-gauge knits can also produce airy structures. Because of their construction, chunky fabrics can be created that are not bulky or heavy – they possess a volume but are still lightweight,

Textured weaves with coarse open surfaces, such as cotton gauze bonded to crinkled paper, promise ultra-absorbency for sports clothes, and especially watersports. Textured fabrics can offer enhanced performance; piqué, for instance, is absorbent and durable. A ribbed fabric can be either knitted or woven and will ensure protection in high-stress areas, such as at knees and elbows – vulnerable body parts where movement is essential. Pleating a fabric can also trap air for better insulation and may also be used for ease of movement and comfort.

Dense weaves can help prevent rain, snow or wind penetration. These compact constructions make a fabric with a firm handle and good performance – they even feel protective. A close-cropped smooth surface often makes for very strong and durable textiles. Microfibre fabrics can protect from the wind, and are frequently used for sportswear linings – sometimes detachable for greater versatility. The future will see more use of these (mainly synthetic) microfibres for moulded, seamless garments.

Ripstop describes a special textile construction which prevents a tear

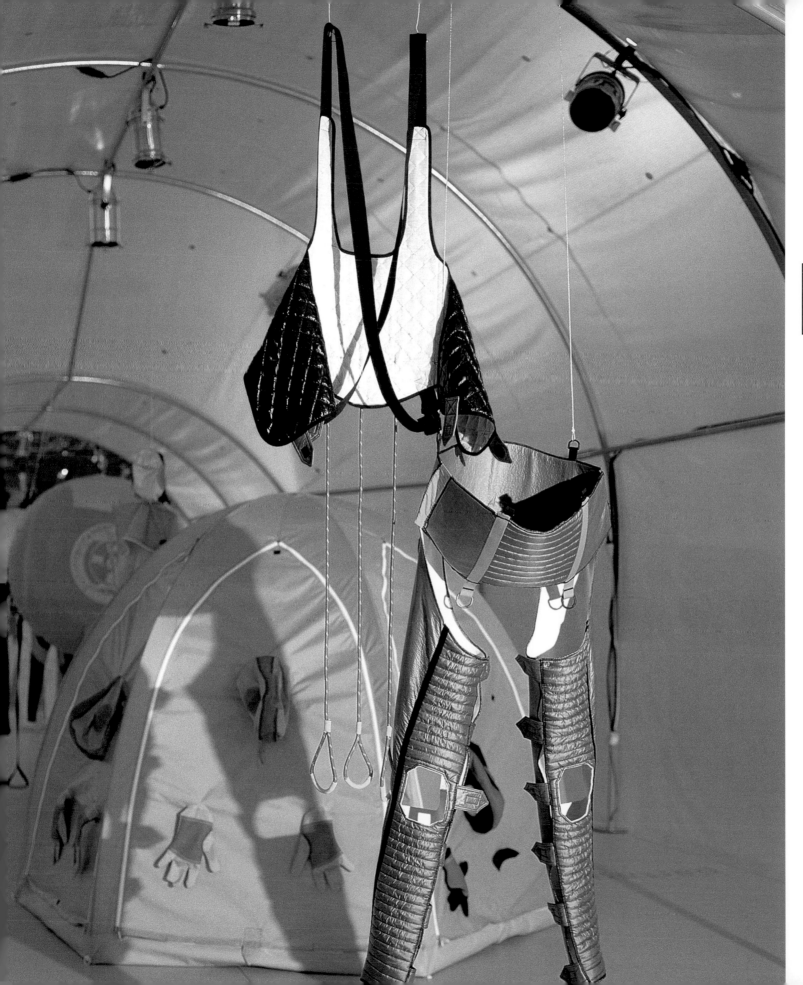

Courtelle Recoil Autumn/Winter 1999/2000. This functional sports knit is made from Courtelle Recoil, a new-generation synthetic acrylic by Acordis. This is often blended with other fibres, natural or synthetic, for an ultra-lightweight textile that feels luxurious. When steamed, it takes on a three-dimensional quality which gives the textile a soft airy texture, volume without weight and insulation. It bridges the gap between traditional knits and the new synthetic fleeces.

schoeller-ComforTemp, produced by Schoeller; ComforTemp is a registered trademark of Frisby Technologies, USA. The three-layer mesh of the fabric can clearly be seen (opposite below). The mesh provides ventilation to allow sweat to escape easily, and when the athlete rests from activity, the mesh insulates the body and helps prevents chilling.

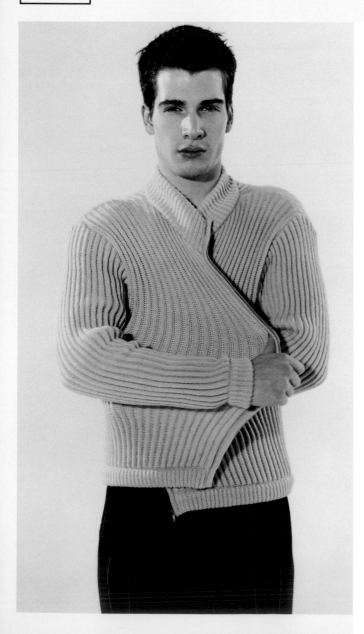

from spreading. A thick yarn used alternately with a thin one gives it its characteristic checked appearance. The fabric is lightweight and has increased strength and resistance – nylon is generally used. A ripstop fabric has many applications, including sports outerwear, linings, sports accessories and equipment.

Dense-pile fabrics play a big part in sports clothing, and cloth with a high pile traps air for insulation, and is very absorbent. Terry is a deep-pile fabric with raised uncut loops, and it is generally used for bathrobes and towels as it is ultra-absorbent and thermally insulating. New developments include a terry-backed polyamide, an absorbent synthetic.

A brushed or tufted inner surface acts as a wick to draw moisture quickly away from the skin, and provides insulation with lightweight volume. Brushed surfaces are often used as an inner lining where they feel good next to the skin. In combination with a highly dense fabric they can provide comfort and performance.

Double-sided fabrics give increased protection, while cellular construction and textured surfaces are more absorbent. Naturals and synthetics, knitted, woven and nonwoven cloth can be double-sided, which makes them very versatile.

The outer surface could be very dense, ultra-smooth and almost like cardboard, and, if a 'bulked', airy or brushed yarn is chosen, the inside face could be soft and warm. A double-sided fleece affords high-quality protection from the weather, and with a soft, brushed back (worn next to the skin) and a smooth outer surface it is windproof and rainproof. Double-weaves or knits trap air effectively, making them particularly good choices for sports activities. Contrasting fabrics can be bonded together; and densely woven wool, cotton or polyamide can be given a fleece or neoprene backing. Bonded polyamide is used for rainproof outer clothes, while bonded jersey can give a knitted cloth improved performance qualities.

Padding of fabrics is primarily for insulation, but its look and soft feel are also attractive. Polyester wadding or synthetic foam is sandwiched between fabrics (a face textile can be quite different from the lining, which gives a garment greater versatility). The quality of the wadding is very important for the performance, and different thicknesses of wadding cater for many different needs. Some wadding is made from synthetic microfibres making it waterproof and breathable, while nonwoven polyester wadding can be combined with many other fibres for greater strength combined with lightness.

Carbon fibre has been incorporated in fabrics and linked to a battery source in order to generate heat – the structure of the carbon fibres makes heat-control possible – with great potential for snowsports. Research and development is currently taking place to introduce a new wadding which offers increased protection against impact.

Foam-backed textiles are shock-absorbing and retain heat owing to their open cellular construction. Knitted fabrics with a foam backing can be very soft, and when blended with elastane have good stretch characteristics, making them suitable for high-action sports.

The choice of textile for a lining is very important, and wind and rain penetration can be virtually eliminated by selecting the most suitable of the latest synthetics.

Linings with a thin back coating of metal, such as titanium, aluminium or silver, will reflect body heat. They provide thermal insulation and protection by helping maintain an even body temperature – used with a weatherproof material they make a good choice for sports in cold and wet conditions. Washable polyester mesh linings are frequently used in sportswear to provide lightweight fabrics that wick perspiration quickly away from the skin, and antibacterial and moisture-absorbing linings are used for high-performance clothing for sports, travel and outdoor wear.

In some sports fabrics, two types of cloth construction (airy and dense) create a 'Differential Porous' (DP) multilayer structure of thin surfaces, which absorbs perspiration and wicks moisture quickly away from the body using capillary action. An added advantage of this system is that it offers good insulation properties because of air trapped between the layers. Next to the wearer's skin is a textile with thicker

denier fibres and a coarse knit, while the outer layer uses finer denier fibres and a densely knitted structure. It helps to keep the wearer warm and dry, even during intense activity in the summer, and it is fast-drying. Some multi-layers use hydrophilic (water-attracting) yarns for high-performance textiles, as in synthetic knits for running, tennis, football and baseball.

With the right choice of fabric, the concept of multilayering is carried through to the clothing itself. A three-layer system is essential in many cases where protection is needed from both the weather and the body's method of regulating temperature by sweating. The textile next to the skin must be capable of wicking moisture away quickly so that the middle and the outer layers can perform at their best. Ranges of highly specialist clothing for the sports enthusiast as well as clothes for leisure wear are being developed based on this layering principle.

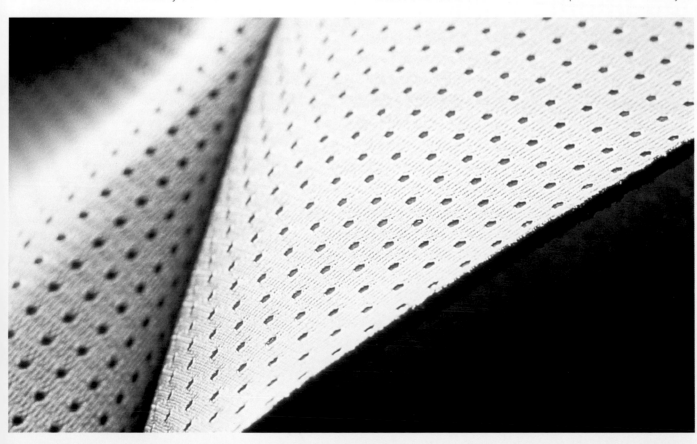

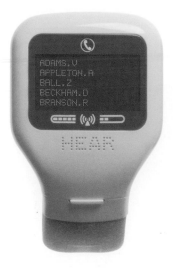

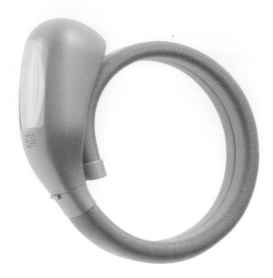

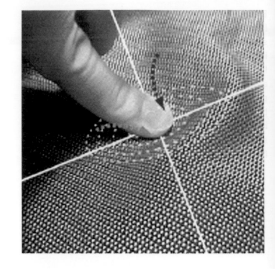

ElekSen Limited, Soft Wrist Phone (above left and centre). This belongs to the Fabrications family of products, designed by Sam Hecht of IDEO for ElekSen, and employing wearable technology. The phone module is connected to a band covered with ElekSen fabric (a blend of DuPont's Lycra) over a steel substrate, available in a variety of colours, textures and patterns. The phone module is soft and functions as a watch when on the wrist; removed and unrolled, it becomes rigid so that it can be used as a phone. It was exhibited at the Museum of Modern Art, New York, 2001, in 'Workspheres' as one of the new products for working lifestyles.

Philips Design, Perfect Performance (below right). The top and shorts are made of a high-stretch textile and have biomimetic sensors to monitor pulse, blood pressure, body temperature, etc., to let wearers know how they are performing. Conductive embroidery and printing connect to an integrated audio device. Copyright Philips Design.

INTERACTIVE TECHNOLOGY

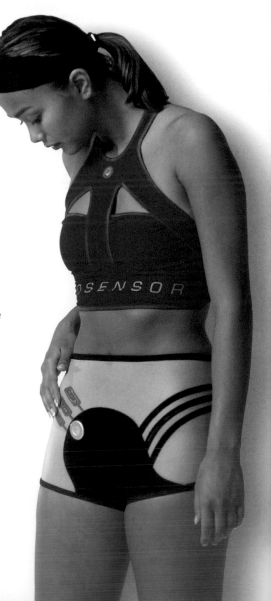

The science of fibres has advanced in great strides, and is developing many functions that were unthought of only a decade ago. Further advances will most probably continue to be made in the first decade of the twenty-first century – changing the look of both sports clothes and fashion and also affecting our lifestyles quite considerably. Intelligent or 'smart' materials, capable of responding to external stimuli, are now meeting our constantly changing needs. Shape memory alloys (SMAs) are a nickel and titanium alloy produced in wire and sheet form and incorporated into the fabric. SMAs remember the wearer's shape, and return to this after washing. At present, the use of SMAs is confined to bra technology and peaked sports caps, but the potential for other sports applications could prove exciting.

Once the problem of incorporating an energy or power supply has been solved, technology will be increasingly miniaturized and ultra-lightweight, while micro-electric components will ensure that future products are interactive and truly portable – almost part of ourselves. Wearable technology could give improved freedom and mobility to people who need to travel light. Microchips are now incorporated into jewellery and accessories, the latest remote controls are soft and a computer can be held in the palm of a hand. As the technology becomes cheaper, it will be more widely accessible; at present it is mainly targeting a young, fashionable audience. The future will probably see portable energy packs and very sophisticated information, communication and entertainment systems. Microscopic computers can be part of the

ElekSen Limited, Pressure Fabric (left). This textile combined with software can sense stimuli which it then converts into digital data. It responds to changes in location and pressure, and has many potential sports applications. Interactive, flexible and washable, its three-dimensional fabric structure includes conductive fibres.

Philips Design, Work Out, Electronic Sportswear (detail right, and below). Jogging pants have an inside pocket with a circuit linked to a conductive printed interface. This connects to a portable audio device entertainment system. The audio controls are worked by pulling cords on the fleece top. Copyright Philips Design.

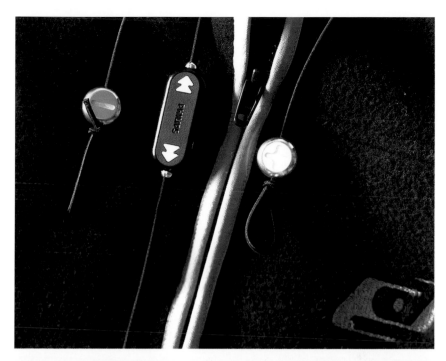

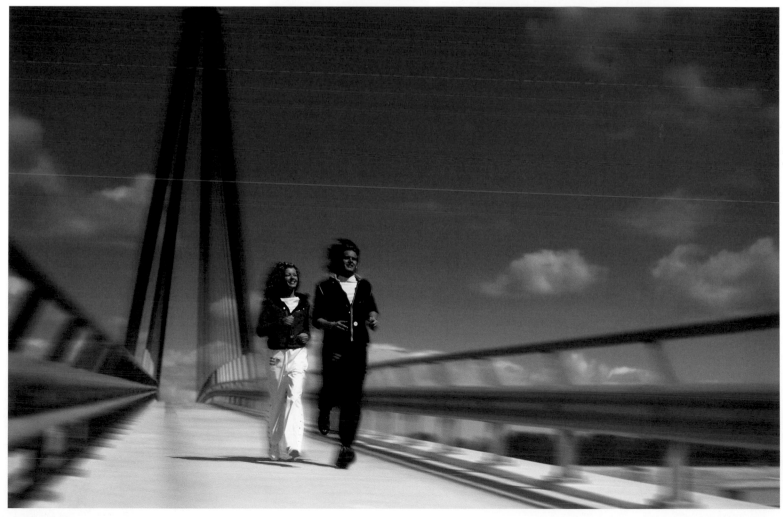

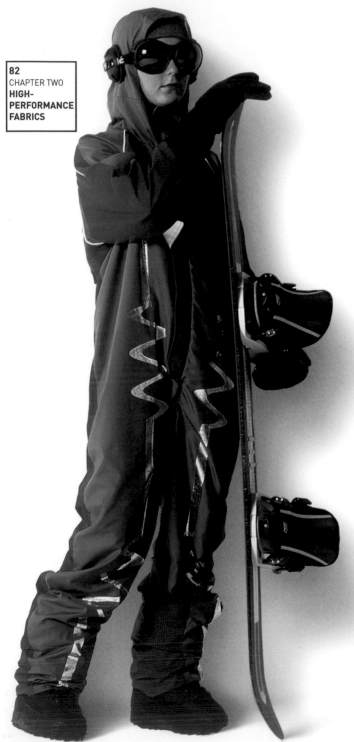

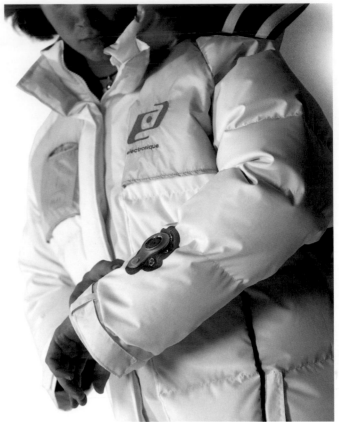

Philips Design, Staying Alive. The padded coat (left and below right) helps protect from hostile environments when cross-country skiing. Integrated GPS (Global Positioning System) enables the wearer's position to be pinpointed. A device on the sleeve (close-up below left) gives the wearer information on position, altitude, longitude, distance and body and atmospheric temperature, and can also receive accurate weather predictions. Copyright Philips Design.

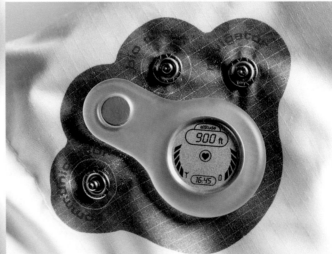

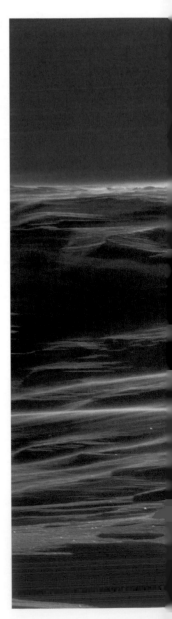

Philips Design, Techno Surfer. This suit for snowboarding or skiing (left) has many built-in devices including: GPS (Global Positioning System); functions for electronic ski passes; temperature sensors; and materials that automatically heat up when the body temperature falls below a certain level. Copyright Philips Design.

fabric and so incorporated directly into clothing or accessories. The idea of flexible circuitry and wearable software is being explored worldwide, fusing developments in the electronics and textile industries.

The latest innovations are 'smart' fabrics that are attractive, soft and warm to the touch, flexible and body-conscious, as opposed to technology's previously hard and rigid materials. Conductive fibres can be integrated into knitted or woven textiles. Concealed wiring can generally be easily removed for washing, but research is under way on wiring that can withstand washing. These interactive materials respond to given information, and, as textiles, are generally lightweight and capable of moulding themselves to the wearer. This could be very useful for sports, and would cater for individual optimum performance capabilities. Already developed is a microchip-controlled stretch fabric that changes with the wearer's movement for a sports bra top. Some 'smart fabrics' measure body stretch for an improved fit; others respond to touch, and can gauge stress and impact. Soft bio-sensors can be integrated to monitor heart and pulse rates, blood pressure, body temperature,

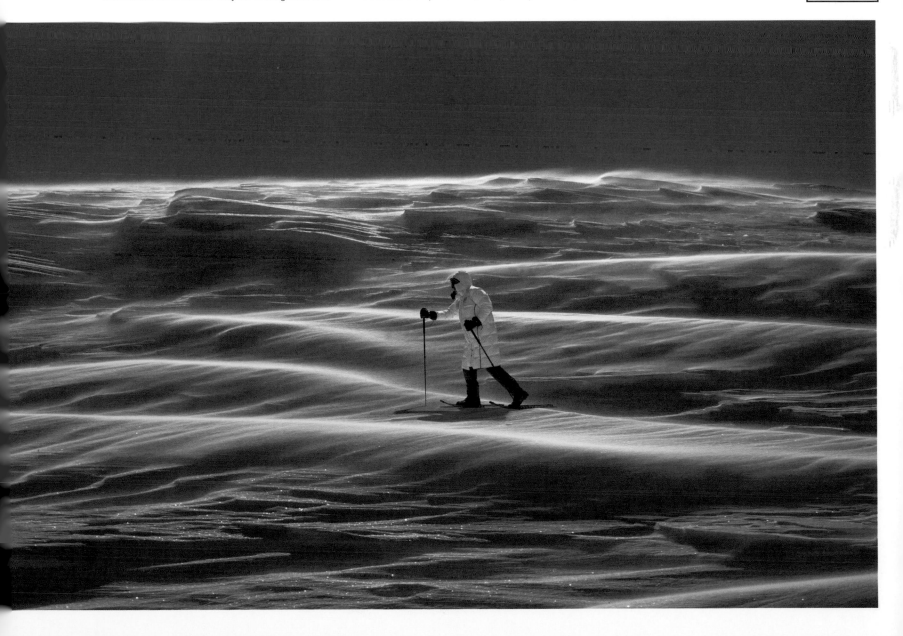

to calculate calories burned, and monitor and protect us from urban pollution. Sensors built into clothes and surrounding the body can help the competitor by checking aim or body position while making a tennis stroke or hitting a golf ball. Borrowing from automotive technology, clothes with air bags could protect the back in a fall. These new textiles offer personal systems that can assess health or professional performance and give immediate feedback.

Our capabilities and limitations are often fully tested when engaged in sports, and the choice of fibre and fabric for a garment or accessory can be fundamental to success in competition. The development of resistant and responsive materials has enabled wearers to perform to their best in comfort.

Functional sports clothing will surely continue to improve. Advances in technology mean that the latest sportswear incorporating interactive systems is moving rapidly from prototype to production. The development of strong, featherweight composites by the textile industry together with increased miniaturization of software have opened the way to these exciting possibilities. Integrated cooling systems in outdoor clothes – gases inside flexible tubes – are in production now. In the very near future, clothes will incorporate temperature sensors and heating materials, and will be able to warm us when the weather cools. We will soon be wearing garments with machine-washable flexible circuitry (as described above) that can be programmed, or that can monitor and respond to our health and well-being. Intensive training for a range of sports will become easier to control, and the wearer will be able to test his or her physical limits fully, but safely. In the future, knowledge from several disciplines, including the textile, science and engineering industries, will combine to benefit both sports professionals and the general public.

Lucy Orta, *Urban Life Guards*, installation commissioned by Expofil 2000. This art work (opposite) takes its inspiration from diving equipment, and comments on ideas of survival and rescue, exploring ideas of garments and shelters. Many high-performance textiles are used, especially chosen for their superior performance properties. They are weatherproof, insulating, absorbent, provide moisture-control and management, and are designed to keep the wearer comfortable and fully protected.

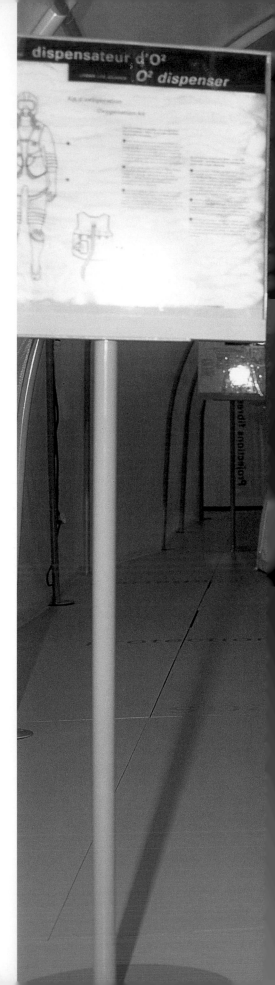

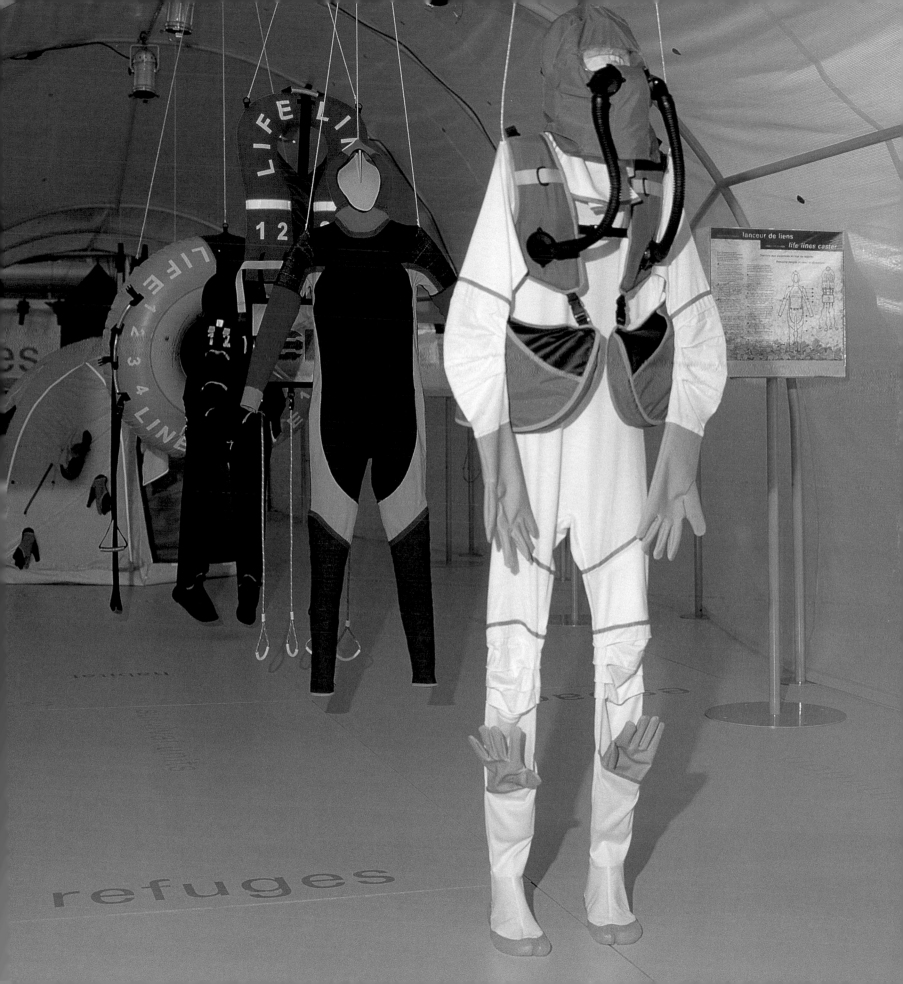

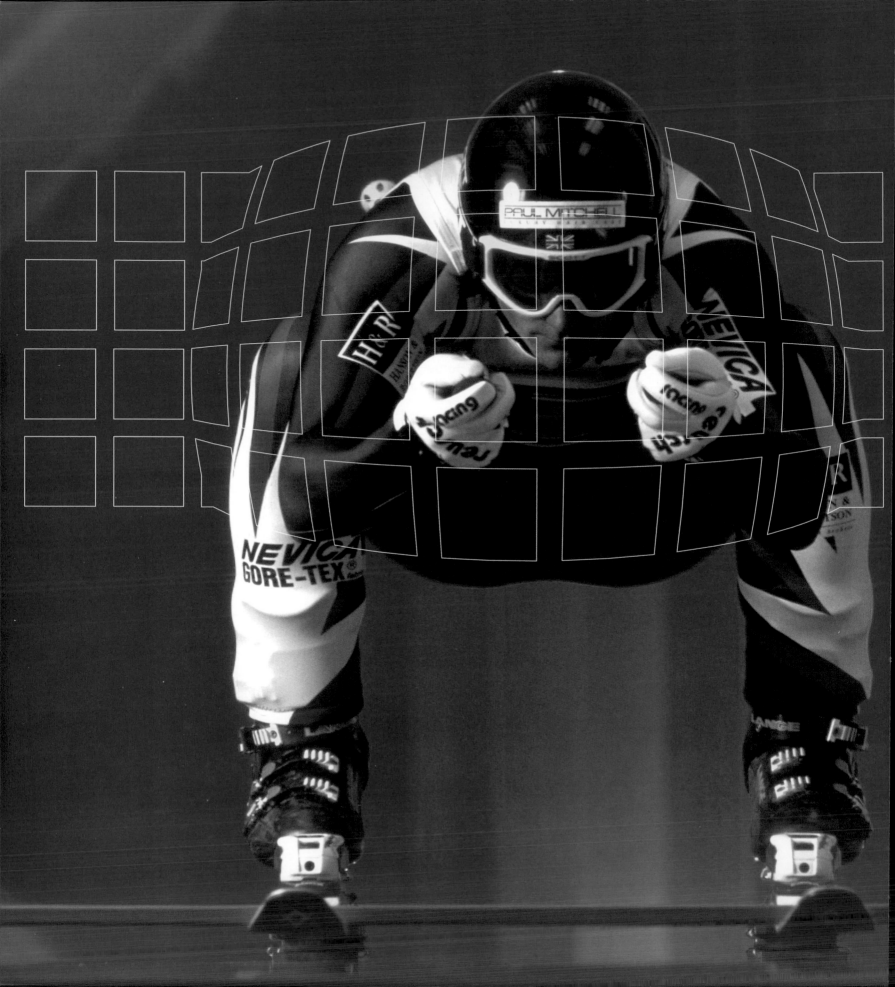

CHAPTER THREE
DESIGNING FOR SPEED AND COMFORT

For today's designer, there can be few areas as challenging as the sports industry. Sport has been responsible for the development of some of the most exciting new materials for over a century. The mass appeal of sport that began in the 1970s and the more recent link with fashion have brought the aesthetic of sports design in line with the high performance already demanded. The two are now inextricably linked. It is no longer enough for sports clothing to perform, it must be actually seen to perform. A 2000 advertisement appearing in *i-D* magazine for Nose shoes listed the performance characteristics of the footwear, with a very small image of a shoe at the bottom of the page. The shoe was the same height as the all-capital typeface. What was actually being sold were the attributes of the shoe, and the product itself had become little more than a tag on which to place them.

Skier Graham Bell of England is undergoing tests in the Jordan wind tunnel to check the most ergonomic position for his body. This type of technology has been developed mainly by the automotive and aerospace industries to record airflow around vehicles so that designs can be altered to create the most aerodynamic vehicles.

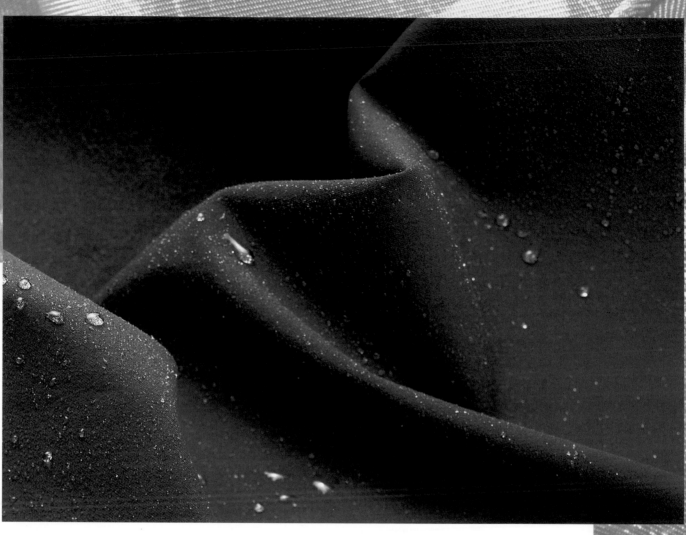

PERFORMANCE

The Swiss manufacturer Schoeller has produced this deodorizing fabric (above), and, as the name suggests, it helps to keep the wearer odour-free.

The fibre used for this Chinon scarf (background) is produced by Toyobo Co Ltd and is made using a milk casein (protein). The handle and lustre are silk-like, and it weighs 10% less than silk. It absorbs and wicks perspiration away from the body and is comfortable to wear.

Sports clothing must and does visually communicate its superiority over rivals. Some garments achieve this by the uniqueness of their design, while others rely on styling. Where the performance is not obvious, the consumer is slow to accept the product. Japanese companies cannot compete in terms of price in natural or ordinary synthetic fabrics with their Asian neighbours, and this has forced them to look at what they can produce that is unique, hence the development of health-giving fabrics. Milk-protein fibre is probably the least beneficial of these, yet, ironically, it is one of the most popular. This is because people like the idea of wearing a fabric made from 'milk'. The other fabrics in the group are appearing in the Western markets very slowly. The fabrics look like regular polyesters or nylon, and there is nothing to indicate that they are providing any additional benefit. In some instances, mini information booklets are already attached to the zipper of the garment in the shops. Ironically, some of these fabrics are bypassing the sports clothes market and are being used by fashion designers who like their sporty image. Vexed Generation have used a wicking fabric in a two-piece women's top and skirt. Wicking, odour-absorbing and other health-giving fabrics are being highlighted by the fashion industry who often use them as the primary fabric for garments, not something tucked away as an undergarment. Taking the

One difficulty in marketing health-giving fabrics is that they often do not look different from ordinary synthetics. Vexed Generation have used a wicking fabric in this powder-blue top and skirt. The 'wicking' function of the fabric means that moisture is drawn away from the body and on to the surface of the fabric where is spreads out across the textile. This keeps the body cool and dry.

lead from their colleagues in fashion, sports clothes designers are now reassigning the potential of these materials.

Sport and fashion have drawn closer in recent years, and there are many parallels between the two, such as the launch of seasonal collections. However, the sports industry fiercely guards its independence, and this allows it to retain a separate identity. If this should change, it is likely that it would lose its attraction as a fashion. This separation gives the sports design industry the freedom to absorb a range of disparate external influences – from the latest fabrics developed for spacesuits, to ethnic clothing designed to protect fishermen from the Arctic climate. No area is hidden from the eagle eye of the sports designer.

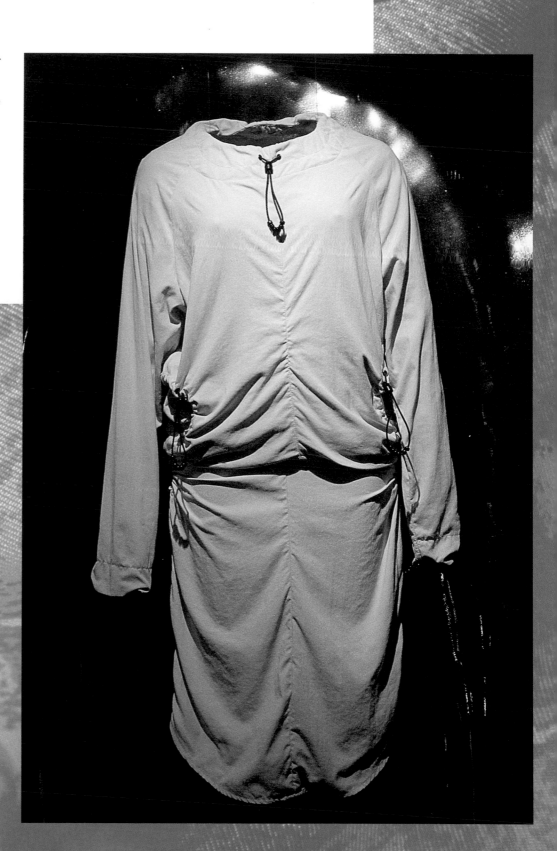

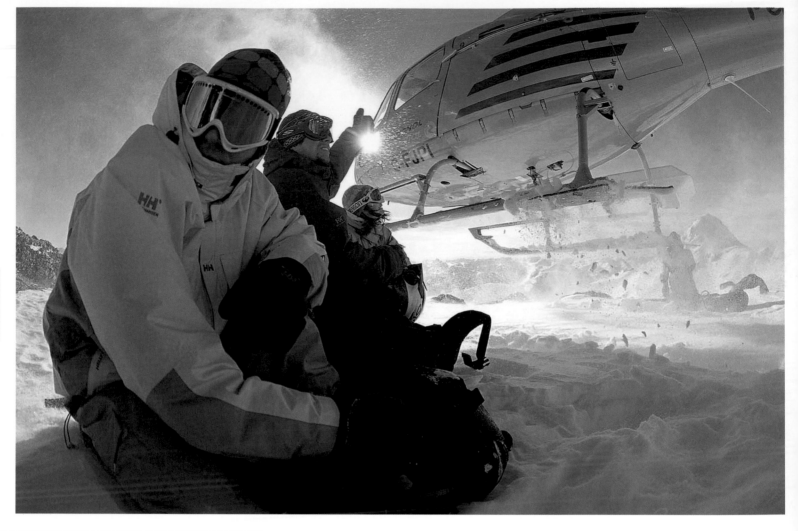

PROTECTION

The most basic function of any clothing is to protect the body from its physical and climatic environment. The extent of the damage caused by the sun to the human body has only been appreciated relatively recently. Clothing is used as a barrier against the sun's harmful rays, and is reasonably effective irrespective of the type of fabric used. A new range of synthetic fabrics, however, have been developed by such companies as Kuraray which provide a more active barrier against ultra-violet rays. Designers realize that it is not enough to use a protective fabric, and the whole garment must be designed to guard against the sun. Helly Hansen's Men's Factor Sun Shirt is one garment that takes its protective role seriously. The main fabric is a Supplex ripstop nylon with a MCS wicking finish and a solar-protection-treatment. The long-sleeved shirt with snap tabs allows the addition of a collar for even more protection. It gives a solar protection rating of 30SPF (Sun Protection Factor).

Fabrics made of natural fibres, such as silk and cotton, are generally considered the most effective in allowing the body to perspire. However, natural fibres are not ideal in that they absorb perspiration but then hold it, so that on cooling the fabric feels damp against the skin. Synthetic materials such as nylon and polyester are traditionally associated with poor absorbency, trapping perspiration on the body. Fibre and fabric engineers are responding to this challenge by developing a range of high-performance fabrics that move perspiration away from the body and keep a dry surface next to the skin. Sportswear manufacturer Cannondale produces a wicking fabric under the brand name Fieldsensor. The fabric is structured so that the fibres decrease in volume from

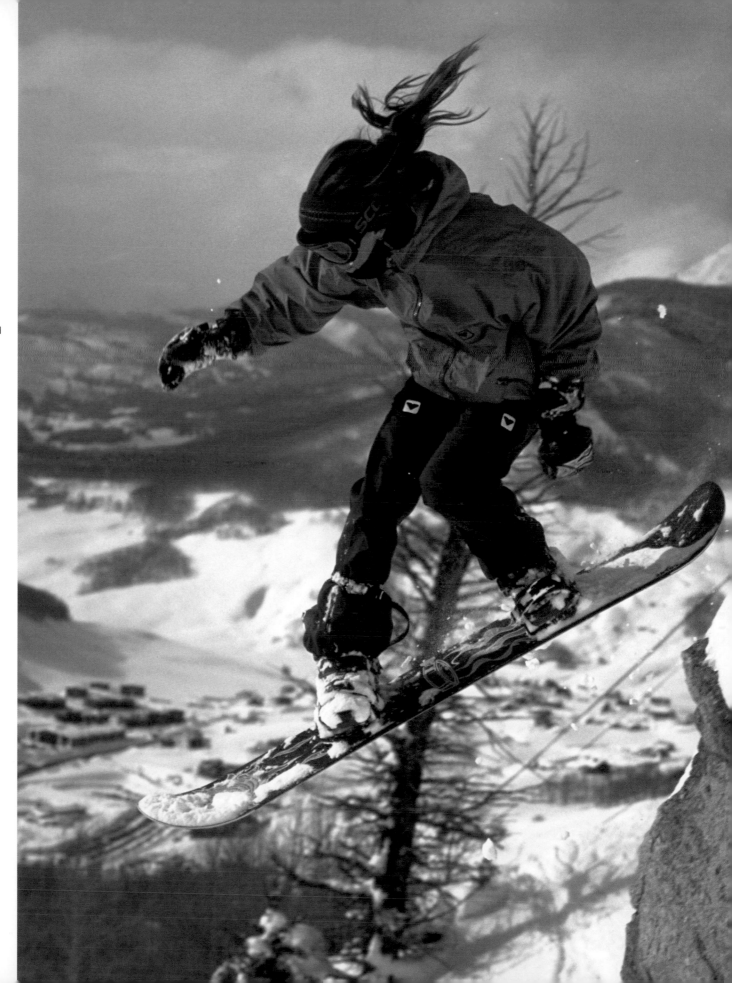

Helly Hansen (left) has gained
a reputation for combining
streetwise looks with no-nonsense
high-performance fabrics and cut.
Much of its clothing is designed
for high-energy winter sports,
but its logos are just as likely
to be seen on the urban streets.

Extreme sports enthusiasts
are among those who demand
the most from their clothes.
High-performance must be
accompanied by strong aesthetics.
Most popular are the specialist
manufacturers whose designers
are often practitioners in their
particular sport, and so understand
the needs and changing fashion
trends firsthand.

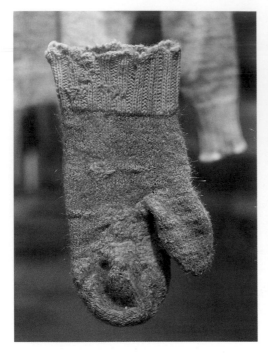

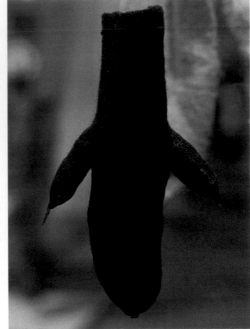

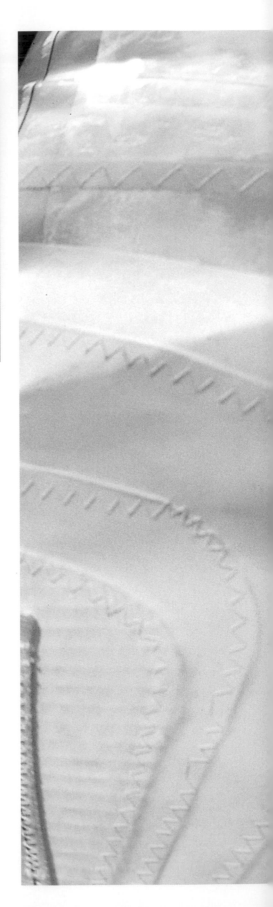

These fishermen's mittens from Denmark's Herning Museum, date from the late 1800s. They were shown beside contemporary sportswear designs at the 2002 exhibition, 'Edge: The Influence of Sportswear', Oksnehallen, Copenhagen. The single-thumb mittens are knitted using human hair to repel water. The double-thumb feature was used by eel fishermen when they fished on ice in winter. One thumb would get wet and extremely cold bringing the eels in, so fishermen then switched to the other thumb.

The UK company, Musto's MPX One Design uses MPX breathable technology and Musto's 3-Layer System. The former is a double-layered fabric where the MPX coating is applied to a waterproof, breathable, abrasion-resistant outer shell.

the inner to outer surface. The high-volume spaces next to the skin absorb moisture, and transport it to the outer surface using an increased capillary action to disperse the moisture for rapid evaporation, leaving the body feeling dry and comfortable.

Protection from rain, wind and snow are equally important, and there is a long tradition of design in this area. Prior to the advent of sportswear and synthetic fibres, ingenious solutions were developed by people living in some of the extreme climates of the world. Sports clothes manufacturers have in the past taken inspiration from the aesthetic qualities of ethnic garments. But designers are now starting to appreciate the lessons in performance and fit-for-purpose garments that can be applied to the design of contemporary waterproof clothing. The Herning Museum in Denmark houses an unusual pair of mittens in its ethnographic collection. They were both designed for use by fishermen. One is knitted using human hair to help repel water. The other mitten has two thumbs so that, after the fisherman had made one wet reaching through the icy water for the eel, he could move his thumb to the dry one once his hand was out of the water.

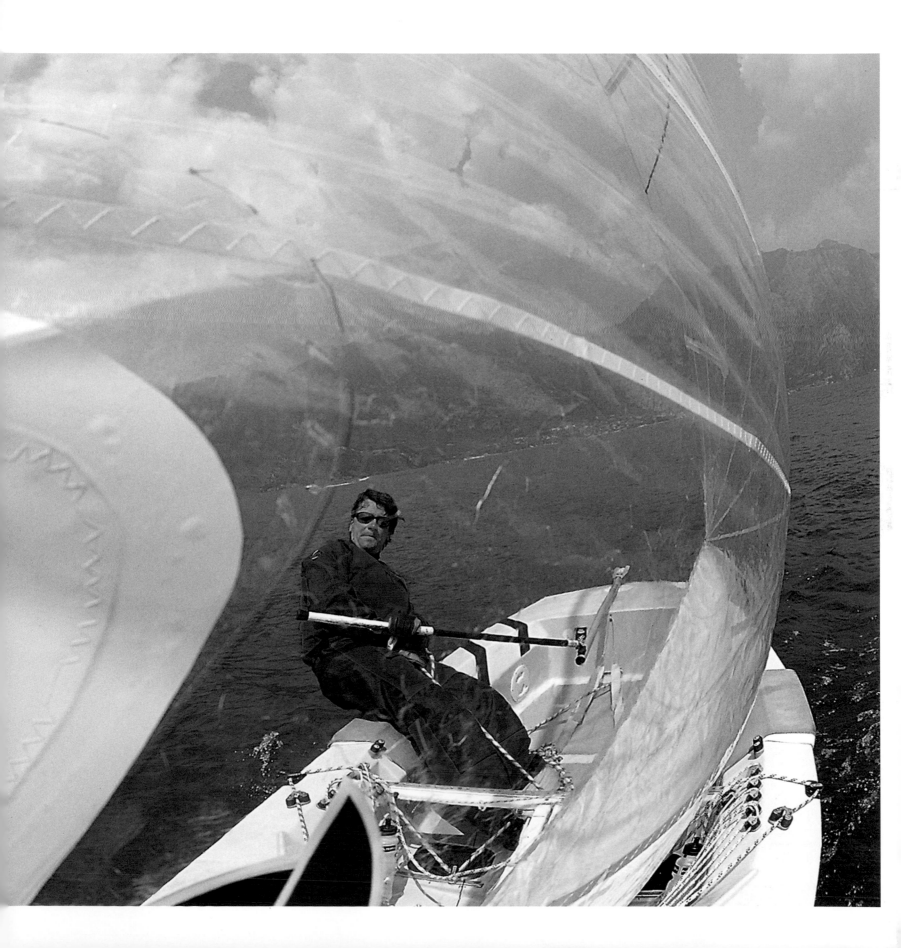

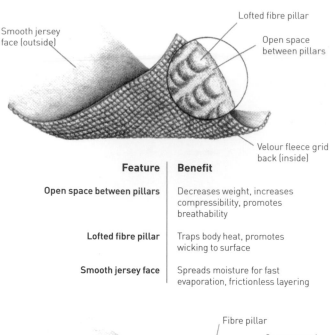

Smooth jersey face (outside)

Lofted fibre pillar

Open space between pillars

Velour fleece grid back (inside)

Feature	Benefit
Open space between pillars	Decreases weight, increases compressibility, promotes breathability
Lofted fibre pillar	Traps body heat, promotes wicking to surface
Smooth jersey face	Spreads moisture for fast evaporation, frictionless layering

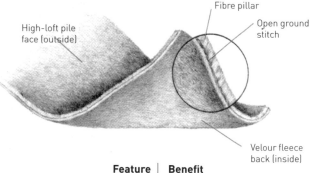

High-loft pile face (outside)

Fibre pillar

Open ground stitch

Velour fleece back (inside)

Feature	Benefit
Open ground stitch	Promotes compressibility
High-loft with low density	Increases warmth, minimizes weight, increases compressibility
High-loft pile face	Maintains its loft for enduring warmth; maximizes moisture movement for a fast dry time

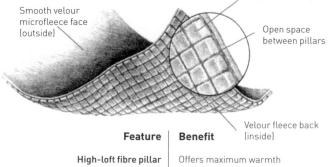

Smooth velour microfleece face (outside)

High-loft fibre pillar

Open space between pillars

Velour fleece back (inside)

Feature	Benefit
High-loft fibre pillar	Offers maximum warmth with less weight
Open space between pillars	Decreases weight, increases compressibility, enhances breathability
Smooth velour microfleece face	Improves wind resistance, increases warmth

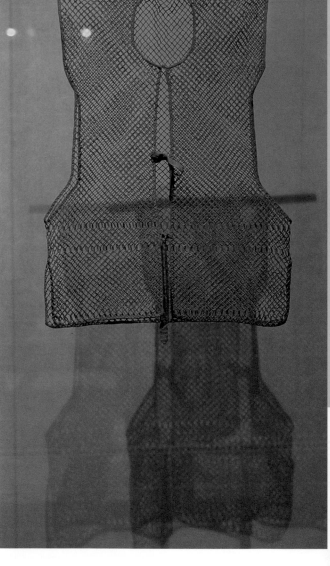

Patagonia's R1, R2 and R3 are the three grades of Polartec Regulator (left), a lightweight fleece that uses a lofted grid structure to trap body heat as well as encouraging wicking of body moisture to the surface of the fabric. The open structure on the underside of the fabric makes it lighter than traditional fleeces and easier to compress. The outer layer is a smooth jersey that allows any moisture wicked away from the body to spread across its surface and evaporate quickly. The fabric structure was inspired by the design of a traditional Chinese bamboo jacket (right) which traps air in its open latticework. The example shown here is from the collection of Linda Wrigglesworth Ltd, London.

Patagonia use a patented EncapSil technology to produce a windproof, water-repellent fabric that is used in a number of their sports ranges, including Velocity shell jackets and vests. The process encapsulates individual yarns with a windproof, water-repellent polymer. This is considered a much more durable alternative to coating the surface of the fabric. The system is flexible enough to be used to produce ripstop polyester (which as the names suggests limits tears in the fabric) without compromising the performance of either process. Burton produce a triple-layered waterproof, breathable jacket for snowboarding. The TriLite jacket uses a fabric of the same name. The garment construction incorporates fully sealed seams, yoke as well as upper and rear arm areas using a stretch TriLite fabric.

The Inuit parka has a rich ethnographic history that includes seasonal variations, inner and outer versions, as well as different styles for men, women and children. Winter parkas are worn with trousers, mittens and boots. All have several layers with the fur of the innermost parka pointing towards the body to act as an air pocket retaining as much air (and consequently warmth) as possible. An example of a woman's inner *amauti* was shown at the British Museum's 'Annuraaq: Arctic Clothing from Igloolik' exhibition, and this was made in

1986 by Zipporah Innuksuk. The fur is turned towards the body and strips of sealskin have been sewn on to the seams for reinforcement and to prevent them from stretching. The fringe trim partly serves a decorative purpose, but also has a practical use preventing the edges from curling or tearing, and cold air from entering. There were also fringes on a young boy's caribou-skin *atajuq*, or combination suit. The hood is separate from the body of the suit, and the decorative fringes around the neck also protect it from draughts.

The parka as well as various aspects of its construction has been utilized by sports and fashion designers alike. It is a garment that has often prompted the wearer to personalize it, so that it assumes a cultural significance. The Mods in the UK in the 1960s wore parkas while riding their scooters, taking meticulous care of both. Their drop-tail design is also used to prevent wind, rain or snow penetration in motorcycling, mountaineering and other sports. The parka itself has undergone several changes, mainly instigated by fashion, but most recently aligned to sport through the use of high-performance fabrics.

The garment has almost become a trademark for British designers Griffin, so much so that when Jeff Griffin asked for suggestions on a name for his first son, his Japanese clients readily replied 'Parka'. His son's name is Parka Rock. Griffin alternates between the use of high-performance fabrics and more traditional coated cotton and linen. The Boar Skin parka from the Autumn/Winter 2001 collection is a woodland camouflage design, and uses a sandblasted cotton/polyester fabric produced in lined and reversible versions. The most

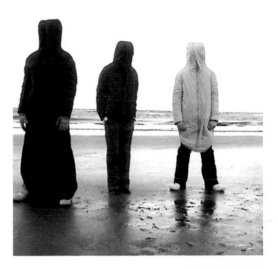

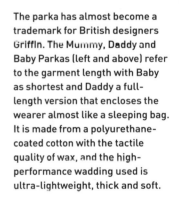

The parka has almost become a trademark for British designers Griffin. The Mummy, Daddy and Baby Parkas (left and above) refer to the garment length with Baby as shortest and Daddy a full-length version that encloses the wearer almost like a sleeping bag. It is made from a polyurethane-coated cotton with the tactile quality of wax, and the high-performance wadding used is ultra-lightweight, thick and soft.

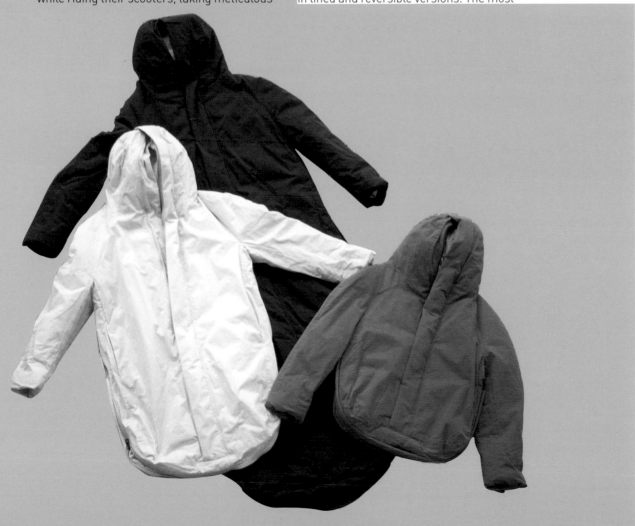

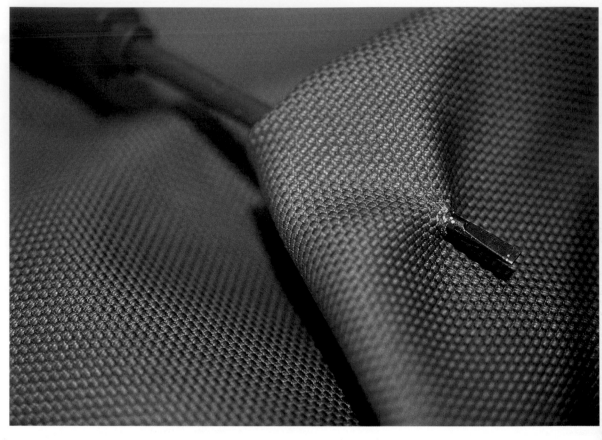

The Belgian textile company Sofinal uses proprietary technology in its unique self-healing fabric (right). The technique combines a special weave and finishing treatment that allows the fabric to repair itself if punctured. The fabric is currently being used in applications as varied as luggage liners and motorcycle jackets.

The challenge in designing protective clothing for sports is to provide designs that combine safety without compromising ease of movement. Italy's Luca Cadalora (opposite) makes full use of his protective kneepads in this qualifying session for the USA Motorcycle Grand Prix held at Laguna Seca, California in September 1994.

intriguing series is a group of three: Mummy, Daddy and Baby Parkas. The titles refer to their length, with Baby as shortest and Daddy a full-length version that encloses the wearer almost like a sleeping bag. The latter is apparently very popular with football supporters and film crews who have to spend long periods of time standing around in the cold. The polyurethane-coated cotton has the tactile quality of wax with a high performance wadding which is ultra-lightweight, thick and soft.

Vexed Generation (Adam Thorpe and Joe Hunter) is London-based and has taken the parka design along a very different route. Hunter describes the importance of fabric: 'Our cloth is as primary as our style. You can't make a shape without having the right cloth.' Most of their fabric suppliers produce high-performance technical textiles for military and protective clothing. This use of over-specified fabric is linked to their concern for personal liberty issues. They want to produce a style

that has a political aesthetic. The Vexed Parka incorporates some classic parka design elements, such as the drop-tail, but they have given it a collar that extends to cover the mouth and nose when zipped up. This references police riot gear as well as pollution-protective masks worn by cyclists.

Nature provides a hard outer layer of protection (an exoskeleton) for some invertebrates, including annelids (such as molluscs) and arthropods (such as insects and lobsters which have jointed limbs). In arthropods, the skeletal muscles are attached to the inside surface of the integument, with many insects relying on the geometry of this hybrid structure for their strength. The combination is particularly important for optimizing leverage and moving objects that are very large relative to the size of the insect. Many insects have more muscle than vertebrates because the exoskeleton affords a larger surface area relative to body volume for muscle attachment than the

internal or endoskeleton. The exoskeleton in nature functions in much the same way as a medieval knight's or Japanese samurai's suit of armour. The demands of high-impact sports, such as motorcycle and luge racing, as well as ice hockey, have seen these competitors increasingly encased in their own artificial exoskeletons.

Protective leathers used by motorcyclists effectively act as exoskeletons, offering a combination of protection and flexibility for ease of movement. Although leather remains the most popular material among motorcyclists, advanced textiles and foams are now being introduced. Early synthetics (like natural fibres), did not perform well in the event of an accident. If the motorcyclist is dragged along a road surface, the fabric rips along with the skin, allowing grit and fabric particles to become embedded in the body tissue. Having these picked out of a wound is not something many motorcyclists are anxious to experience.

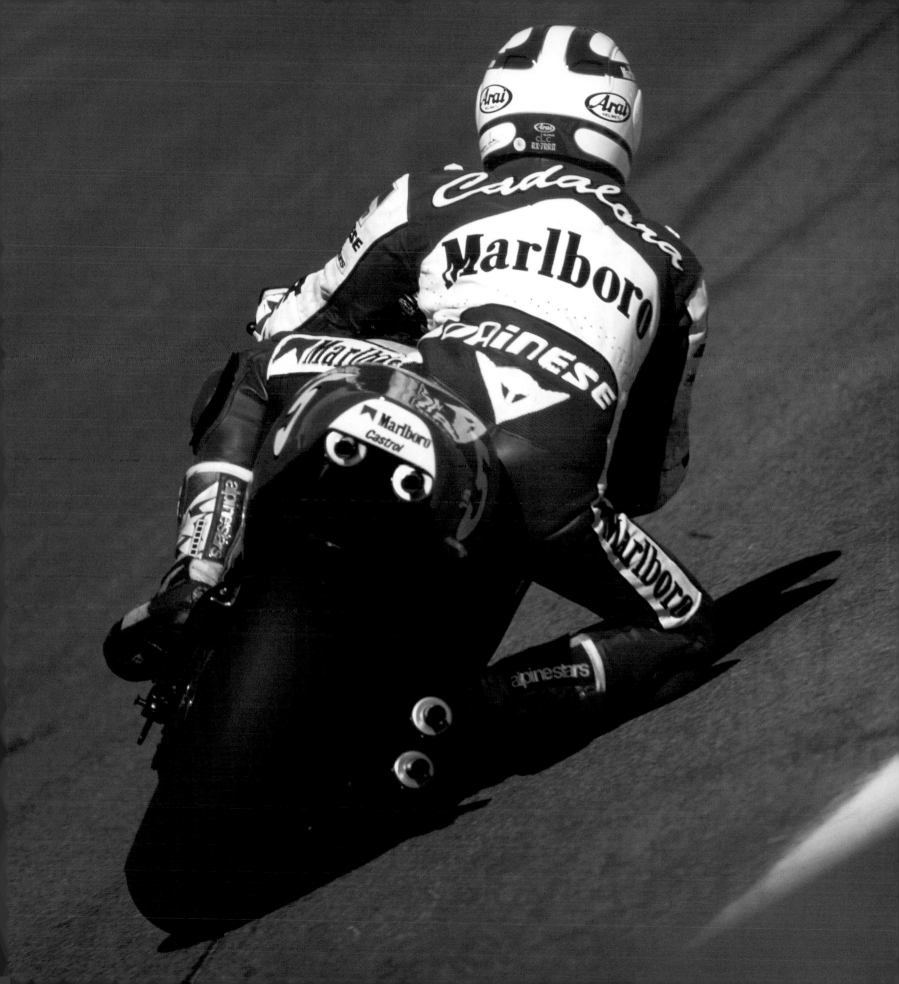

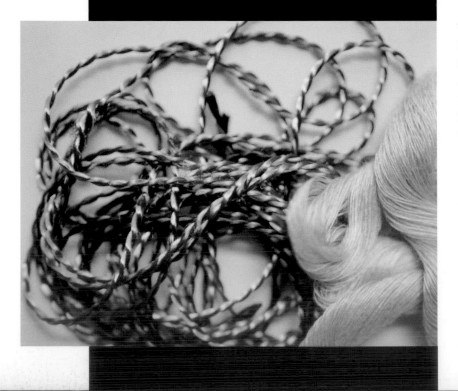

The new range of performance fabrics being used in sports clothes – aramid, carbon and glass fibre – have usually come via the space, military or even sports equipment industries. Each of these disciplines is very demanding, so the materials bring with them this rich source of performance data. Such fabrics are most commonly used in combination with leather to add reinforcement in specially vulnerable areas, such as the elbow, knee, and back. They can also be used on their own or with other synthetic fabrics. One problem in using them on their own is that they need a protective coating to stabilize them, and another is the difficulty in colouring these yarns. Carbon and aramid fibres are only available in black and yellow respectively, and glass fibre is usually manufactured white, occasionally black. Where colour is added, it is generally included in the coating. Motorcycle designers have overcome these aesthetic limitations either by covering the materials with leather or using them in their natural state.

While performance has always been implicit in the design of motorcycle clothing, it is now becoming explicit in the way that it is communicated through the use of colour, pattern and the design itself. Manufacturers SPIDI have designed motorcycle gloves that highlight the areas that have been reinforced (such as the knuckles) through the use of a black-and-yellow (carbon and aramid) zigzag pattern. Reinforcement is no longer confined to the interior of the jacket and the trousers. It is becoming increasingly common to make flexible systems with sleeve or Velcro systems that can accommodate additional protective pads. Italian motorcycle clothing manufacturer Dainese, have worked with the British designer Mark Sadler to develop its 'bap' protector. The design provides a hard protective shell that acts like an exoskeleton

Advanced manufacturing techniques allow designers to use fabrics as alternatives to heavier materials, such as metal. In some instances, the two are combined to bring together the strength of the metal, with the flexibility of the textile: an aluminium-coated glass fibre produced by Tekson GmbH (above); a selection of 100% stainless steel and synthetic/metal blended yarn and thread from Bekintex NV (below).

High-performance materials such as carbon fibre are now being used in many different areas of clothing, product and vehicle design. Woven, knitted, nonwoven and braided structures are becoming increasingly common as manufacturing technologies have caught up with fibre developments, and costs are beginning to come down. These images show a range of braided structures from Siltex, where carbon fibre is used on its own (black), with glass fibre (black and white) and with aramid fibres (black and yellow). Each has its own unique performance characteristics determined by the mix of yarns.

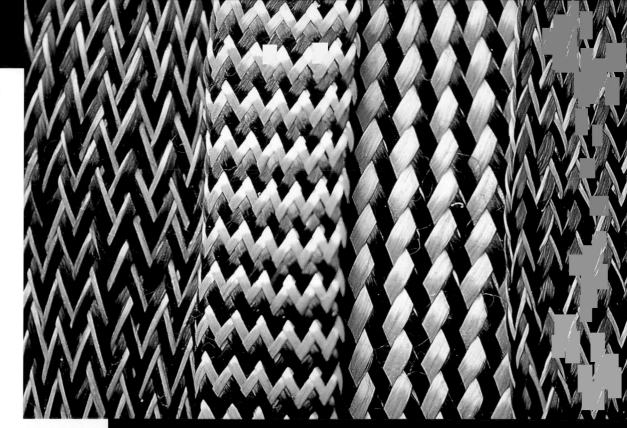

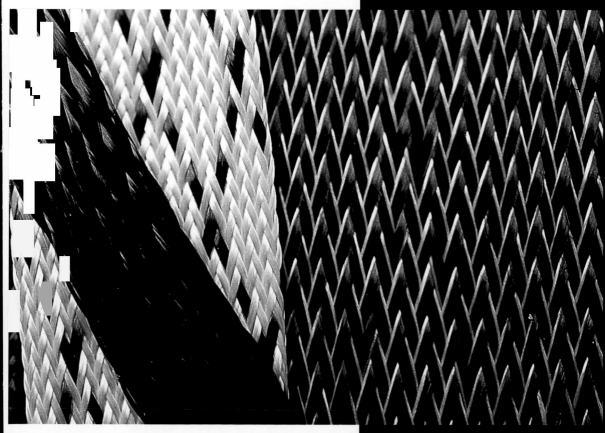

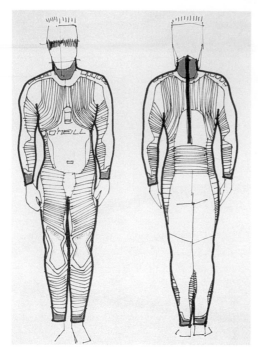

protecting the spine, elbows, knees and other vulnerable areas. The bap-like protective pads can be strapped on using a Velcro or elasticized mechanism so that it leaves the rest of the body freedom of movement. The aesthetic of the garment is one of extreme protection, with its performance worn on its sleeve – literally. Though considerably lighter, more flexible and comfortable to wear, it remains a modern equivalent of the medieval suit of armour.

There are some sports where protection and self-preservation are synonymous – ice hockey for example. In this fast-moving game, when players collide, it is with some force. Protective pads are essential for all, but it is the cage-like attire of the goalie that stands out. Goalies typically wear about a quarter of their body weight in protection which covers every inch of their body. The end result is an intimidating form that looks not unlike a samurai warrior or robot. During the game, the ice hockey goalie can lose up to 3 kilograms (7 lbs) through sweating, so that his equipment feels even heavier. The protective pads absorb much of this perspiration. Those used to be made of leather, but manufacturers are now changing

to a lighter synthetic and making use of antimicrobial fabric developments. Bauer's Supreme 5000 series pads all use an antimcrobial liner and the Vapor 10 pants and gloves use a quick-drying silver lining material. Even the socks are quick drying, while the Gripliner lining keeps the foot in place. The clothing must protect and allow movement at the same time. The Supreme 5000 shoulder and elbow pads rely on moulded polyethylene caps for rigid areas, using asymmetrical shapes for bicep protection. A softer gel protection is used between these caps to allow some body movement. Bauer's Reactor 6 leg pads use anatomical knee and shin cradles for a better fit and to prevent the pads rotating. The calf wing is raised to give better stability when the goalie is in the butterfly position, while Flexx Darts allow a full range of knee movement without compromising protection. But it is the mask that is the goalie's most distinctive, and personalized piece of equipment. Top goalkeepers have a cast taken of their head then the mask is made to fit exactly using fibreglass or an aramid such as DuPont's Kevlar. Pro-Masque Inc. make their Pro-Masque and PM-2000 Millennium masks by hand using wire jigs. The materials used are amongst the strongest, most rigid yet lightweight available: a multi-directional, triaxial Vectorply fibreglass, Kevlar, carbon graphite and Vectran (this was used by NASA to make the air bags that protected the lunar Rover on Mars). The cage protecting the face can be made of polished stainless steel, with the company offering to plate cages with chrome or gold.

Not all protection is quite so extreme. O'Neill teamed up with the California design consultancy, Vent Design to create the Animal wetsuit. O'Neill, the pioneer of wetsuit design, has always been aware of customer needs and the far from idyllic weather conditions that have to be endured. Surfers in Cornwall and California alike, can get cold waiting around for the surf

O'Neill teamed up with the California design consultancy, Vent Design to create the Animal wetsuit (right, and patent drawing for the design, left). The wetsuit is designed to allow ease of movement, particularly around elbow and knee joints, without loss of thermal insulation. One of the innovative characteristics is its utilization of the O'Neill Expansion System. The moulding system produces bellows-like sections for use in high-flex areas forming accordion pleats for ease of movement. Before this, closed-cell neoprene had not been moulded in this manner.

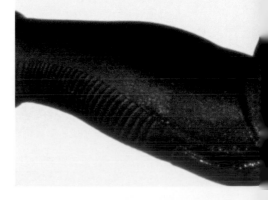

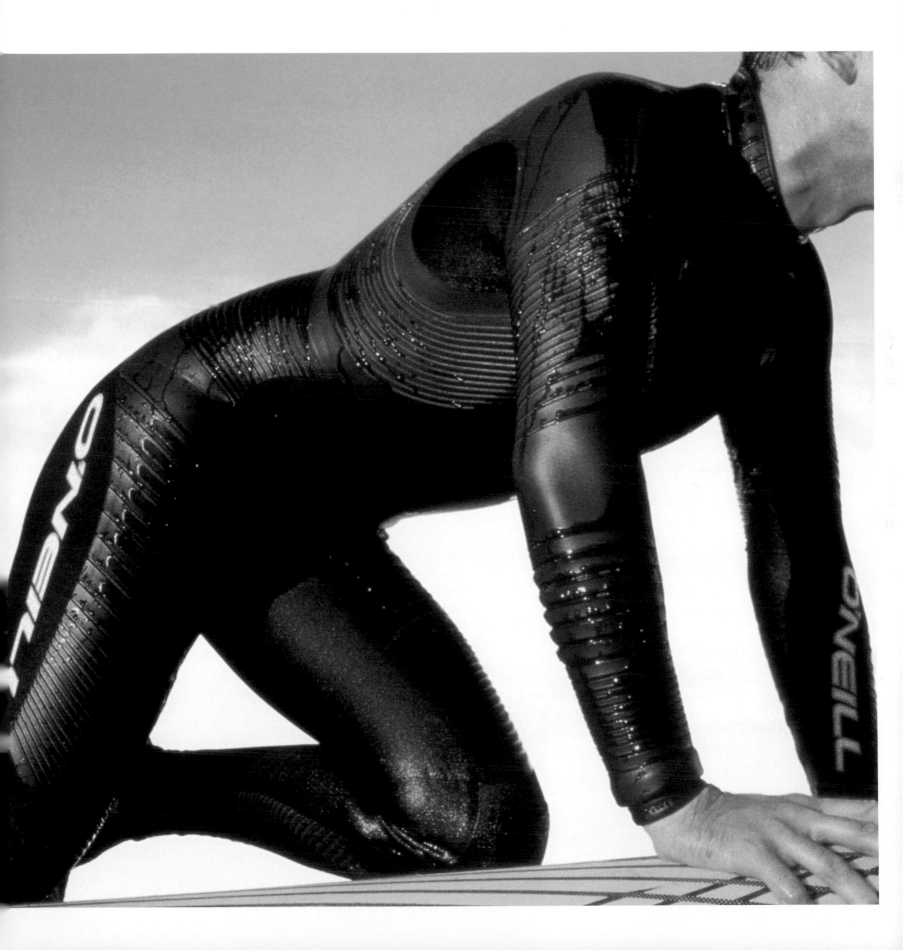

Nature makes abundant use of folds and pleats for many different reasons. Some add structural strength, while others perform valuable functions. The fan-shaped leaves shown here, are growing in California. They are angled towards the sun and their pleated form serve to channel precious rainwater down along the leaves and stem, towards its roots.

to be just right. Once in the water, they want to be able to move easily and to keep cool, so that thicker neoprene is not the simple solution. The brief set by O'Neill for the design of the Animal wetsuit included the need for freedom of movement, particularly around elbow and knee joints, without loss of thermal insulation. The finished appearance is quite unlike any traditional wetsuit design that uses a smooth matt neoprene. One of the innovative characteristics (apart from its appearance, which is, as the name suggests, like an animal), is that it utilizes a production technology that is more often associated with product design. Despite the use of such a high-tech material, the human element remains very much in evidence in the production process. Each garment

takes a hundred and twenty man-hours to assemble.

The extraction of good design from nature is called biomimetics or biomimicry. This approach transcends different design disciplines, and is being used by engineers, architects and product designers alike. This allows designers not only to draw on nature for inspiration, but also look at how designers and engineers from other areas approach a similar problem. Using nature in this way, biomimetics forms part of a growing trend towards multidisciplinary design practice and thinking.

The correlation between weight and strength is one that poses problems for the engineer who needs to make the aeroplane or car

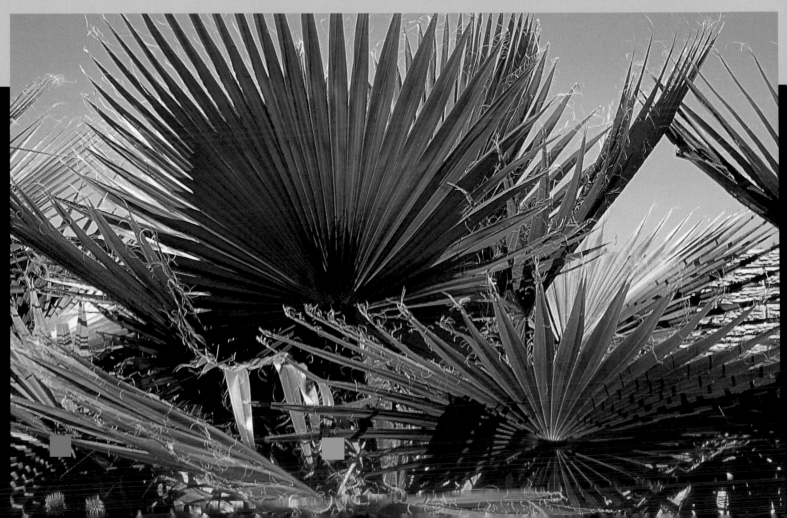

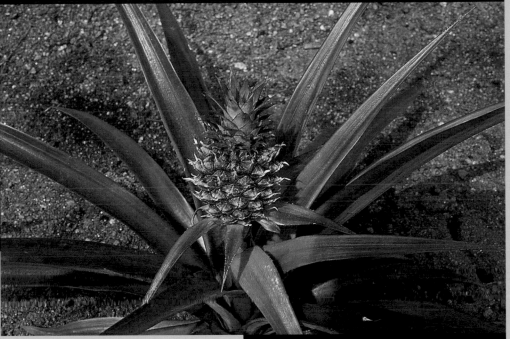

The growth pattern of pineapples and pine cones has inspired the design of a folded Pineapple or Ananas pattern, a name chosen by Biruta Kresling and Nathalie Malliard at the University of Reading's Department of Biomimetics. The expansion capabilities and flexibility of the pineapple structure can be adapted for textiles using a paper template (as shown below). Traditionally the fabric would have been shaped using stitching techniques, such as smocking; however, the fact that thermoplastic fabrics can be permanently shaped using heat has created many more possibilities and greater use of this structure in sports clothes.

lighter so that it uses less fuel in transit. It is also a problem for the designer of sports shoes who has to develop soles that will provide the necessary support, but with the minimum weight. The materials used in these instances can allow some weight saving. To see any significant improvement, however, it is necessary to use the materials in a different way. This is where biomimetics plays a role. Nature uses the minimum amount of material, relying instead on clever design, one example of which is its use of folded or pleated structures.

The shell of the abalone is scarred and covered with barnacles on the exterior, but inside is a smooth mother-of-pearl lining. Researcher Mehmet Sarikaya at the University of Washington has made a study of the shell's structural properties, and describes the abalone as being 'twice as tough as any ceramic we know of – instead of breaking like a man-made ceramic, the shell deforms under stress and behaves like a metal.' The secret of this high strength lies in the protein chain, which folds into a zigzag forming an accordion-like pleated sheet. While researchers still struggle to create a ceramic along the same principles as

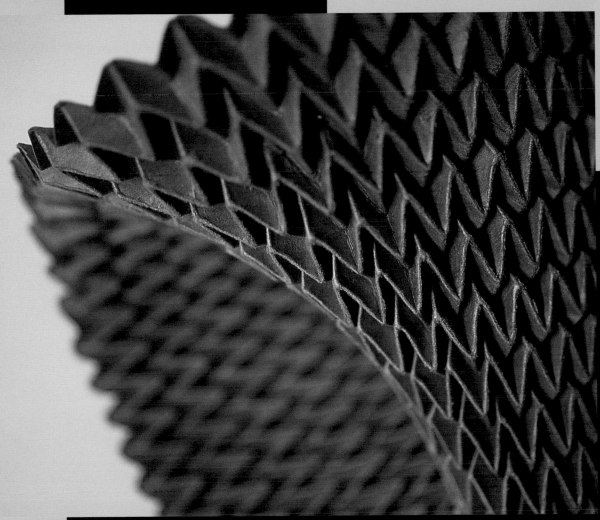

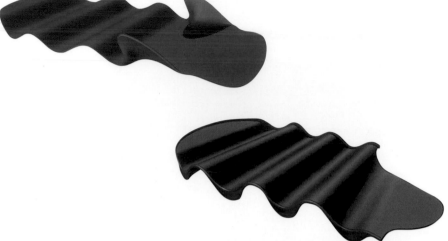

The engineering behind Mizuno's Wave technology is a pleated, origami-like structure. While more traditional midsoles rely on flat materials that simply absorb energy at the point of impact, Mizuno Wave disperses the force of the impact uniformly over the length and width of the midsole.

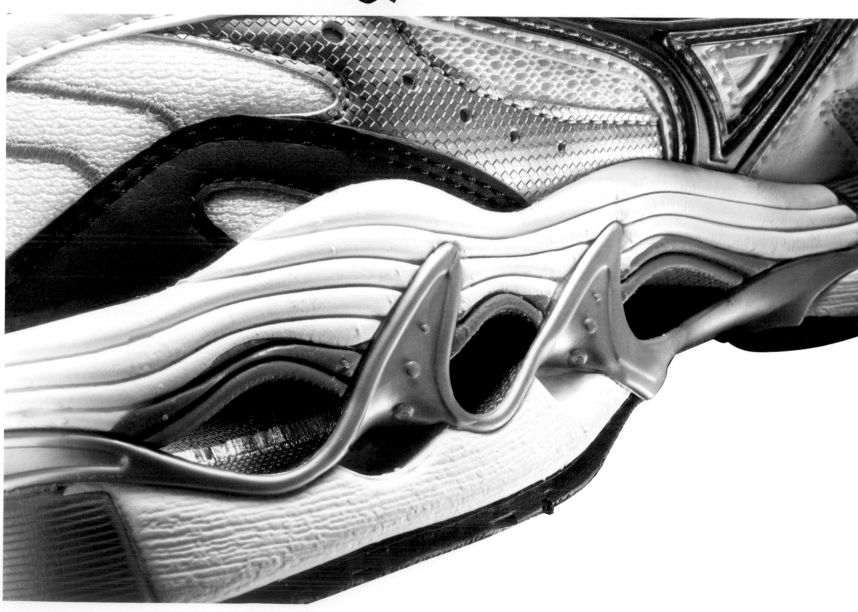

Mizuno have used their Wave technology for footwear with very different requirements. Shown here (left to right) are a golf shoe, a football boot with moulded studs, a baseball/softball shoe and a running shoe.

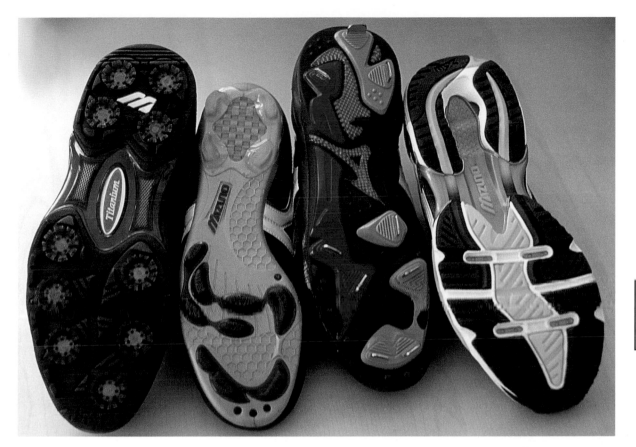

the abalone, engineers have adopted the general principle of folding structures with some success.

While this interest from engineers is relatively recent, the structural and dynamic properties of folds in nature have inspired Japanese craftsmen for centuries. The paper art of origami has evolved as a decorative art in Japan, and, at its most basic, contracts or expands a large surface by simply pulling two opposing corners apart. Origami possesses qualities that can provide inspiration for other designer disciplines.

The Japanese sports clothing and equipment manufacturer, Mizuno, has developed a Mizuno Wave design for use in sports shoes. The design is pleated, origami-like, but the support mechanism was inspired by the movement of waves against the seashore. While more traditional midsoles rely on flat materials that simply absorb energy at the point of impact, Mizuno Wave

disperses the force of the impact uniformly over the length and width of the midsole. As the foot falls, there is a slight rolling motion (hence the name) that provides motion control and relieves stress on the ankle and knee joints. The biomechanically engineered technology can be used in many different types of sports shoe, including the golf and baseball shoe. Each sport has its own particular demands, and the technology is adapted and augmented for each.

The sole of the Mizuno Wave golf shoe consists of several layers to form a composite structure. The midsole uses a layer of compression-moulded EVA foam to provide cushioning. Mizuno Wave technology allows the golfer's foot to move properly during the swing, a movement that causes the foot to be simultaneously twisted and raised. Then comes the outer sole. The design uses another of its specially developed technologies, AutoTrax, for the spike system. This reduces the overall weight of the shoe

and maximizes traction. A bonus to the golf course is that it is also more gentle on the greens.

Requirements for the baseball shoe are rather different. Although the baseball player also performs swinging motions, he must throw the ball and run as well. Mizuno's Chipper 9-Spike (mid/low) shoe for baseball is designed to enable the player to perform all these activities with ease. The midsole uses a full-length contoured compression-moulded EVA footbed to disperse impact and provide stability and cushioning for the foot. The VS-2 Form Board is placed underneath the insole to provide cushioning that can be customized for each player, while a Parallel Wave Plate is inserted in the heel. The outer sole includes a pressure-dispersion platform to dissipate any pressure from the cleats themselves. The Pebax spike plate is contoured and the company's 9-Spike configuration combines strength and flexibility.

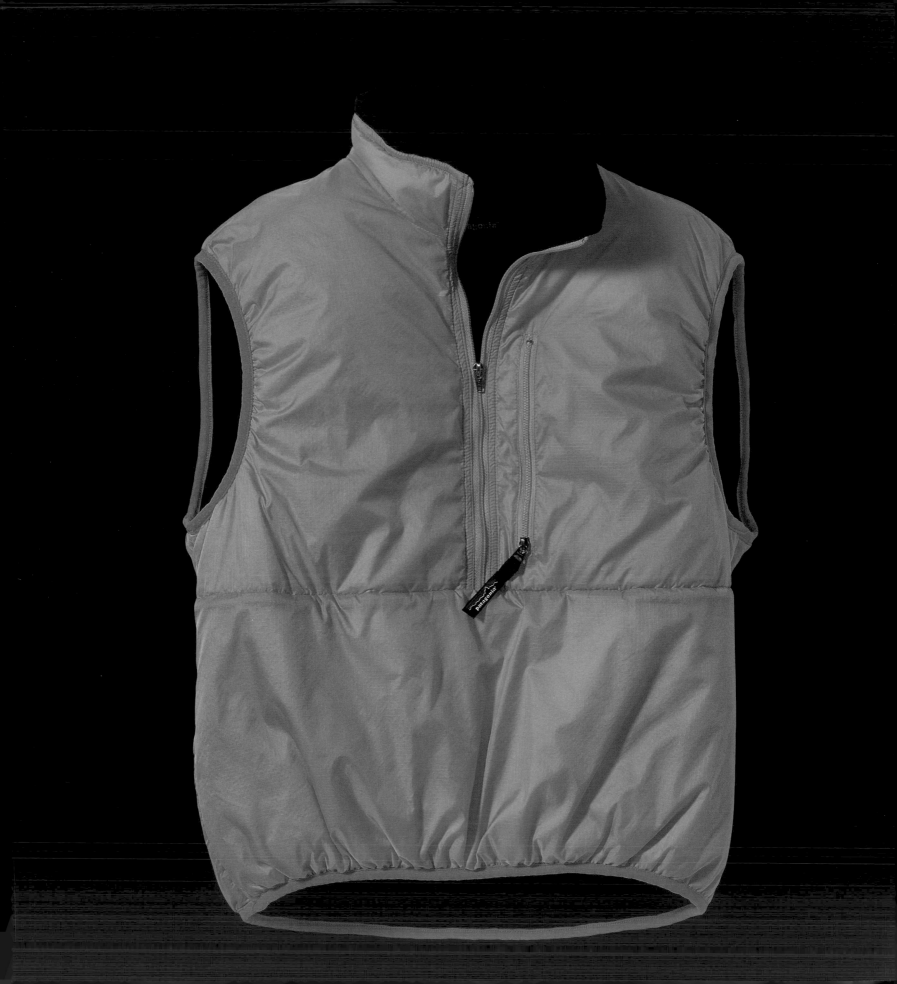

Patagonia's Puffball jackets and vests (opposite) don't need constant pampering to keep them dry and they retain their insulating qualities even when wet. They're also lightweight, compressible (they can be stuffed into their own vertical zippered chest pocket), wind-resistant and add warmth as part of a layering system. The polyester shell and nylon ripstop lining slide easily over or under layers.

Examples of ripstop nylon from Carrington (right). The fabric can be produced in a range of weights, colours and finishing treatments that include fluorocarbon proofing and polyurethane coatings.

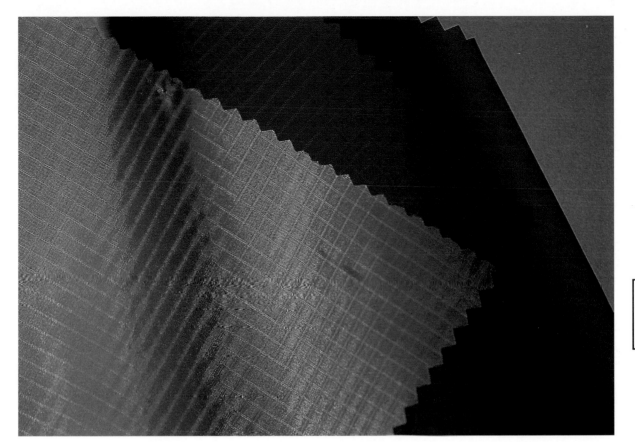

COMFORT

The word comfort implies a passive state, but the demands of sports clothes are such that for them to function properly it is often necessary to include an adaptive or active material or design. For most activities, clothing to be comfortable should keep the body dry and at a pleasant temperature, and should not be too tight or loose. Flexibility can be provided in the fabric where it is essentially a 'smart' or intelligent material that can detect changes in the environment and adapt accordingly. Designers are also producing garments that are functionally gradient, using rigid materials where protection is needed but otherwise employing softer fabrics that work easily with movement. This can also extend to designs where a single garment can be modified for different conditions, or through the use of a layering system. Good design and the use of high-quality materials matter in making comfortable sports clothes.

Designers are continually refining ways of layering clothing, with new ideas appearing on the market each season. Snowboarding and yachting are particularly demanding because high activity takes place in a cold or wet environment. Waterproof breathable fabrics are a basic necessity and W. L. Gore's range of Gore-Tex fabrics are among the most popular. But the fabric is just the beginning, and designers must devise ways of making seams and pockets watertight while creating larger vent areas that can be opened to allow air to move around the body. With layered clothes, the wearer must still be able to move with ease. Articulated elbow and knee joints are one solution to this, and zip-away hoods are becoming another industry standard. Competition is tough, particularly in the snowboarding and mountain sports market, so designers cannot be complacent. The result is that innovation is constant and good design gets better.

Patagonia's waterproof breathable Ice Nine jacket uses a 3-layer Gore-Tex XCR (Extended Comfort Range) composite of mini-ripstop nylon that has been bonded to a Gore-Tex XCR membrane. A polyester scrim, treated with a durable water-repellent finish, lines the jacket, and further reinforcement has been added to vulnerable areas using a nylon and Gore-Tex XCR membrane laminate. Elbows have been articulated for ease of movement, and zips are made extra-long with double sliders and stay-open wind-flaps for ventilation.

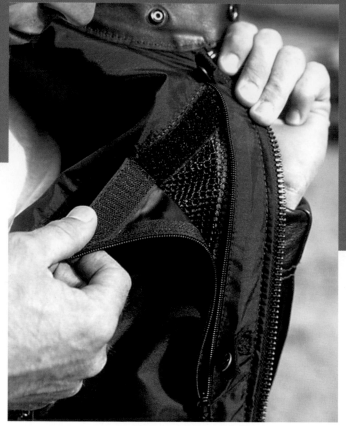

Vanson's Avenger Vent System provides the largest controllable vent area of any Vanson jacket. In this elegantly simple system two panels on the front of the jacket fold down to expose perforated leather panels behind. This cooling method distinguishes itself from other venting systems by preventing the jacket from ballooning and changing size with each vent opened.

The Vanson patented Air Curtain inside the lining allows the wearer to regulate the amount of air flowing through the competition weight PROperf ventilated front, offering many different degrees of ventilation.

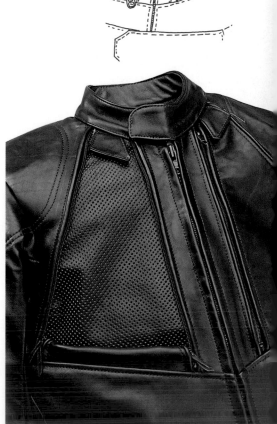

Burton's AK snowboarding jacket and vent pants also use three layers of Gore-Tex fabric with sealed seams. The lightweight clothing is designed for extreme weather conditions. The jacket is equipped with chest-mounted cargo pockets which have mesh-backed venting zips. The underarm venting zips have double storm flaps, while an inner snow skirt has pant attachment loops. Ease of movement is a priority, and an articulated design has been used for the arms of the jacket and the AK Vent pant legs. The pants also have venting zips that run from the waist to the knee area.

Helly Hansen is another company that provides serious protection for snowboarders. Articulated arm and leg designs are common in many of its garments, as are ventilation pit zips. Helly Hansen's women's Luxor pants include additional comfort features. A brushed microfleece lining and 3M's Thinsulate nonwoven in the seat and knee areas give extra warmth without adding any noticeable weight.

Some of the most sophisticated vent designs have been developed for motorcycle and luge suits. Vanson Leathers are best known for their motorcycle leathers but also produce a range of luge suits with some innovative vent design features. The Avenger vent is a system whereby two panels on the front of the jacket fold down to expose perforated leather panels behind. This method prevents the jacket from ballooning and changing size when a vent is opened. A variation on this is the company's Air Curtain Vent (used in its Cobra jacket). Here the front of the jacket is perforated but has an airtight membrane behind. Within the membrane are panels that can be zipped up or down then folded into pockets that allow air to flow through the jacket to be released through exit vents at the back. By having the vents on the inside, graphics can be applied to the front of the jacket, something that is not possible with the Avenger vent. Both systems are patented. Vanson has also designed a vent system for use in the sleeve

Vanson's Cobra jacket uses Vanson's Air Curtain technology to provide an internal air curtain that folds down to let cooling air flow inside for summer riding, or zips air tight for cooler days and early morning rides. The Competition Weight PROperf front is the key to this new riding technology, the same leather used on Vanson's AMA approved race suits. An adjustable waistband is concealed inside the jacket to allow the wearer to add clothing with comfort.

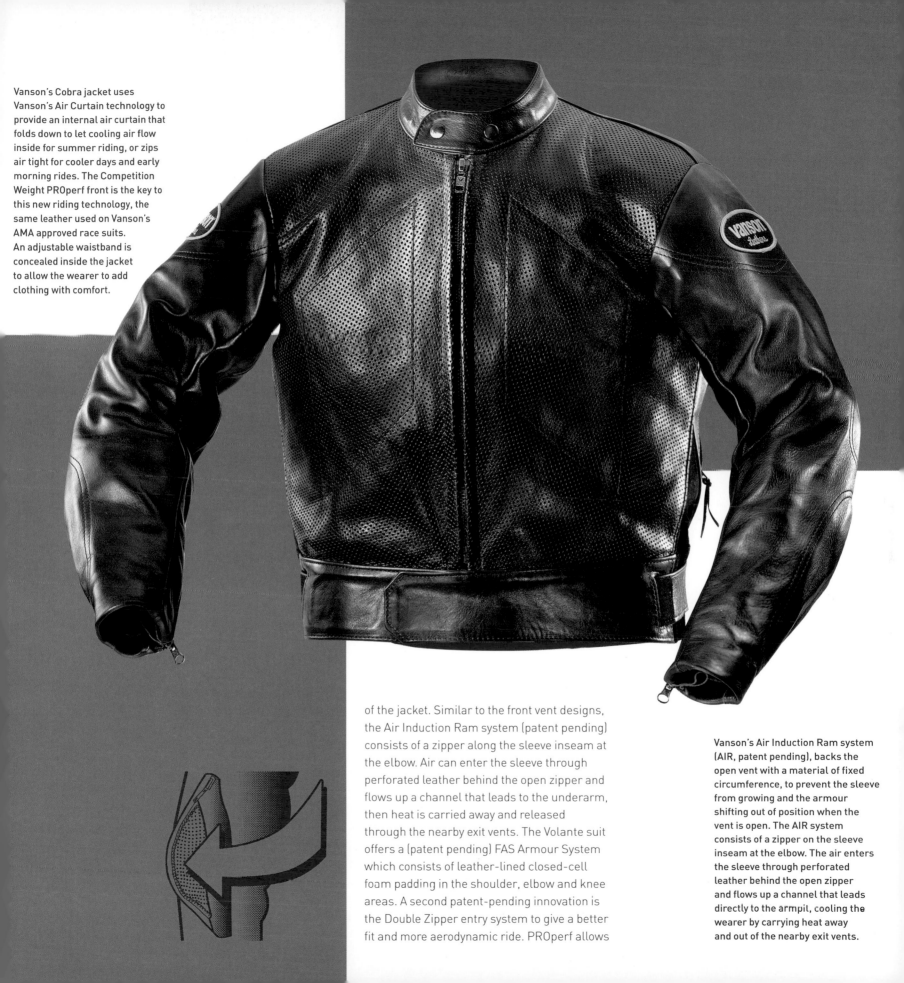

of the jacket. Similar to the front vent designs, the Air Induction Ram system (patent pending) consists of a zipper along the sleeve inseam at the elbow. Air can enter the sleeve through perforated leather behind the open zipper and flows up a channel that leads to the underarm, then heat is carried away and released through the nearby exit vents. The Volante suit offers a (patent pending) FAS Armour System which consists of leather-lined closed-cell foam padding in the shoulder, elbow and knee areas. A second patent-pending innovation is the Double Zipper entry system to give a better fit and more aerodynamic ride. PROperf allows

Vanson's Air Induction Ram system (AIR, patent pending), backs the open vent with a material of fixed circumference, to prevent the sleeve from growing and the armour shifting out of position when the vent is open. The AIR system consists of a zipper on the sleeve inseam at the elbow. The air enters the sleeve through perforated leather behind the open zipper and flows up a channel that leads directly to the armpit, cooling the wearer by carrying heat away and out of the nearby exit vents.

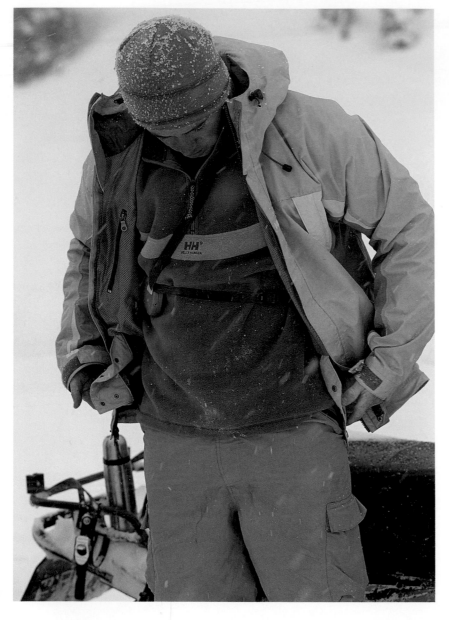

Helly Hansen's Cortex jacket (left) uses Helly Tech fabric, a waterproof breathable double-layered laminate that is combined with fully taped seams for added weather-resistance.

The HPX fabric from Musto (right) combines waterproof, breathable technology with durability. The fabric is made up of a liner, a Gore-Tex ePTFE membrane, outer shell and oleophobic coating.

Musto's MPX Gore-Tex Coastal jacket and trousers (far right) include such design features as a hood spray channel to deflect water from the face and neck, a double storm flap with drainage channel covering a two-way zip and double cuffs that can be adjusted to give virtual drysuit cuff protection.

activity. The design allows the garment to combine ease of movement with breathability, flexibility and warmth. There are various outer jackets available as zip-in designs. The Women's Hidden Peak Parka is waterproof and breathable in a Gore-Tex lightweight taffeta two-layer fabric, with further reinforcement on the shoulders, elbows and sides for protection against abrasion. The seams are hot-taped with Gore-Seam for added protection, and the lining is made of a brushed synthetic mesh (which helps moisture-vapour transfer) and a nylon taffeta.

Musto have developed a 3-Layer System to keep yachtsmen dry and at a comfortable temperature at all times. The base layer is worn next to the skin and serves to wick moisture away from the body. The company uses a polyester fabric that absorbs less than 0.5 per cent of its weight in water. Musto's middle layer uses a Gore-Tex fabric to wick moisture away from the body but protect it from larger water droplets coming through. This garment effectively provides an insulating layer of warm dry air close to the body. The outermost layer must also be waterproof and breathable, again Gore-Tex or a hydrophilic fabric. When Gore-Tex is used, it is treated with an oleophobic chemical to prevent oil-based spillages clogging up the microscopic pores and reducing breathability. Musto has developed its clothing for survival in extreme conditions. When round-the-world

single and dual-ventilated leather panels around the suit, and a back-expanded variation to allow ease of movement. The back pad is articulated and the DuPont aramid, Kevlar, provides added protection for vulnerable areas. Finally, a wicking fabric is used for the lining to move perspiration away from the body.

The North Face and other companies are starting to combine garments using a zip-in design system. This allows such combinations as jackets and vests to be zipped into each other with cuffs secured with a loop and snap-

closure system, creating one garment that combines insulation with weather protection. Garments that can be combined are given a zip-in compatible icon to let customers know which can be worn together. The individual components are also designed for maximum comfort. Vests in the North Face range that can be used in this system include the Stretch Windstopper. This uses a windproof stretch fleece in a design that includes two core-vent openings for ventilation and access to internal jackets. The vents are located around the chest area, which is considered to be the most effective position for dissipating heat during

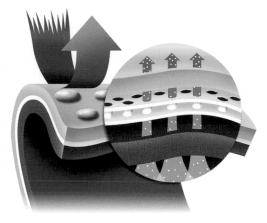

yachtsman Tony Bullimore's yacht capsized in 1997, it was Musto's clothing that he was wearing and that undoubtedly helped save his life.

Without customizing, however, there will always be a limit as to how well a garment fits. Manufacturers are recognizing this, and including flexibility in their design so that users can make their own adjustments. Much of this comes down to detail: the articulated elbow areas and gusseted cuffs all help to make the garment more comfortable. One of the most significant improvements that affects both comfort and performance is seam technology.

Textile manufacturers such as W. L. Gore strictly monitor how their fabric is produced and used. It is not enough that the textile itself is waterproof if the seam lets in water. Stitching is a very low-tech process in comparison with the technology applied to fibre and fabric production, yet it need not be. The Etholen Collection at the National Museum in Helsinki and the ethnographic collection at the British Museum both house very fine collections of Inuit waterproof clothing for ordinary and ceremonial use. A pair of Inuit waterproof sealskin boots in the British Museum are made from shaved sealskin, and, to ensure the maximum water-resistance, the stitching at the seams only extends half-way through the skin. The sewing-needle used is smaller in diameter

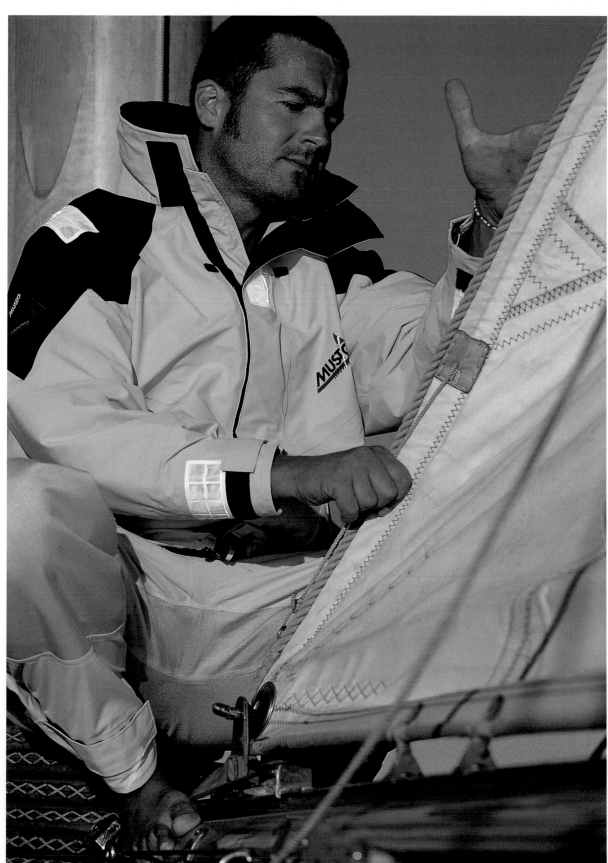

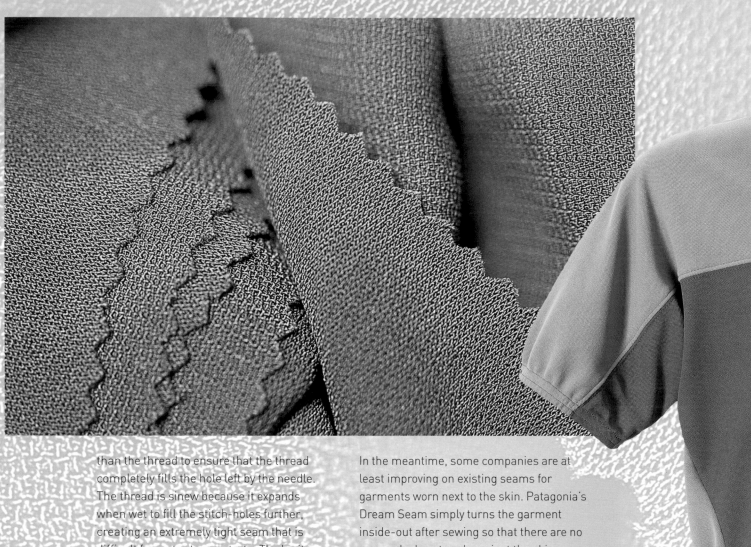

than the thread to ensure that the thread completely fills the hole left by the needle. The thread is sinew because it expands when wet to fill the stitch-holes further, creating an extremely tight seam that is difficult for water to penetrate. The Inuit peoples have developed ingenious ways of making seams watertight using very limited materials. Fishskin is sewn with beach grass. The grass swells up when wet to form a secure seal that keeps water out.

Sinew and beach grass are unlikely to be employed by sports designers, but they have developed some innovative solutions to the problem of seams. W. L. Gore has developed its own special seam technology, Gore-Seam, for use with its waterproof breathable fabrics. A number of garment manufacturers are finishing stitched seams with an adhesive bond, and using double storm flaps to protect pockets and zips. Seamless garments are already available in lingerie, but are slow to find their way into the sports market.

In the meantime, some companies are at least improving on existing seams for garments worn next to the skin. Patagonia's Dream Seam simply turns the garment inside-out after sewing so that there are no exposed edges to rub against the skin.

Intimate apparel for sports has always been an important consideration for men, while the needs of women were largely ignored. This changed dramatically in 1977 when athlete Hinda Miller grew frustrated with what was available on the market, and with Lisa Lindahl set about designing the Jog Bra. The basis for their first design was in fact the jock strap which had been invented for male athletes a century before. The first Jog Bra was constructed from two jock straps that were reassembled and sewn together. Twenty-five thousand were sold in the first year and around forty million two decades later.

Researchers at the University of Wollongong in Australia are developing a SmartBra which

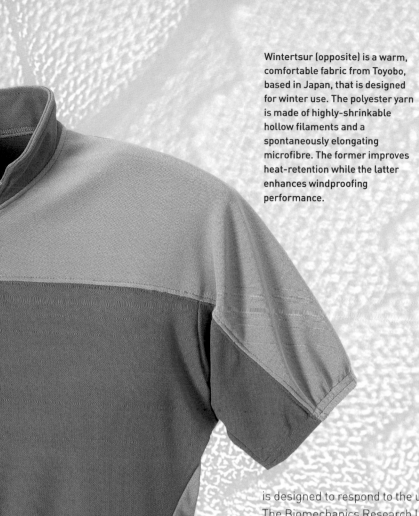

Wintertsur (opposite) is a warm, comfortable fabric from Toyobo, based in Japan, that is designed for winter use. The polyester yarn is made of highly-shrinkable hollow filaments and a spontaneously elongating microfibre. The former improves heat-retention while the latter enhances windproofing performance.

Patagonia's Capilene top (centre) uses an Airius high-performance endurance fabric to help keep the wearer cool and ventilated during summer activity. Almost 50% polyester, a polymer sheath encloses the fibre to move moisture away from the body, performing a wicking function.

Toyobo's Triactor polyester fibres combines filaments both hollow and Y-shaped in cross-section (right). The result is a fabric that has good absorption, is quick-drying and keeps the wearer cool and comfortable.

Toyobo have developed a range of highly engineered polyester and nylon fibres and yarns. Air cube is one example, where, as the name suggests, the nylon fibre has a square-shaped hollow core. With less bulk the fibre is lightweight and the air inside insulates.

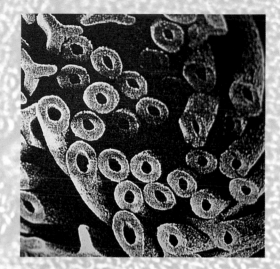

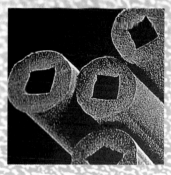

is designed to respond to the user's needs. The Biomechanics Research Laboratory have attached sensors to the straps and midriff of a bra which transmits data to a computer using a telemetry system as the wearer moves. Information gathered from tests will be stored on a tiny microchip that will ultimately become the 'brain' of the smart bra, signalling the fabric to expand and contract in response to the user's movement. The product is still under development, but the university is in discussion with lingerie manufacturers.

Insulation has a major role to play in creating comfortable garments, and air is one of the best insulators available. Hairs on the skin of the human body rise to trap air and therefore warmth. The penguin's feathers can open like valves to allow ventilation, or, alternatively, can use their density to restrict the movement of warm air away from the body. Underneath the distinctive white fur of the polar bear, its skin is black. The hairs are actually translucent and serve to guide infra-red light towards the skin where it is stored and heats the body. The fur and air trapped around each of the hairs serve as insulation and prevent the heat from dissipating quickly.

Textiles have been designed to manipulate airflow for centuries. The Chinese bamboo jacket traps air in its delicate latticework, a design that has been copied in the Western string vest and more recently by Patagonia. Yvon Chouinard, the owner of Patagonia and the driving force behind the company's philosophy, owns an impressive collection of ethnographic garments. A selection are displayed at the company head office in Ventura, California, where they serve as inspiration for new performance fabrics. Included in the collection is an example of a Chinese bamboo jacket, and parallels can be drawn between its design and that of Polartech Regulator fabrics (illustrated on p. 94). The company developed this range with its long-term partner in fabric development, US-based Malden Mills.

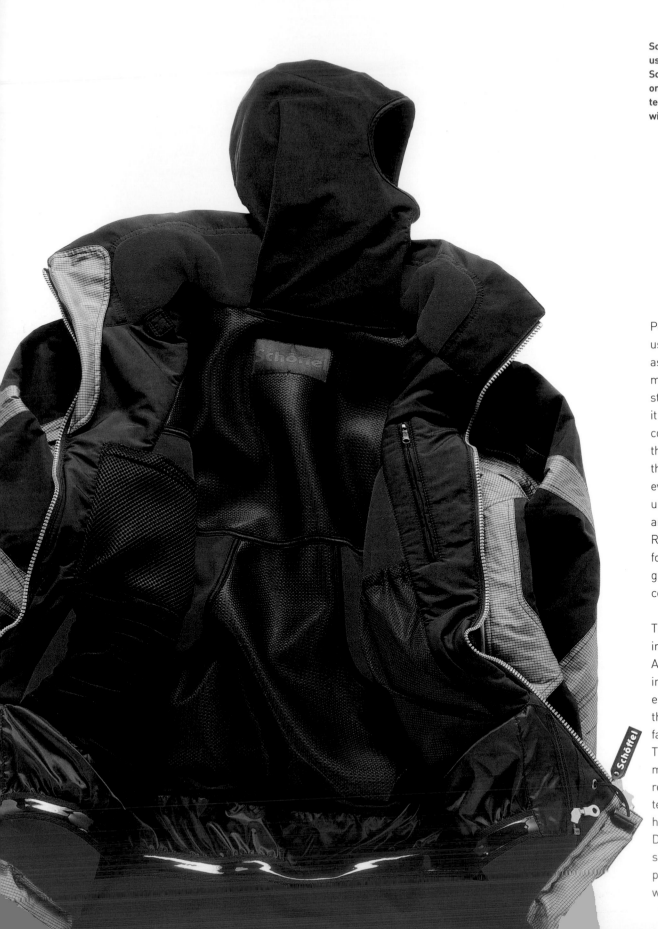

Schoffel's Project 3000 ski jacket uses a ComforTemp fabric from Schoeller. The textile is based on phase-change material technology, to protect the wearer without compromising comfort.

Polartec Regulator is a lightweight fleece that uses a lofted grid structure to trap body heat, as well as encouraging the wicking of body moisture to the surface of the fabric. The open structure on the underside of the fabric makes it lighter than traditional fleeces and easier to compress. The outer layer is a smooth jersey that allows any moisture wicked away from the body to spread across its surface and evaporate quickly. The fabric is used in underwear, sweaters, jackets and trousers in any season with different grades available. The R1 grade is the lightest and most breathable, followed by the R2 which is warmer. The third grade, R3, provides the greatest insulation coupled with wind-resistance.

The North Face use a different Polartec fabric in its Free Climb fleece jackets. The Polartec Aircore fleece uses hollow fibres to trap air inside the actual fibres. The company estimates that this provides the wearer with the warmth expected of a two-hundredweight fabric, but with a 15 per cent weight-saving. The structure of the woven or knitted fabric means that usage can crush the hollow fibres reducing their effectiveness. The Japanese textile company, Toyobo, produces a polyester hollow fibre with a cross-section called Dialegato. The internal structure acts as scaffolding when the fibre is put under pressure, moving to displace the load without losing the airpocket.

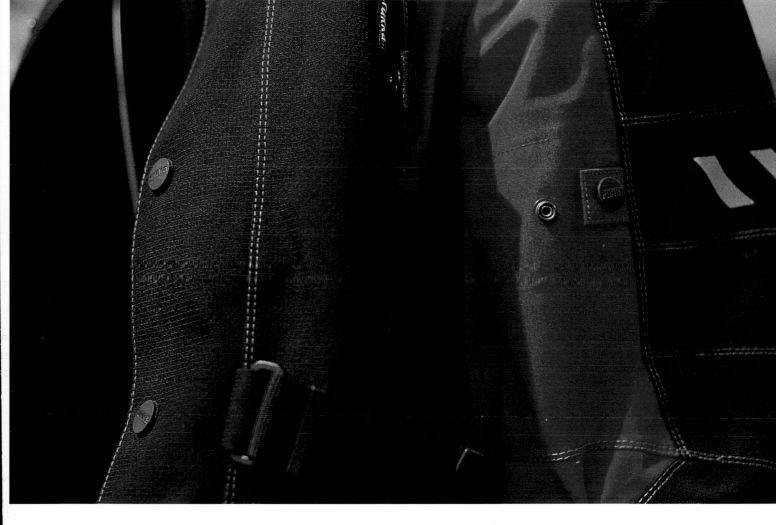

The Armatech range of clothing from Finland's Rukka has been specially developed for sports and touring motorcycle enthusiasts. Both jacket (shown here) and trousers are waterproof and breathable in Gore-Tex 3-layer ARMACOR laminate technology. ARMACOR combines aramid and polyamide fibres for protection and comfort. The lining features Outlast Phase-Change Material (PCM) which offers the wearer an individual microclimate, adapting to changes in climate and activity. The retro-reflective printing technology from 3M ensures visibility at night.

There is an increasing demand from consumers for multi-performance clothing where the benefits can be incorporated into the minimum number of materials. The difficulty is that with each additional function there is a danger that another may be cancelled – how many coatings before the fabric ceases to be breathable? Textile and sports clothes manufacturers are managing to respond to this demand, and are producing some exciting developments.

The Swiss textile manufacturer Schoeller has developed ComforTemp, a phase-change material (PCM) where the PCM is incorporated into a foam. It has also managed to add a number of additional functions without compromising its temperature-regulating properties:

active breathing; moisture regulation; odour-absorption; UV protection; weather-, washing- and crease-resistance. This allows designers to reduce the number of layers in their garments so that the performance of the fabric can have a direct impact on the design of sports attire.

Athletes have little choice about where they compete and the climate they may have to adapt to. Ideally they will arrive seven to ten days in advance of the competition, in time to recover from any jet-lag and become acclimatized to local conditions. This is not always possible, however, so some researchers are looking at alternative ways of encouraging the body to adapt more quickly, in particular to heat and humidity. Reducing the skin temperature before endurance

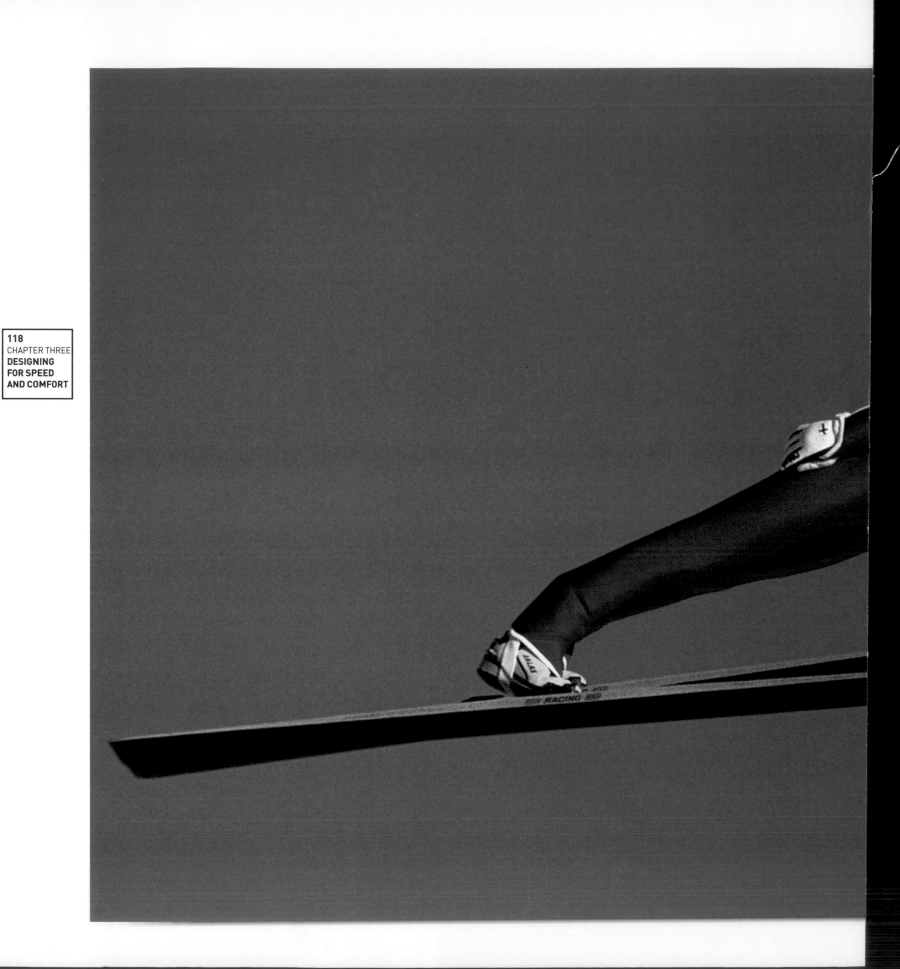

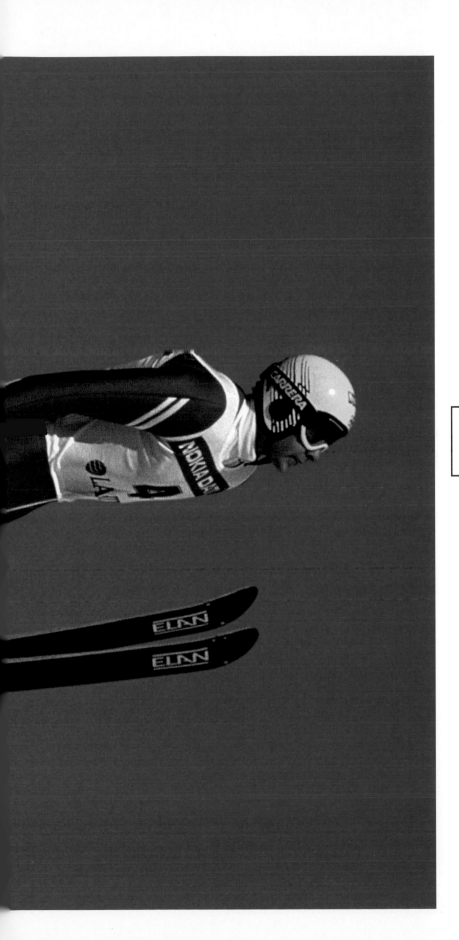

No aspect of a competitor's performance avoids scrutiny. In such sports as skiing, swimming and cycling the position of the body is constantly monitored to ensure that the competitor is adopting the most ergonomic position at all times. Matti Nykanen of Finland in action (left) in a practice ski jump in Finland in February 1989 for the World Nordic Combined Ski Championships.

ERGONOMICS

Presented with a dimpled baseball bat, not unlike a dimpled golfball, that would reduce aeronautic drag and produce a faster swing, the major baseball leagues declined to adopt it. In contrast, new advances in sports clothes go largely unchallenged by the sporting authorities. At the 2000 Sydney Olympics there was some grumbling about the potential advantage that Speedo's Fastskin bodysuit might give swimmers, but it was ultimately allowed. Races are being won by fractions of seconds, so that every advantage is critical to the competitor. The result is that every aspect of a competition is analysed, from the posture of the athlete, to the aerodynamic properties of the singlet fabric. This analysis of sport is concentrated in two scientific processes that are themselves linked – anthropometry and ergonomics. Anthropometry is the study of the range of human physical dimensions, such as height and shoulder width, and the distance between anatomical points on the body. From this, information can be deduced to define human limits in terms of body dimensions

Ironman Wetsuits are made from a super-light, super-buoyant, closed-cell neoprene. The smooth rubber skin has a special multi-coated slick surface to minimize friction. Shown here is a range of the company's wetsuits including its VO2 'stealth' technology which was developed in conjunction with the University of Calgary, Canada. The technology affords the hydrodynamic wetsuit such advantages as buoyancy, reduced drag, and water elimination, but without requiring the increased metabolic cost and restricted breathing capacity that is usually encountered with triathlon wetsuits.

Every aspect of the speed cyclist and his equipment is optimized to have minimal drag: bicycle, helmet, clothing, shoes and, of course, the position of the cyclist's body all combine to offer minimum wind-resistance. The British cyclist, Chris Boardman, is shown opposite during his 1993 attempt to break the One Hour Cycling Record in Bordeaux, France. He did, in fact, break the record with a distance of 52.270 kilometres.

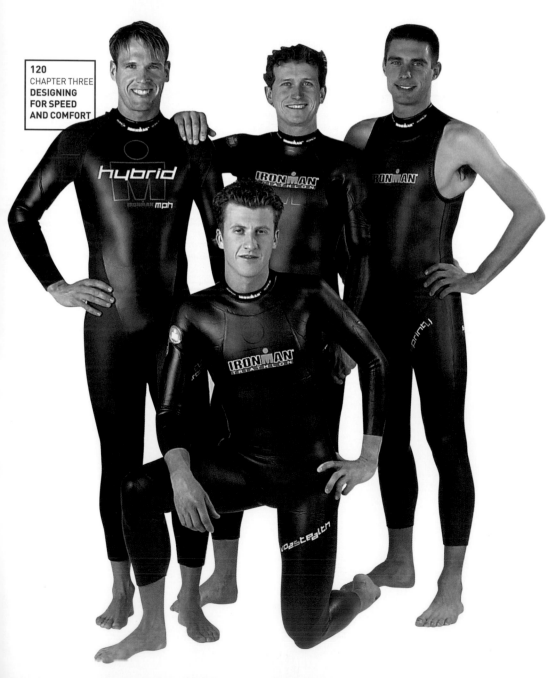

and optimum fit between people and their environment. This data is being applied to the study of ergonomics. Ergonomics is no longer a science that is reserved for the automotive or aerospace industries. Sport is also using the technology for analysis.

Wind tunnels are most commonly used to test the aerodynamic properties of new vehicles. Every new car that rolls off the factory production line is put through this process to check for any weak points in the design. Skiing and cycling are two sports in particular that have been making good use of wind tunnels in training as well as clothing and equipment assessment. The British Speed Ski Team has been training in the University of Glasgow's wind tunnel which is located in the Department of Aerospace Engineering. The racer's changing position is continuously assessed to ensure that the body is in the most aerodynamic position, and moves at one with the equipment at all times during a race. The ski equipment is also designed to be as aerodynamic as possible: helmets are made of Kevlar and glass fibre, and fitted to each individual racer. The design allows a smooth flow of air over the head and shoulders. A polyurethane-coated Lycra fabric is used for the ski suit, with mandatory back protection bonded into the material.

While there are very few diploma and degree courses at colleges for the design of sports clothing, with many designers coming from

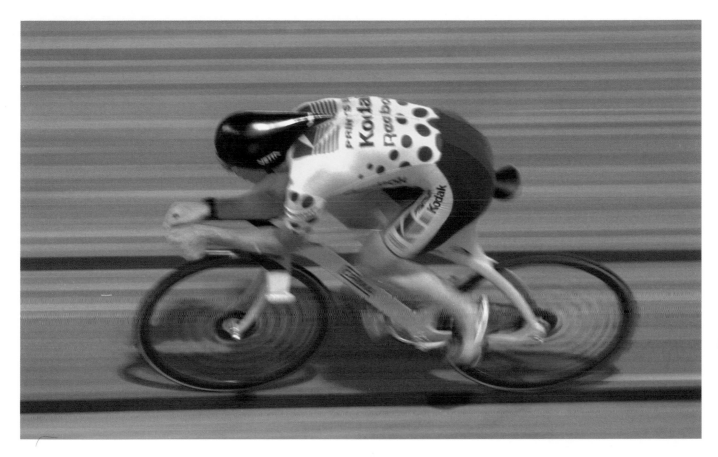

a training in textile or product design, the science of sport and performance is very well served across the globe. Boston's Massachusetts Institute of Technology (MIT) is home to the Laboratory for Sports Innovation, part of the university's department of Aeronautics and Astronautics. It is seen as a natural extension of the department's function, which is concerned with aerodynamics and the effect of wind on the body or object being used – MIT's Wright Brothers Wind Tunnel, built in 1937, is capable of generating winds of up to 200 miles per hour (320 km an hour). This is being used to examine performance in a variety of sports from bobsled racing to downhill skiing and cycling. Researchers use a trail of water vapour to study how air flows over the bike and the rider. The cycling-monitoring system measures not just wind speed but also aerodynamic drag (friction caused by the wind), the power with which the cyclist pedals and the heart rate. The rider is able to monitor his own performance and adapt posture

accordingly as the data is transmitted to a head-up display unit mounted in the helmet. The Laboratory for Sports Innovation is developing a microscopic sensor that can be attached to in-line skates in order to measure their instantaneous and average speed. It will also look at the difference between the speed when the skater pushes off and when coasting afterwards. This information will be given to the skater undergoing the test using a device attached to the wrist.

The Human Performance Laboratory at the University of Calgary includes sport techniques and performance as well as orthotics (studies in foot support), sports shoes and sports surfaces in its research areas. Biomechanics is central to this research, and is challenging existing wisdom on the best attributes of a running shoe. High-speed tripod-mounted cameras are also used here to record and measure the different phases of a shoe's contact with a force-sensing platform. The department's

director, Benno M. Nigg, has conducted research indicating that running on a hard surface produces no more injuries than on soft surfaces. This extends to comparing the effect of high-impact sports, such as basketball and running, with low-impact sports, such as swimming. The director claims that high-impact sports do not result in more degenerative joint diseases – osteoarthritis, for example – than low-impact sports. His studies show that just before ground contact, muscles become tense to counteract soft tissue vibrations. The body wants to generate some vibration, and adding further cushioning in the running shoe interferes with this natural tendency. Researchers in Britain are starting to investigate evidence that this may also be true of motorcycle and bicycle helmets. In Britain and British Columbia Sikhs are allowed exemption on religious grounds from wearing motorcycle helmets, which cannot be fitted over the turban. The closely wrapped turban provides protection and, unlike regular helmets, allows some flexibility.

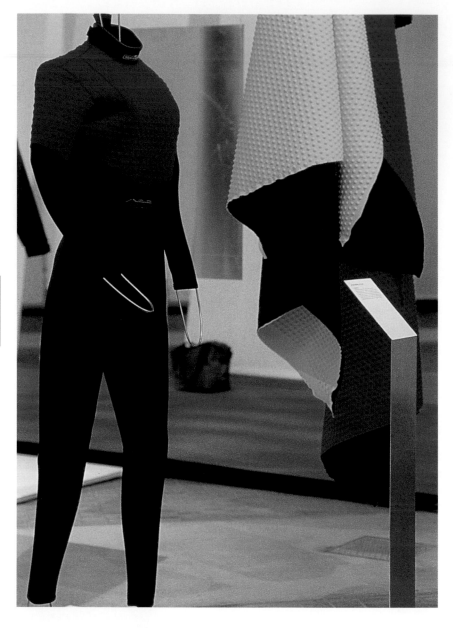

Developed by the British company, Microthermal Systems Ltd, Stomatex (shown left and right) is a neoprene as well as being a smart material. It removes perspiration by mimicking transpiration in nature. Tiny curved chambers in the material behave as miniature pumps to move moisture away from the skin when the body is active. The moisture is removed through tiny pinhead exit pores in the centre of each domed surface. The neoprene is sandwiched between two layers of jersey knitted fabric.

This new approach to sports shoe design is also being investigated by designers and manufacturers. Nike is reconsidering its attempt to control pronation in running shoes. Pronation is the flattening-out of the arch when the foot hits the ground, with the inner side tilted slightly lower than the outer side of the foot. It also describes the process of shifting weight from one side of the foot to the other. The opposite is referred to as supination. In an interview in *Scientific American Presents* (Volume II, Number 3), Mario Lafortune, director of Nike Sport Research Laboratory, described the use

of rigid devices, such as dual density mid-soles and footbridges, as 'like trying to stop pronation with a brick wall'. Researchers at the company are now looking at ways in which pronation can be slowed down rather than suddenly blocked.

Designers are now trying to find ways in which the running shoe will give athletes the ergonomic experience of running barefoot while offering protection against the ground surface. Recent research suggests that support for the foot is best provided by the foot itself. If a shoe or other support system does

the job instead, then the body's natural inclination is to be lazy. Running barefoot or giving a minimum of protection around the foot has precedents in earlier civilizations. In ancient Greece, a warrior wore a sandal only on his left foot, leaving the right bare. This was to allow him to lead with his left foot (assuming he was right-handed), when he would extend it along with his shield towards the enemy. His left foot also served as a kicking foot, acting as an extra weapon in battle. On social occasions the warrior was careful to enter the home of a friend with his right (friendly) foot first.

Scuba-diving fins prove much more effective under water that the human foot on its own. Most designs mimic the movement of the fish fin, making the diver more hydrodynamic while swimming. They are flexible enough to move in water, but the individual components on the fin are usually fixed rigid. Bob Evans Design Inc in Santa Barbara have designed a flexible blade so that the tip of the fin can move independently, affording better movement and control. The suitably titled Extra Force fin also has whiskers placed towards the tip of the fin to allow a two-stroke kick cycle which creates better water channelling and diminishes recovery resistance. Comfort is not discounted, with an open-toe design to reduce the danger of toe or foot cramps. As the diver moves the fin to a down, or power stroke, the Extra

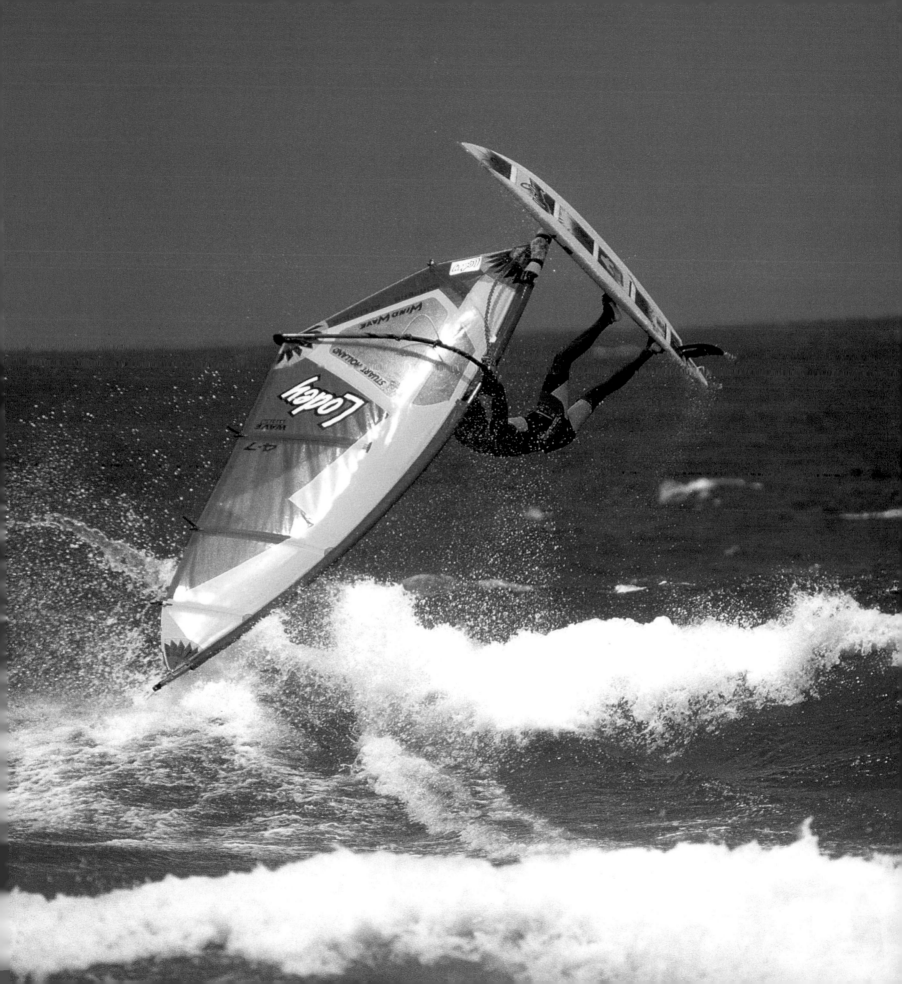

Speedo's Fastskin bodysuit is inspired by the shark, or rather, it is based on its skin. The shark's body shape is not considered very hydrodynamic and should make it slow-moving. A series of tiny ridges on the skin manages to counteract this disadvantage, and it is this pattern that is the basis for Speedo's design.

This Coloured Scanning Electron Micrograph shows the scales from the skin of a shark (opposite). These sharply pointed, placoid scales are also known as dermal teeth because they give the shark's skin a sandpaper feel. The tip of each scale is made of dentine overlaid with dental enamel. The lower part of each scale, which anchors it into the skin, is made of bone. Shark's scales considerably reduce the water-resistance around the skin of the shark.

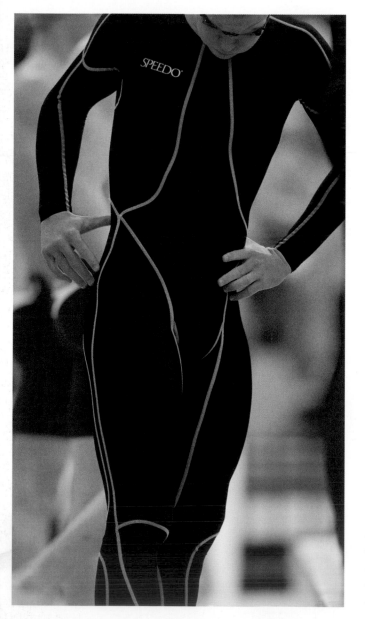

Force fin flays out for a maximum surface area. This utilizes the front muscles of the swimmer's leg which are the strongest. The blade then returns to its original position when moved to the up position and this thrusts the swimmer forward.

Until 1969 it was believed that in swimming, pulling the arm through water with force produced an opposite force of equal intensity, propelling the swimmer forward. This followed from Newton's Third Law. Swimming coaches therefore encouraged swimmers to pull their arm straight back in a stroke. Underwater film footage showed that the best swimmers did not pull their arm directly back, instead they curved it slightly. In 1971 James 'Doc' Counsilman (coach to Mark Spitz) revised this view, and suggested that the lift forces that keep an aeroplane in the air were an appropriate analogy to the swimmer's propulsion in water. This was adapted from classical physics, specifically Bernoulli's principle. Applied to swimming, the theory is that water will travel more quickly over the knuckles than the palm of the hand, and it is the difference in pressure between the two sides that will generate propulsion. The US Olympic Committee has funded an engineer at Honeywell Engines and Systems to analyse the ergonomics of swimming. They have designed computer software that examines the velocity at which water flows over the limb, pressure changes in water

and how these affect the forces of lift and drag. The technology has been likened to a wind tunnel in a computer. Findings to date indicate that the paddle effect based on Newton may be closest to being correct, although some lift would seem to be involved as well.

Speedo's Fastskin bodysuit is based on the shark, one of the fastest fish in the sea. Or rather, it is based on its skin. The shark's body shape is not considered very hydrodynamic in itself, and should, in fact, make it quite slow-moving in water. A series of tiny ridges on the skin manages to counteract this disadvantage, and it is this pattern that is mimicked by Speedo. A three-dimensional body-scanning process ensures that competitive swimmers get a swimsuit that matches the contours of their body, and can align muscles with the seams to provide tendon-like tension. The Federation International de Natation Amateur (FINA) approved use of the swimsuit in time for the Sydney Olympics. Controversy has emerged because reducing drag and enhancing performance (as Speedo claim in promotional literature) is seen by some as violating FINA's own guidelines which ban any accoutrements that give a competitor an advantage. The matter was referred by the Australian Olympic Committee to the Court of Arbitration for Sport in Switzerland, who ruled in FINA's favour.

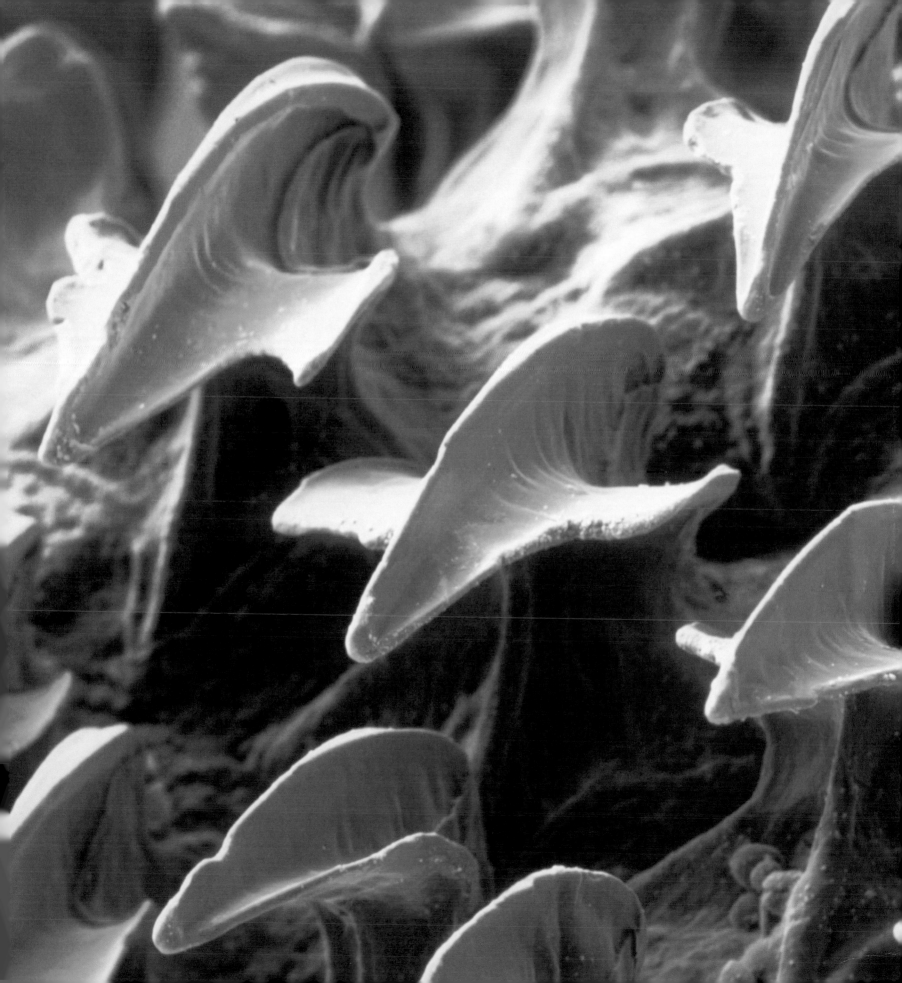

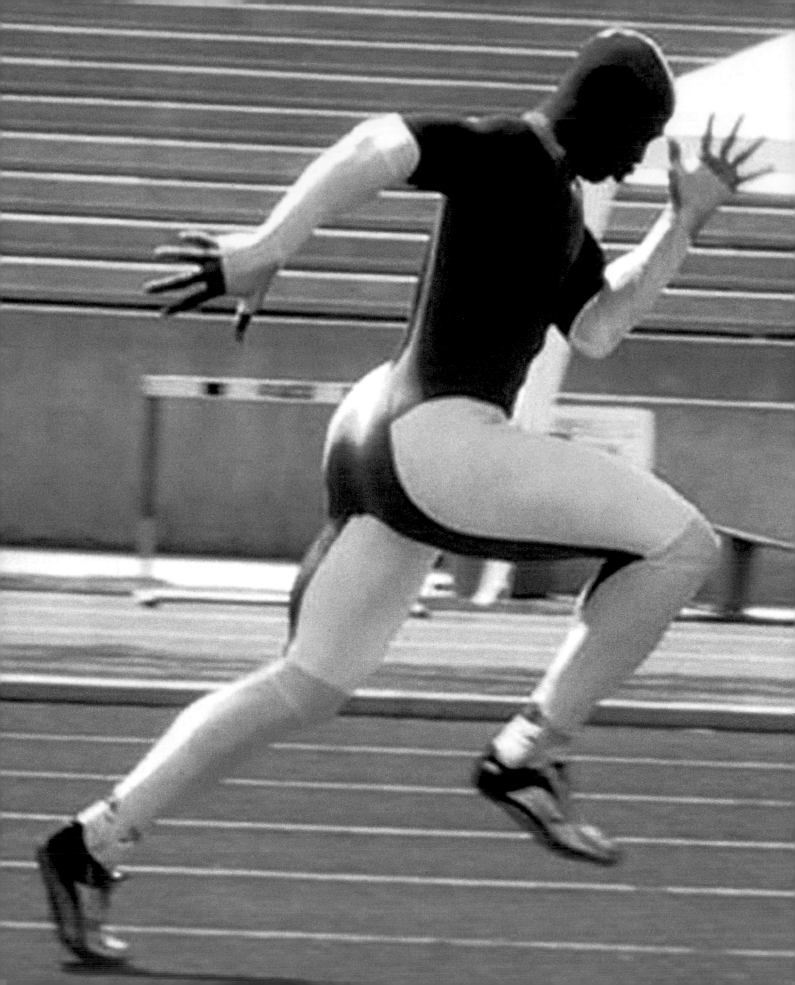

Nike's Swiftsuit is shown below at concept stage and opposite worn by Maurice Greene. One of the unusual features of the suit is that it leaves very little of the body exposed, even covering the head, to avoid wind-resistance caused by the athlete's hair.

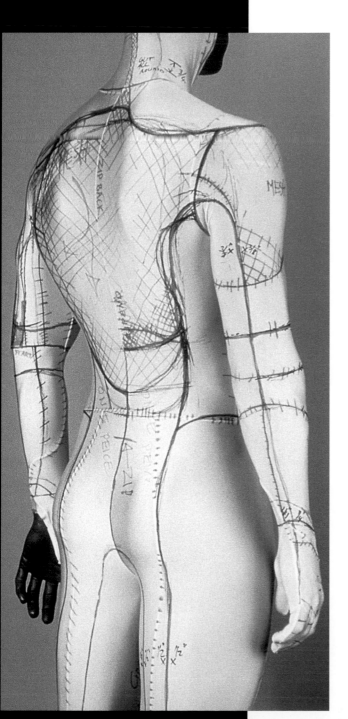

The Swift Suit is Nike's aerodynamic solution to the problem of drag in track events. As a full bodysuit it covers the hair and even the hands, where a low-friction coated fabric is used. The designers assigned to each part of the body a Reynolds number based on its velocity and size. The Reynolds number is a measurement of a fluid (in this instance air) flowing over a surface. An appropriate fabric has been assigned to each segment, taking account of additional needs, such as insulation: the torso features a polyester/spandex microfibre tricot fabric; the head (hood) area is a combination of nylon/spandex mesh and textured polyester/spandex tricot; the upper leg region is comprised of a polyester/spandex microfibre tricot and a three-layer textured polyester/spandex tricot; the hands and stirrups use a polyurethane-coated nylon/spandex tricot. Wherever possible, the seams have been moved to the back of the garment to reduce drag, and those at the front have been carefully positioned in the direction of airflow. All seams are cut to be horizontal when at maximum velocity. This is not a simple garment, and it takes two machinists two days to assemble one garment.

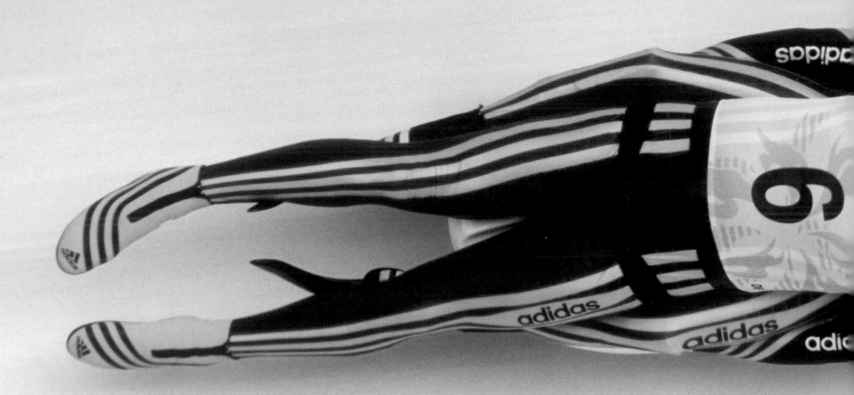

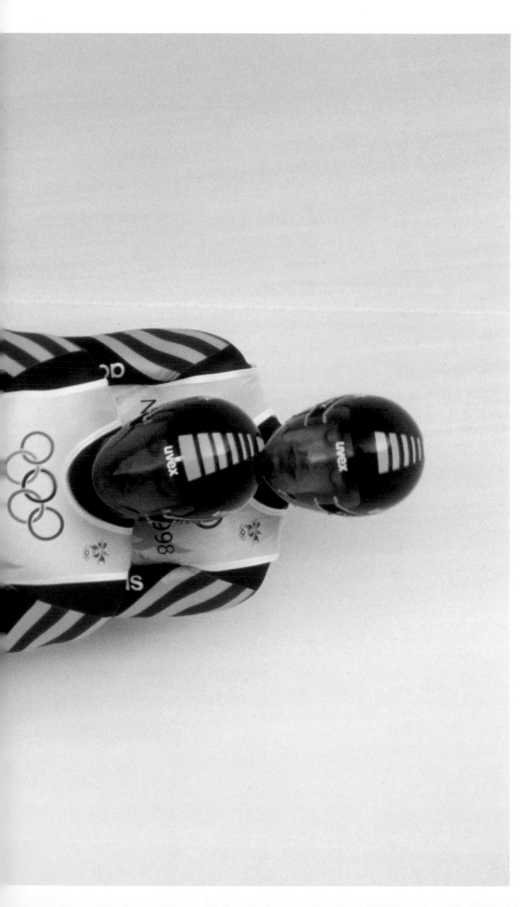

The basic design of luge suits is not unlike motorcycling leathers, and many manufacturers produce both. Stefan Krausse and Jan Behrendt of Germany are shown here competing in the men's double luge during the 1999 Winter Olympic Games in Nagano, Japan.

While other areas of design move towards simplicity, it is noticeable that sports attire has become increasingly complex. This is partly a production issue. While it remains financially insignificant for manufacturers to use more than thirty different pieces of fabric, foam and trim on the uppers of a pair of track shoes, there is little incentive for them to reduce this number. The benefit of such complexity to the consumer is one of performance. In competition this may save vital seconds and mean the difference between winning and losing. It may also prevent serious injury, although this raises the question as to whether such risks would be taken without the safety factor afforded by hyper-protective clothing.

Many design disciplines have courted multidisciplinary design practice, but sports clothes manufacture is one of the few to embrace it so successfully. This may be in part due to the fact that many designers have trained in related areas of design, such as product and fashion, and so are more open to other ways of thinking. The changing demands of the sports themselves, and the umbilical link to the world at large, will undoubtedly maintain the vibrancy of sports design.

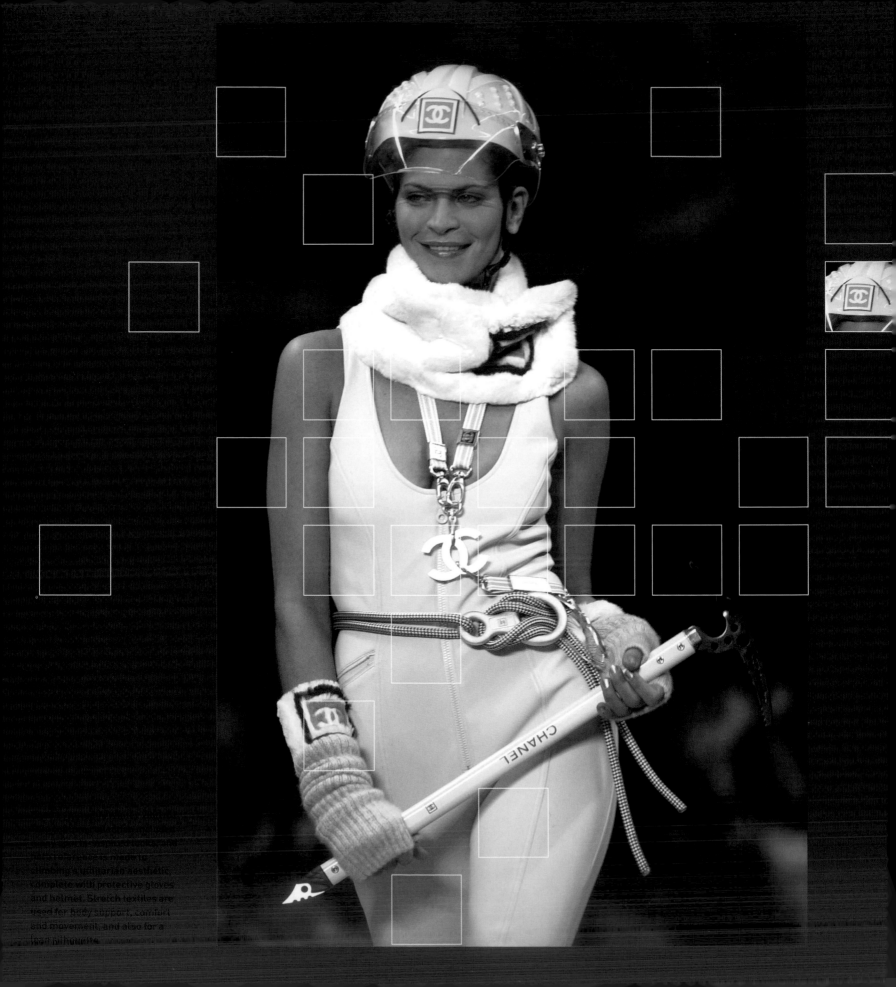

... orted... to
climbing a utilitarian aesthetic,
complete with protective gloves
and helmet. Stretch textiles are
used for body support, comfort
and movement, and also for a
... silhouette.

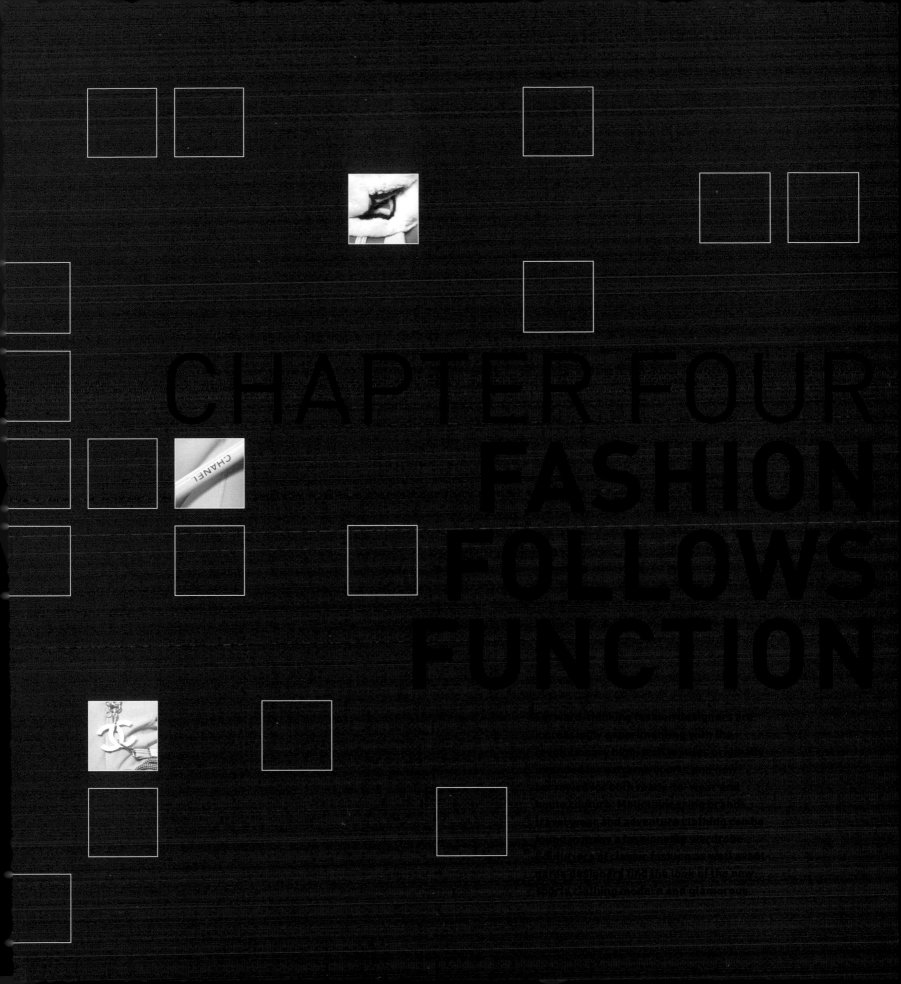

CHAPTER FOUR FASHION FOLLOWS FUNCTION

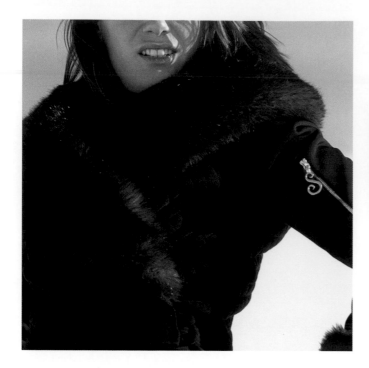

LIFESTYLE

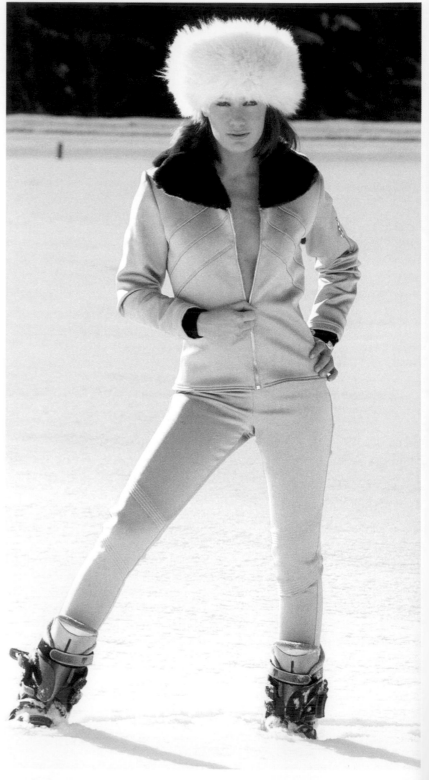

Sport is recognized as one of the biggest lifestyle influences, reflected in our preference today for utilitarian, comfortable clothing. For city dwellers, sport redresses the balance, encouraging inner serenity as well as bodily fitness. Yoga and the martial arts provide a mental as well as physical challenge, and are increasing in popularity – it is accepted that an active mind and body are beneficial for health and beauty.

The latest designer sports labels are aimed at the 18–34 age group, with the result that anyone wearing them can seem young, healthy and active by association. Sports-inspired fashion advertisements suggest links with a clean-living active life: sport is fashionable, and sporty references give collections a contemporary edge.

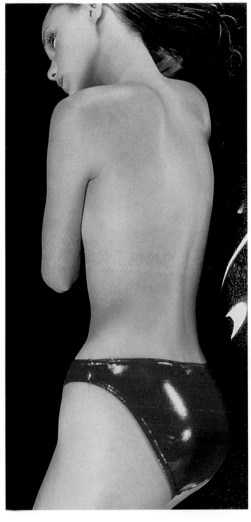

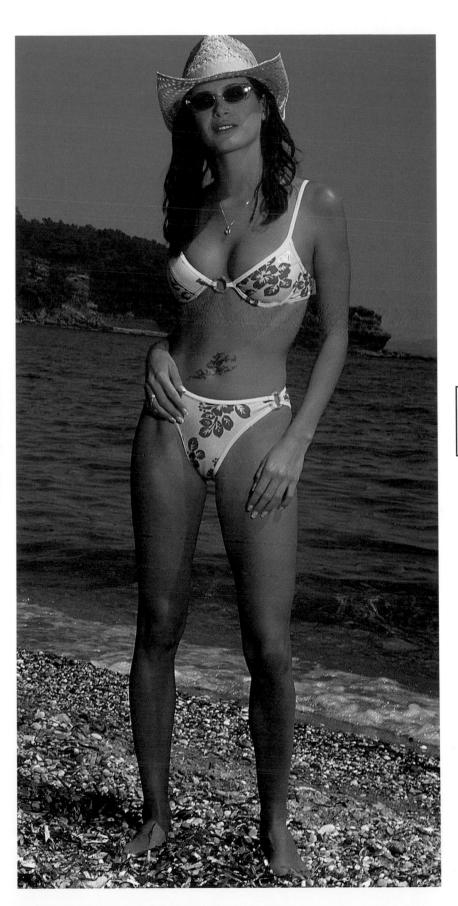

Sam de Terán, Pussy ski suit (detail), worn by British society celebrity Tara Palmer-Tomkinson, on the slopes above Klosters in Switzerland (opposite, top left). A Schoeller textile with WB-400 membrane has been hand-quilted, and the wrap-around collar and cuffs are of fake fur.

Joelynian, Cherry High Gloss, designer swimwear, Spring/Summer 1999. Fashion duo Joelynian uses a polyamide and Lycra (DuPont) mix fabric which has been given a high-gloss fabric finish for this 'wet' look.

Sam de Terán, iridescent blue ski suit with fake fur hat, worn by Tara Palmer-Tomkinson, Klosters (opposite right). This Schoeller textile with its WB-400 membrane and Lycra (DuPont) provides stretch, softness and protection. The suit keeps the wearer warm in cold temperatures, and it is machine-washable.

Quiksilver, Roxy Life collection, Loverboy bikini, Spring/Summer 2001. The collection, aimed at the modern active woman, is inspired by 1970s surf culture and psychedelia, and there are also ethnic influences from Africa and Asia. Swimwear fits like a second skin in a fabric of polyamide and Lycra (DuPont).

Quiksilver, Roxy Life collection, Autumn/Winter 2001/02. The jacket is reversible and made from a water-repellent nylon with natural down and feather padding. The bodywarmer and skirt are in a water-repellent lacquered fabric with contrasting lining (synthetic fleece with polyester padding in the bodywarmer and brushed poplin in the skirt). The model line-up includes professional surfers and snowboarders.

Technical, sports-specific clothes are frequently appropriated by those who would like to associate themselves with certain sports, such as basketball, BMX-riding and skateboarding, and these clothes have made a strong impact on young urban streetwear. Cult surfer style is taken up by non-surfers keen to share the image, and has entered ready-to-wear for both men and women – surf-style shops have opened up inland, far from the sea, to answer this growing demand. Snowboarding, now as hip as surfing, attracts the same kind of enthusiastic cult following.

Diffusion ranges are aimed at the youth market, often ahead of the mainstream trends, and they incorporate sporty and functional elements for an edgy look. High-performance protective clothing for outdoor sports, such as synthetic fleeces and weatherproof jackets, have been readily accepted over the whole spectrum from sports professionals to the non-active. The new technology allows wearers to customize clothing to create their own expression of individuality, and urban clothes often combine sports detailing with other references.

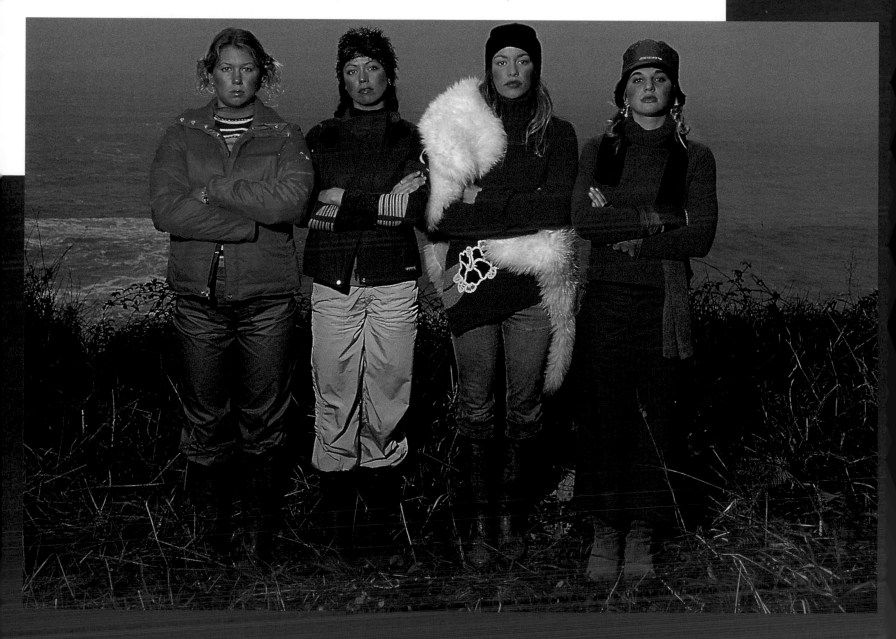

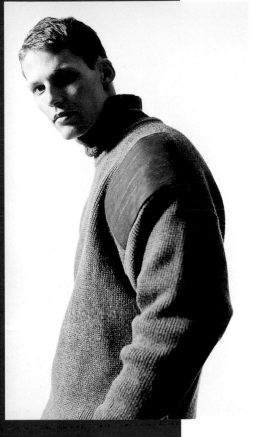

Holland & Holland, Menswear, Autumn/Winter 2001/02. The sweater (left) is made from extra fine merino wool which has been given a Teflon (DuPont) finish to make it water- and stain-resistant, with large shoulder-pads where rain is likely to beat down. Inspired by fishermen's jerseys, the cashmere sweater (below) provides extreme softness and comfort as well as protection, and the trousers are made of cotton moleskin, a traditional brushed textile. The cape (right) is made of cotton with a polyurethane coating for protection against the weather.

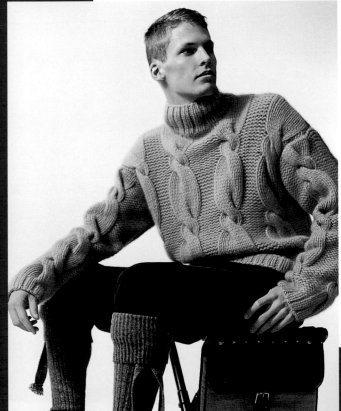

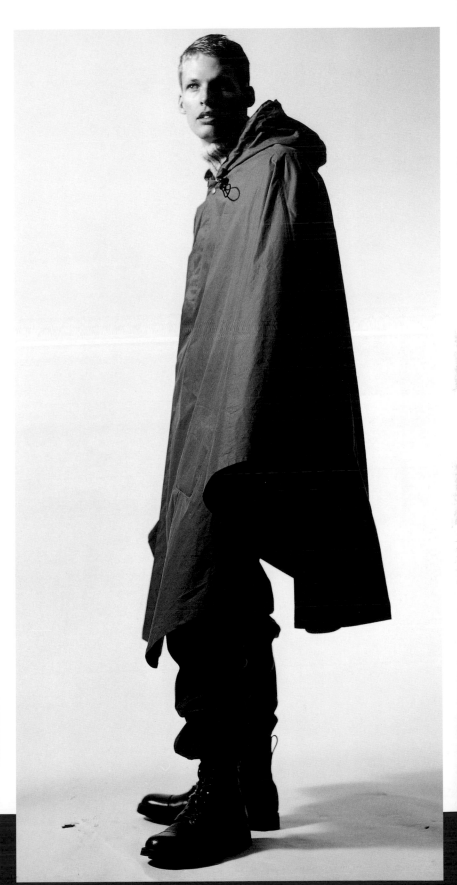

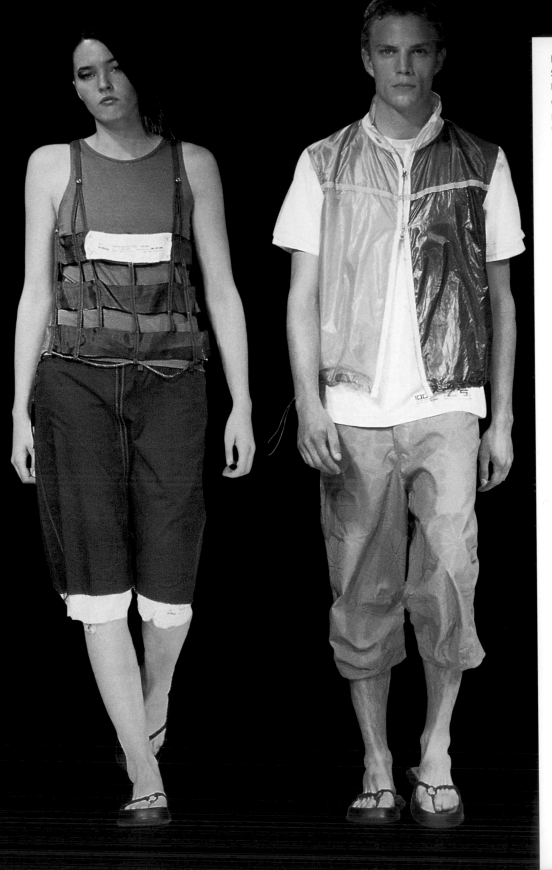

Michiko Koshino, 100s, Spring/Summer 2001. This is a limited edition (100) of unisex clothing inspired by military parachutes. The garments are taped and over-stitched and reference utilitarian clothing.

Other factors are influencing our preference for sports-inspired clothes. Many people now work from home, and clothing is generally becoming more relaxed and less formal. City workers want adaptable clothes that will do for office, gym, restaurant and club – versatile clothing for busy and complicated lives and for most kinds of weather. The revolutionary new sports textiles are beginning to erode the distinctions between menswear and womenswear, and between sports clothes and fashion, with the emphasis instead being on lifestyle. Both the Parisian Coco Chanel and the American designer Claire McCardell were important precursors of the de luxe sports attire aesthetic. McCardell inspired the whole 'sports/fashion' look by using fabrics such as polyamide and stretch textiles in the 1940s, influencing many contemporary American designers, such as Ralph Lauren, Donna Karan and Calvin Klein. The USA leads the way, and many fashion names have launched their own separate 'sports' diffusion line, designing garments and accessories for the city, taking sports clothes as their point of departure and creating a luxury version, choosing the most advanced technical textiles for a new and functional aesthetic.

Ralph Lauren, Autumn/Winter 2001/02. This designer often fuses a romantic vision of Britain with American sports clothing for a look that does not date. A well-tailored jacket and jodphurs complete the classic equestrian look.

Effi Samara, Autumn/Winter 1999/2000. Reference is made to equestrian clothing. Here, a full-length nylon skirt is teamed with a skinny cashmere cardigan, and a backless, polo-necked cashmere top is worn with slim-cut white trousers.

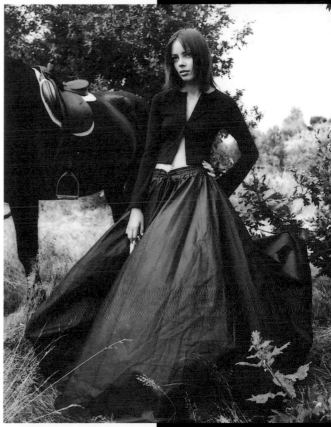

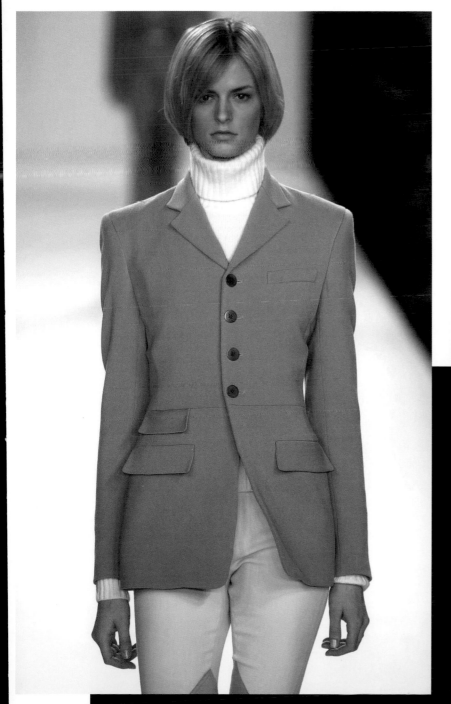

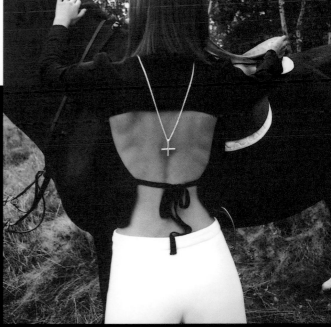

Samsonite Blacklabel, Womenswear and Accessories Collection, Autumn/Winter 2001/02. The fine jersey top and wide-legged trousers (below) are practical and elegant. References are to leisure pursuits.

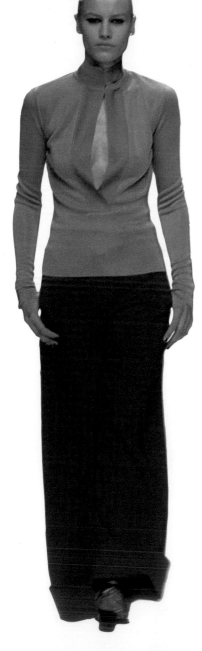

Stone Island, Spring/Summer 2001. This waterproof parka is made from a transparent nylon bonded to a cotton lining with polyurethane coating. White thermo-tapes on the seams are visible through the fabric. Welt pockets and the central closure have concealed stud fastenings.

The streamlined yet relaxed aesthetic of 'utility chic' is most visible in the choice of fabric. Fashion designers choose the new high-tech fabrics for their original appearance and sensual texture – their high-performance properties are an added benefit. Some of these fabrics appear light and even delicate, although they are strong, durable and fully weatherproof. These sophisticated fabrics suggest alternative approaches for fashion designers.

The years devoted to research and development are often reflected in the cost of a textile, but demand and worldwide competition are bringing down the price of such fabrics, allowing both the established and the more experimental designers to use them in their collections.

Manufacturers are also realizing that the future lies with advanced fabrics. High-performance textiles originally developed for sports are used in bodywear and hosiery for their moisture-management properties and comfort. For both menswear and womenswear the new fibre blends and cloth finishes suit the more informal style. Textiles with optimum stretch are as popular for the new fashions as for sports. The new techno-naturals and the advanced synthetics are usually breathable and allow perspiration to evaporate rapidly, while protecting the wearer from the elements.

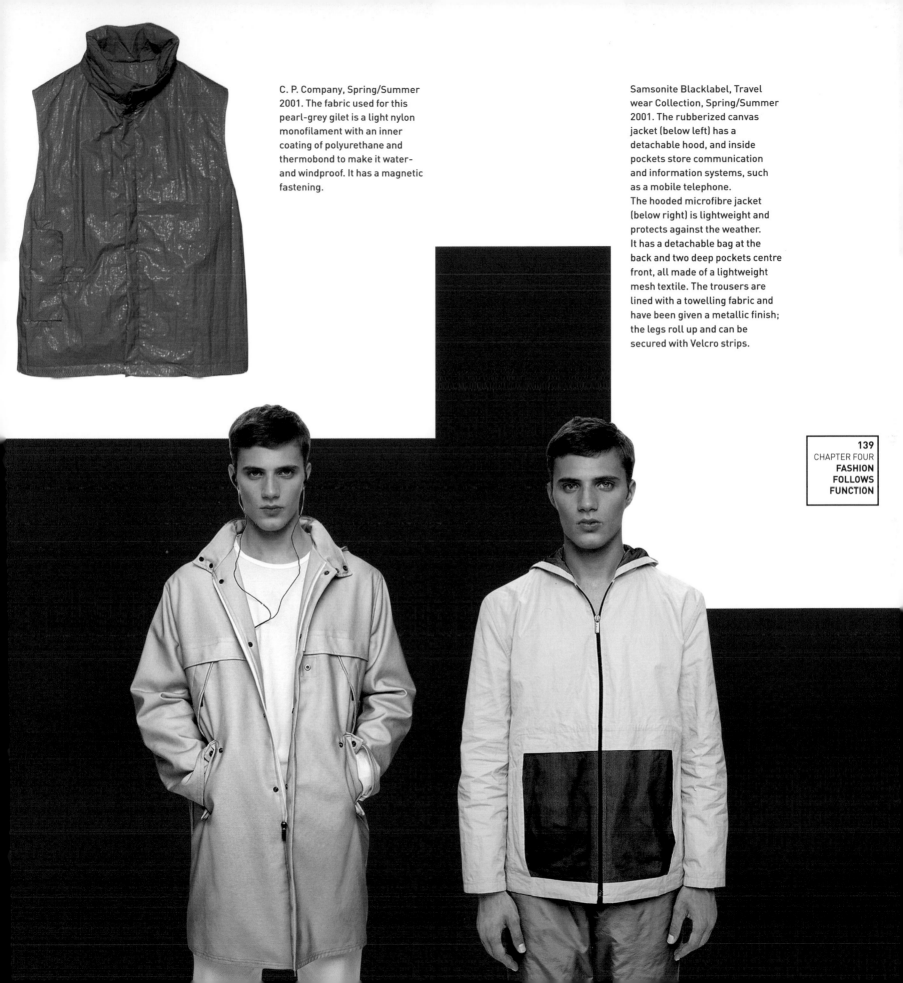

C. P. Company, Spring/Summer 2001. The fabric used for this pearl-grey gilet is a light nylon monofilament with an inner coating of polyurethane and thermobond to make it water- and windproof. It has a magnetic fastening.

Samsonite Blacklabel, Travel wear Collection, Spring/Summer 2001. The rubberized canvas jacket (below left) has a detachable hood, and inside pockets store communication and information systems, such as a mobile telephone. The hooded microfibre jacket (below right) is lightweight and protects against the weather. It has a detachable bag at the back and two deep pockets centre front, all made of a lightweight mesh textile. The trousers are lined with a towelling fabric and have been given a metallic finish; the legs roll up and can be secured with Velcro strips.

Mandarina Duck, Fiberduck
Jacket, Spring/Summer 2000.
Mandarina Duck's patented
paper-like fabric Fiberduck
originates from the car industry
where it is used for seat linings.
It is lightweight, protects
against wind and rain, is abrasion-
resistant and machine-washable.
Fiberduck has a silicone and
rubber treatment that repels
water and makes it crinkle-free.

The new textiles work well in the city, and provide practical, easy-care clothing that packs and travels well. Another great advantage is that advanced synthetics are almost dry when they emerge from a 30°–40°C (86°–104°F) machine wash, and need little ironing. Synthetic closed-cell foam is chosen by fashion designers for its attractive look and soft, warm feel as well as for its lack of weight and insulating properties. Other functional fabrics that are crossing over to fashion include the latest antimicrobials; fresh-smelling and non-irritant, they are often chosen for general daywear.

The new microfibres and advanced finishing treatments give a wide choice from many different visual and tactile effects. There are unusual blends – cotton corduroy is generally associated with leisure wear, but when cotton is combined with cashmere, it produces a corduroy with a very soft look and handle, suited to luxurious urban wear. Nonwovens can result in papery textiles with a crunchy, crackly texture. Textiles coated, fused or bonded are very stylish as well as providing extra comfort and performance.

Hybrid clothing – between sports clothes and pure fashion – is where action clothing, prêt-à-porter and the rarefied world of haute couture meet. Fashion also influences sports clothes in its turn, and sports collections are becoming more glamorous. Track runners can now wear aerodynamic one-piece garments in low-resistance synthetics; beaded stretch tulle may be used for sports

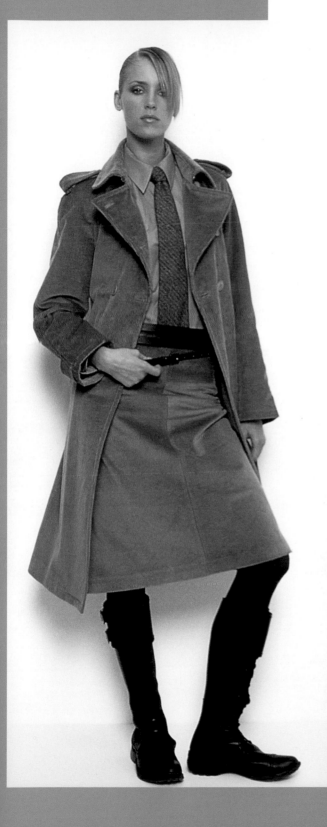

tops, and sequinned hotpants for running. Practical and decorative, they are suited to action and fashion alike. There are even such playful details as frills, fringes, embroidery and cut-out shapes. Clothes worn for golfing these days include fewer traditional Madras patterns and checked knits, and favour natural colours and technical textiles (stretch and weatherproof while being breathable).

Today's fashion designers enjoy working with textiles that are high-performance, using them for both face fabrics and linings. Synthetic fleece, for example, is used for lining collars and pockets. Made from 100 per cent polyester, the ubiquitous 'fleece' has been a tremendous success in fashion collections. For a new look and texture, this fleece can be laminated to synthetic foam.

Samsonite Blacklabel, Travel wear Collection, Autumn/Winter 2001/02. Corduroy is used here (left) to give an Italian look of relaxed elegance. The sturdy leather boots are both utilitarian and fashionable. The designer, Gigi Vezzola describes this collection as 'Sport'ly: sportswear Made in Italy'.

The shirt-like corduroy jacket (below) is soft and unstructured, and demonstrates the relaxed look inspired by Italian leisure clothes. Knitted sleeves allow freer movement. This collection was inspired by the book *Bobos in Paradise* by David Brooks, which describes the 'Bourgeois Bohemian', who wants high-performance utility clothing.

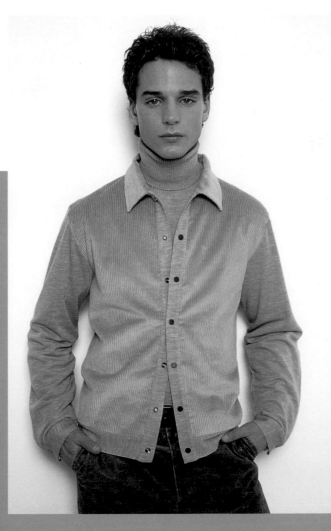

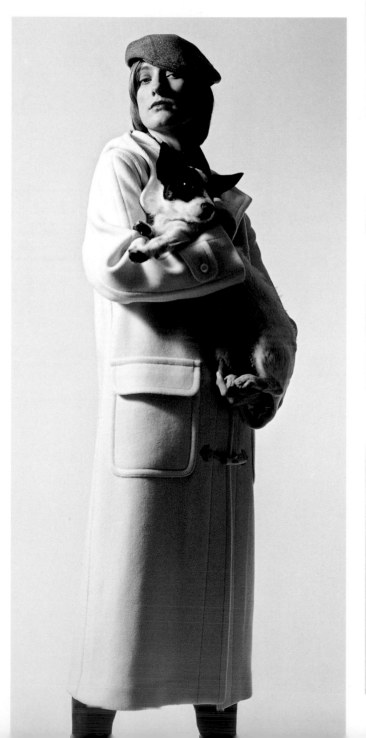

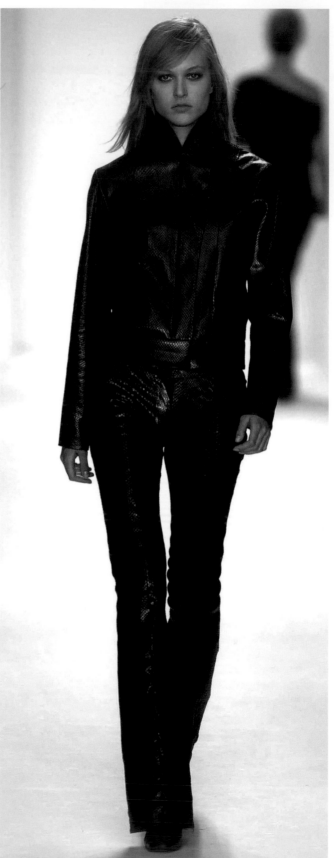

Holland & Holland, Autumn/Winter 2001/02. The duffle coat (far left) is both fashionable and practical. Here it is worn with a sporting country cap. The duffle, or duffel, favourite of 1950s students, is now a classic with its deep pockets, hood and toggle fastenings. It was traditionally made from a coarse, thick woollen cloth from the Belgian town of Duffel; this design uses pure new wool with a waterproof Teflon (DuPont) coating to make it even more functional.

Calvin Klein, Autumn/Winter 2001/02. This black leather outfit makes reference to motorcycling. Leather has been used as a protective outer layer for many years, and new ways of tanning allow for toughness with softness. The jacket and trousers are protective, but the look is glamorous.

Quiksilver, Roxy Life collection, Boomerang jacket, Autumn/Winter 2001/02. The bright yellow jacket, worn by the US surfer Veronica Kay (opposite), is made from mixed wool flannel with a neoprene bonding which takes surf culture into everyday clothing. Its protective properties are increased by the concealed fastening.

Low-resistance synthetics, including silicone, are often used for sports. Techno-naturals offer a natural look and feel, together with the benefits from improved performance. Leather and sheepskin are now lean and ultra-soft, and leather can be made into a stretch fabric or a mesh.

Super-stretch fabrics with a high percentage of Lycra (DuPont) are a popular choice for fashion of all kinds. Mixed with other fibres, both synthetic and natural, even a small proportion of Lycra can give stretch performance. Very much in demand internationally for fashion clothes, Lycra provides a 'well-being' factor – comfort is now just as important as appearance. Lack of weight and bulk means that they can easily be layered – tube dresses over trousers, for example. These clothes are great fun and they are also versatile – they can be pushed up or pulled down for several different looks. Lycra-mix leggings, originally made for sports of all kinds, were taken up by many non-sporty individuals for easy, comfortable dressing.

In the fashion world, Lycra was made famous by the Tunisian-born fashion designer, Azzedine Alaïa. This synthetic rubber now appears in both ready-to-wear and haute couture collections. Another synthetic rubber, neoprene, also appears on the catwalk, and is chosen for its softness and warmth and its protective qualities. When mixed with silk, neoprene can take on unusual looks and textures, and when bonded to fleece becomes a new high-performance textile. Since it is thermoplastic, neoprene

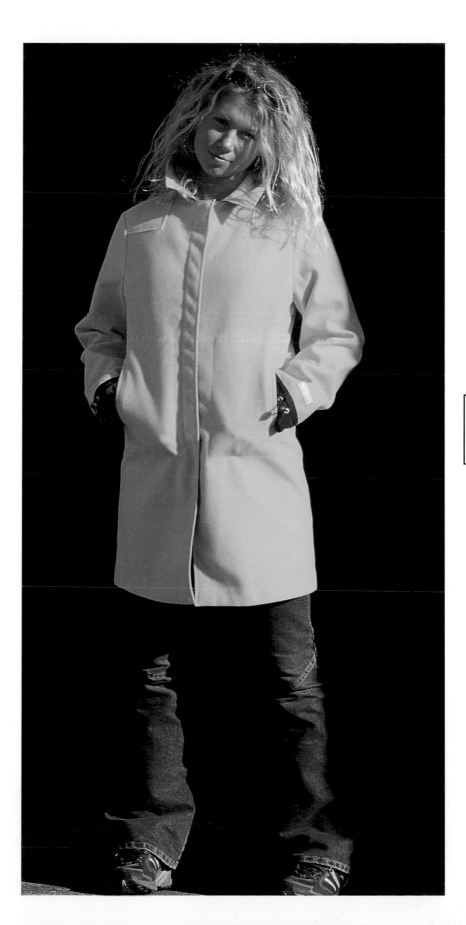

Quiksilver, Alex Goes, Spring/ Summer 2001. The name of this range suggests unisex wear and action. Technical fabrics are often used in Quiksilver collections for functional, fashionable clothing. Styling is kept simple and detailing reflects sports influences. The skirt (left) is made of a silk and polyester blend with a CoolMax (DuPont) mesh lining for high performance and comfort.

Michiko Koshino, Autumn/Winter 2001/02. YEN Jeans makes reference to a Japanese aesthetic, but fuses this with a Western look. The jeans are of denim woven on original 1940s looms, and a vintage wash adds to the aged appearance. A shirt with a busy, bright print is worn over a mesh vest. Mesh is ideal as a base layer as its structure traps air but also allows the skin to breathe.

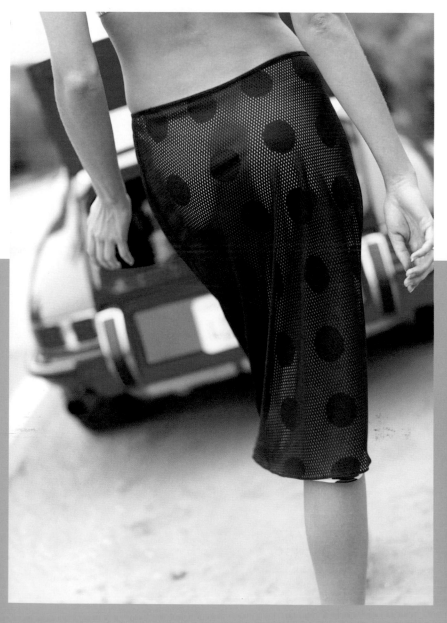

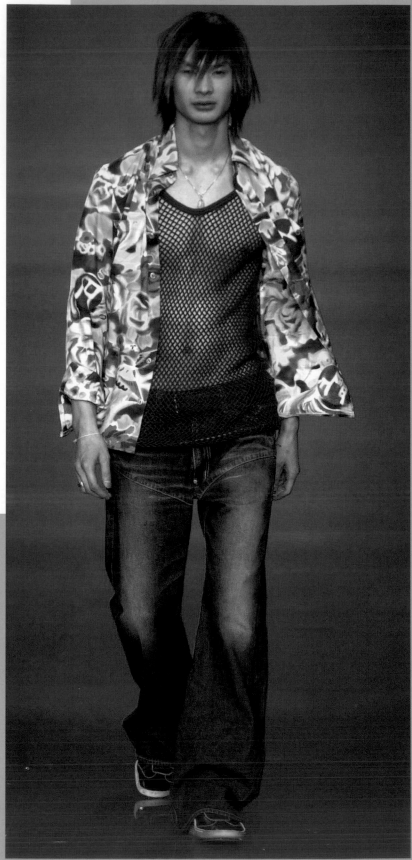

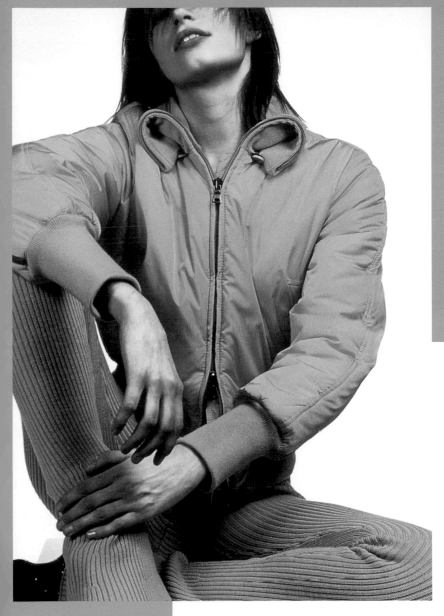

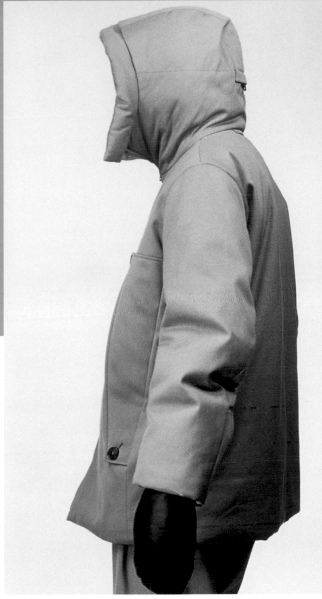

Prada Sport, Womenswear, Autumn/Winter 2000/01. This jacket is made of an ultra-compact double nylon microfibre with feather wadding, and the leggings are of merino wool. Both have been treated with Teflon (DuPont) to make them showerproof and stain-resistant.

can be heat-moulded into completely seamless garments and permanent contours, an example being pre-formed T-shirts in doubled jersey neoprene. Comfort should accompany elegance – the new softer and lighter textiles can make this easier to attain for fashion designers. Foam fabrics when bonded are usually bulky, but they have a protective volume and can be cut or combined with other materials for ease of movement. Ultra-lightweight mesh or laser-net fabrics provide ventilation for underwear, for linings, as panels or inserts, or as accents or trim.

Performance can be built in. The transfer of technology from other design disciplines has yielded new flexibles – weaves and nonwovens – and 'smart' fabrics. Finishes can transform a substrate, and reflective textiles, originally developed for high-visibility safety wear, are now being used for general outdoor wear and footwear.

These sophisticated materials with their new aesthetics and textures are a completely new development, and frequently perform better than fabrics previously on the market.

Prada Sport, Menswear, Autumn/ Winter 2000/01. The jacket and trousers are made of a Teflon (DuPont) treated cotton with polyurethane resin, making them showerproof and stain-resistant. The extended hood gives protection from the rain whether in the mountains or the city.

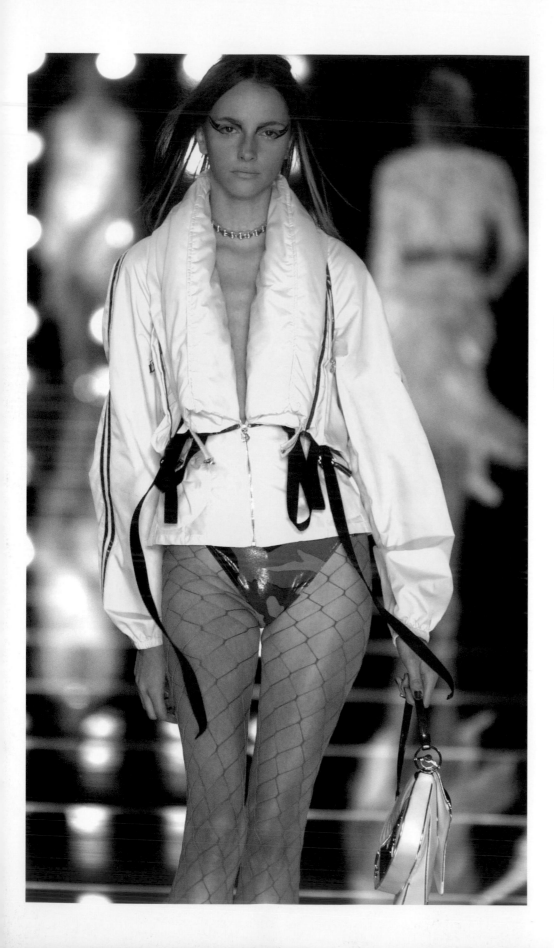

Christian Dior, Spring/Summer 2001. This bright yellow jacket echoes the style of life jackets with the safety colour, padded collar and front, tabs (to pull in case of emergency) and sporty stripes on the sleeves. Worn here with camouflage knickers and mesh tights, the look is part-functional and part-provocative.

COLOUR AND PRINT

High-visibility colours, 'safety yellow', for example, are vitally important for those working in poor light, but fashion designers also favour them. Shocking colours and bright sportsclub hues are very popular on the catwalk. Blocking of colours (fabric in different colours seamed together) is often taken from sports' dynamic images – a signal-red stripe on black to give a sense of speed, for instance. As for details, visual accents or highlights in electric yellow, turquoise, magenta or lime-green are used on outdoor wear. Monotone black, grey and navy can be brightened with light-reflecting surfaces of silver and bronze metallics. Colour contrasts can be playful and practical, as in the use of reflective trims for both sports and city clothes. For the sports look in contemporary fashion, however, neon-brights are no longer considered essential, and colours are often less brash. One-colour or two-tone jackets are common, cut in a streamlined, minimalist style, and with subtler trim and logos.

Prints, used in sportswear as accents, engineered prints or all-over prints, are often appropriated by international fashion. With the recent advances in printing technology, rollers or screens are no longer necessary,

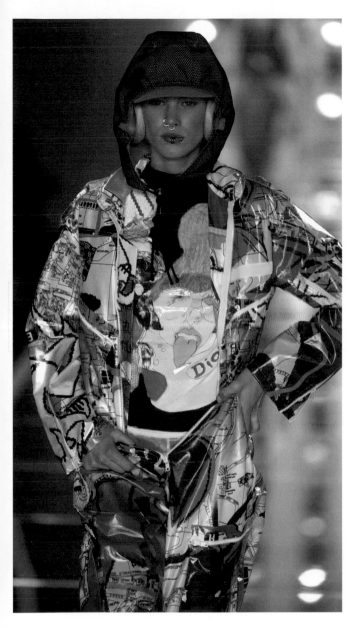

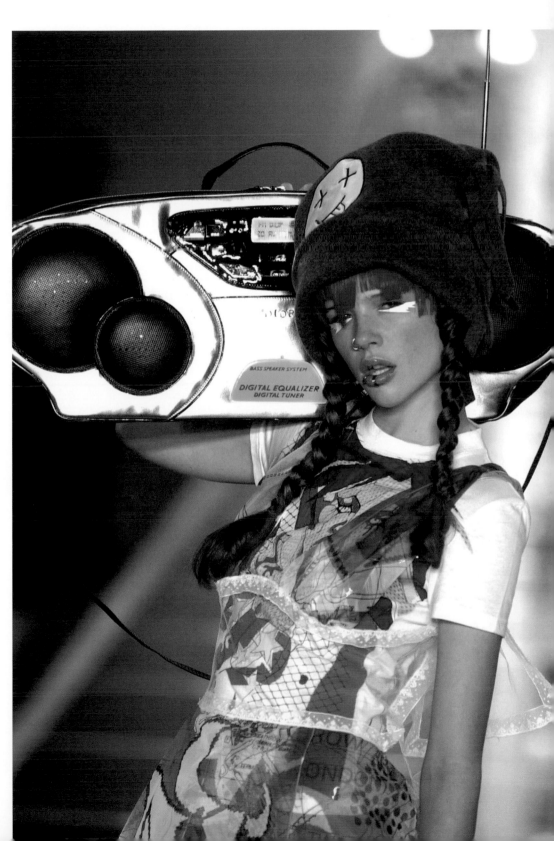

Christian Dior, Autumn/Winter
2001/02. Bright sports-inspired
colours make for eye-catching
designs (above). Styling is
functional, with hooded garments
and a relaxed cut.

Christian Dior, Autumn/Winter
2001/02. A streetstyle influence
is often emphasized in the
international catwalk shows
(right), and here Dior shows very
bright, even fluorescent prints
for a powerful fashion statement .

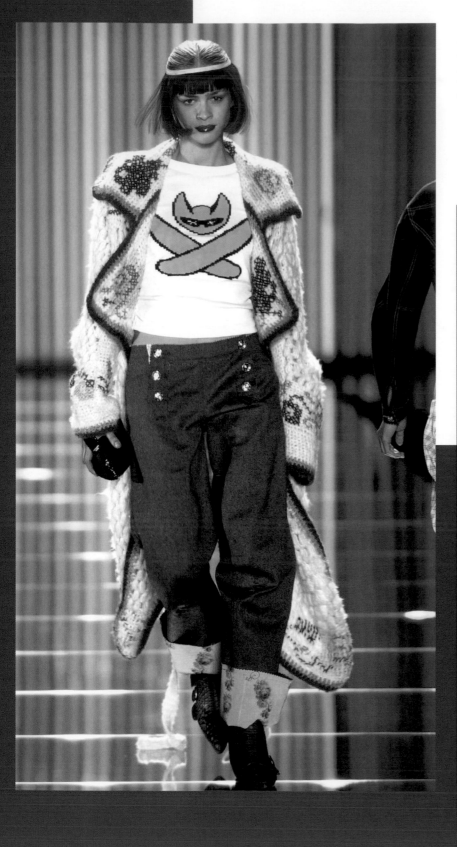

Galliano, Autumn/Winter 2001/02. Sports-inspired logos and ample cutting give this outfit a relaxed, active street look. Low-slung trousers have deep and decorative turn-ups.

Jean Paul Gaultier, Autumn/Winter 2001/02. This body armour takes ideas from protective motorbike wear, using traditional leather but with intense colour blocking and inventive cutting featuring many zips; parts are merely linked to allow for extreme movement.

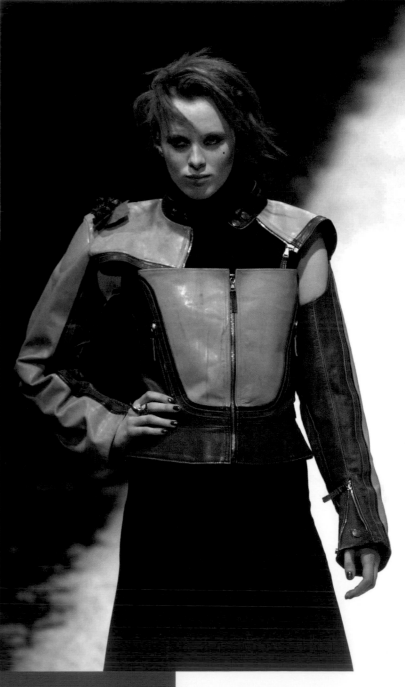

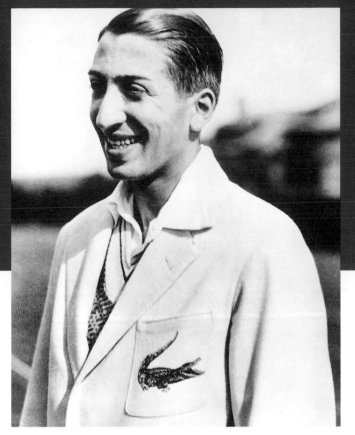

The French tennis star, René Lacoste at the US Open in 1927, wearing the 'alligator' logo. Lacoste, who was promised an alligator suitcase if he won an important match for the French Davis Cup team, also owed his nickname Alligator to his tenacity. The embroidered logo promoted his polo shirts for tennis and golf.

The Lacoste company now makes functional sports clothing as well as good quality sports-inspired fashion for men, women and children. Lacoste is an international name, and this Lacoste boutique (below) opened in Tokyo in August 2000, selling a wide range of goods, from classic polo shirts to sports bags.

and heat-transfer prints and digital print technology can create a new look.

Attention-grabbing graphics, logos and labels are often a major component of sports and leisure wear, and are a big influence on urban fashion. In the sports world, instantly recognizable colours and logos help with team identification, and in the city they are often used for the recognition of social groups. There are entire publications on the graphic designs that can be incorporated into sports and streetwear. These are sometimes the only decorative element on very purist, functional clothing, and references are drawn from Japanese and American comics, or suggest a military inspiration. Surfing, skate- and snowboarding cult wear is frequently an influence, its eye-catching and often controversial imagery showing the power of street culture.

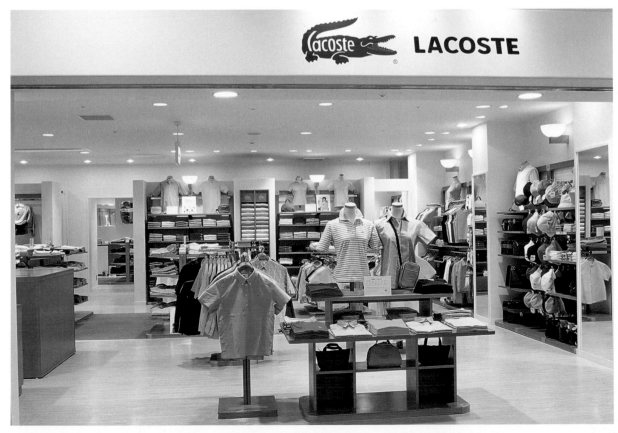

Joanna George, University of Derby, MA Performance Sportswear Design, Climbing Suit. Line drawings by climber Joanna George show a two-piece climbing suit with functional detail and fabrication. She now works freelance for Troll, Rab and Mountain Range, among other companies.

Mari Mattila, University of Derby, MA Performance Sportswear Design, Motorcyclist Clothing (far right). This shows the vulnerable areas of the body, and suggests appropriate abrasion-resistant, durable and flexible textiles. Mari Mattila was sponsored by DuPont and has worked with Rukka, a Finnish company which specializes in motorcycle clothing and extreme outdoor sports clothing.

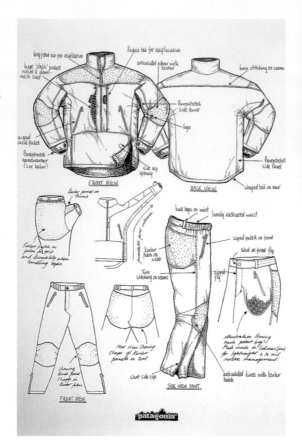

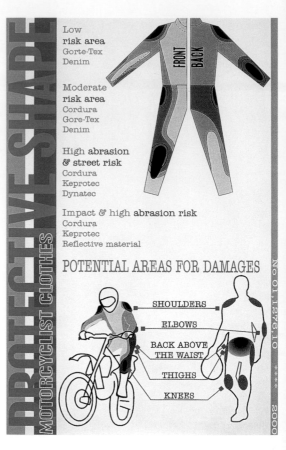

CUT AND CONSTRUCTION

The new textiles allow the fashion designer a great deal of flexibility – less cutting, seaming and shaping is necessary with stretch fabrics, for example. It is the combination of the right fabric with cut and construction techniques that makes the garment successful. Sophisticated yet practical chic is the new urban look that is simultaneously glamorous and casual.

The characteristics of high-performance clothes have significantly influenced the modern silhouette. Aerodynamic, anatomical cutting makes use of ultra-fine, super-lightweight, supple textiles. The new versions of leather and sheepskin can give a cleaner silhouette, maximum comfort, great tactile appeal and good looks.

A refined shape focuses attention on the textile, and gives a streamlined silhouette for contemporary clothing.

Pattern-cutting in sports clothes needs to make generous allowance for movement, and clothing is being cut in more comfortable widths for a sense of freedom. This is reflected in urban fashion where today's relaxed feel is a contrast to the rigorous tailoring of the 1980s, and shows a freedom in design which is now seen internationally. Men's fashionable tailoring, in particular, in spite of its very conservative and traditional reputation, has taken on the sports influence very directly. It is often deconstructed and softer tailoring is employed for a distinctly 'active' look.

Clothing inspired by skateboard wear is generally unisex, and its baggy, casual styling is very influenced by the street. Low-waisted trousers and skirts look relaxed and feel comfortable. Fashion also takes its cue from training tops, skirts, trousers and bodysuits.

Asymmetric cutting gives a new look for both menswear and womenswear. Relaxed and ample cutting often leads to 'cocooned' or 'wrapped' clothing, and keeps the wearer warm by generously wrapping fabric around the body – this is used for coats, jackets and dresses. Wrapover designs frequently use Velcro for fastening and give a sense of being enveloped – life in the city can be tough, and the 'protection' look is very popular.

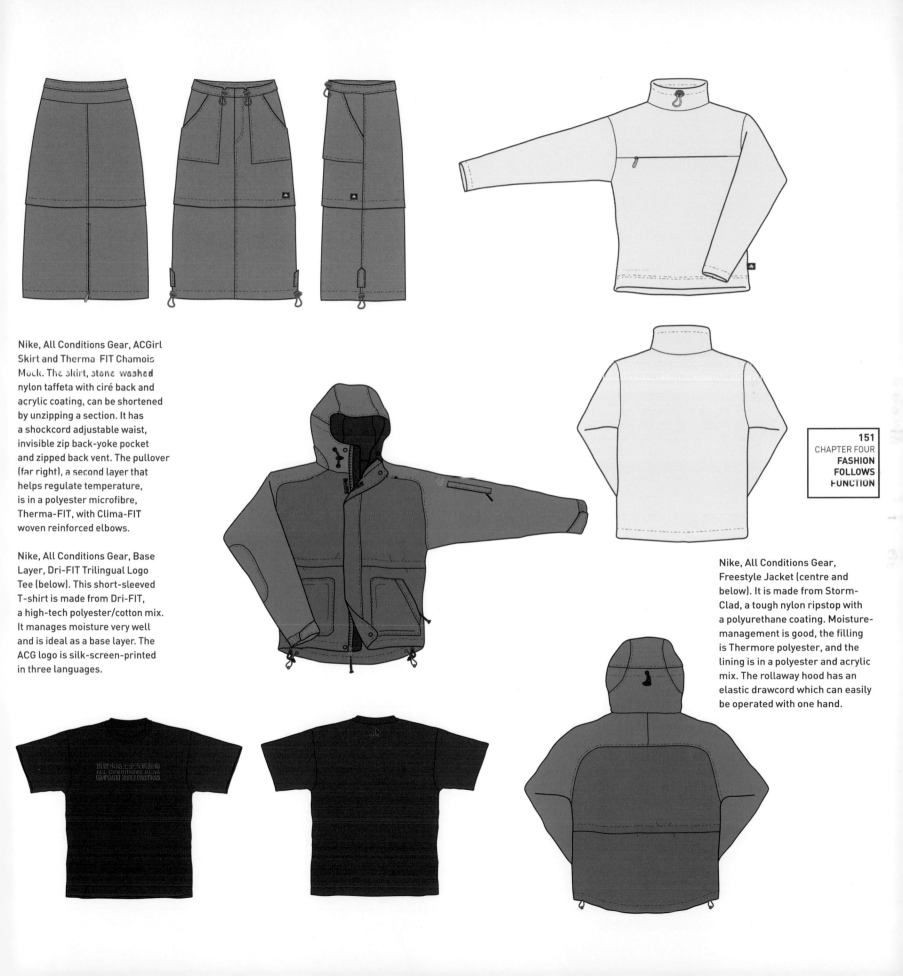

Nike, All Conditions Gear, ACGirl Skirt and Therma FIT Chamois Mock. The skirt, stone-washed nylon taffeta with ciré back and acrylic coating, can be shortened by unzipping a section. It has a shockcord adjustable waist, invisible zip back-yoke pocket and zipped back vent. The pullover (far right), a second layer that helps regulate temperature, is in a polyester microfibre, Therma-FIT, with Clima-FIT woven reinforced elbows.

Nike, All Conditions Gear, Base Layer, Dri-FIT Trilingual Logo Tee (below). This short-sleeved T-shirt is made from Dri-FIT, a high-tech polyester/cotton mix. It manages moisture very well and is ideal as a base layer. The ACG logo is silk-screen-printed in three languages.

Nike, All Conditions Gear, Freestyle Jacket (centre and below). It is made from Storm-Clad, a tough nylon ripstop with a polyurethane coating. Moisture-management is good, the filling is Thermore polyester, and the lining is in a polyester and acrylic mix. The rollaway hood has an elastic drawcord which can easily be operated with one hand.

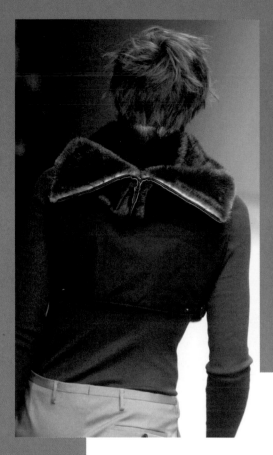

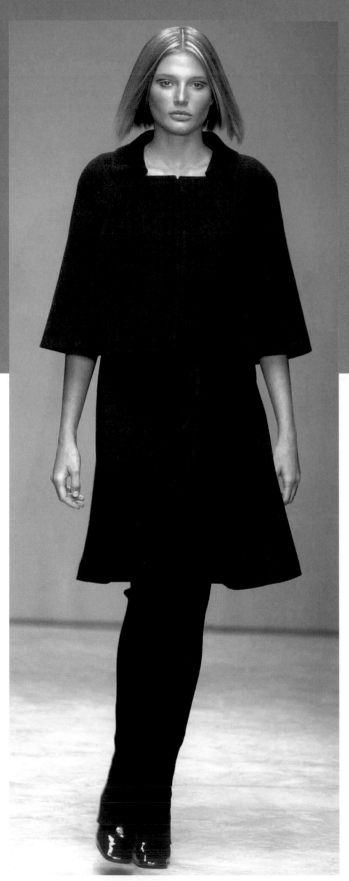

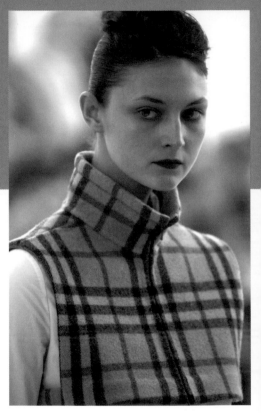

Prada, Autumn/Winter 2001/02. A leather and sheepskin-lined hooded top is worn over a slim knit (right). The hood can be unzipped down the centre to lie flat when not needed.

Prada, Autumn/Winter 2001/02. Elegant and designed for urban streets, this cape (right) covers the shoulders and shields the upper arms. The silhouette is understated and very wearable.

Burberry, Autumn/Winter 2001/02. The traditional British house Burberry went into functional clothing decades ago when Burberry coats were worn for early mountain sports. The signature beige, red, black and white plaid is updated for the protective outer layer (far right) which allows the wearer to move easily.

Many clothes specifically styled for sports are seen in modern fashion. Hooded garments (suit jackets in the city), cagoules, jumpsuits, sweatshirts, pedal-pushers and hotpants are highly fashionable. Capes which pull over the head to sit on the shoulders protect the most vulnerable areas, such as shoulders, upper torso and arms. They borrow from foul-weather clothing, and, by varying the material, can look very glamorous. Bodywarmers provide an extra, non-restrictive layer; for these, bulky fabrics, such as the thicker sheepskins or heavily padded or quilted materials, can be used,

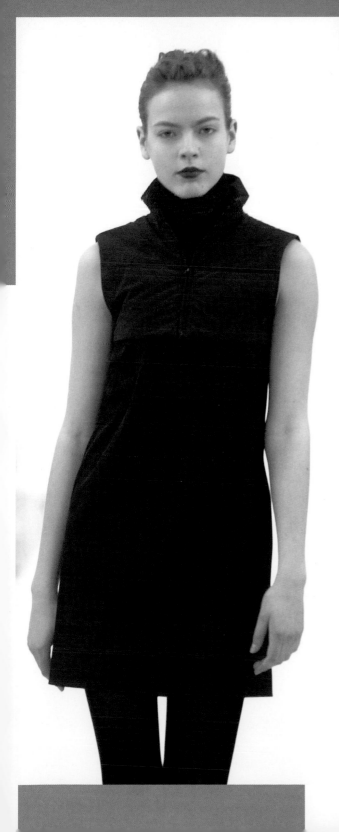

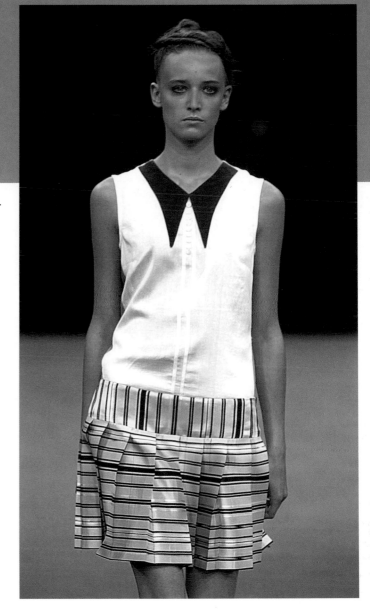

Burberry, Autumn/Winter 2001/02. A zipped funnel neck and a functional sports aesthetic is combined with a conservative navy pinstripe fabric (left) merging the sporty and and the city look.

Dries Van Noten, Spring/Summer 2001. This Belgian designer draws inspiration from gentler sports, such as tennis. A white body with black collar is distinctive and classical, whereas the pleated skirt gives ease of movement. The aesthetic recalls leisure wear from the 1920s and 1930s.

and will keep the wearer warm while still allowing a wide range of movement. The shellsuit comes directly from clothing worn after athletic activities. Quite futuristic, it was nevertheless hated by most fashion aficionados, and was taken up by people more interested in its comfort.

The US 'sneaker dress' is a casual garment influenced by sports, the street, and the way 'down-dressing' is being incorporated into the workplace. These sneaker dresses are intended for work, and are made of high-tech performance (usually stretch) fabrics which allow for maximum movement and shape-recovery. They are worn with sports footwear for a modern 'on-the-move' look. Sports-influenced fashion is now acceptable at work, and is already blurring the distinction between ready-to-wear and sports clothes. Dresses give a more streamlined look than separates, are practical and more comfortable to wear all day. Tube-dresses made of high-stretch textiles were very popular in the 1980s and are again in vogue. They are good for travelling as they are crease-resistant and roll up into the tiniest of spaces.

Vexed Generation Clothing Limited, SABS collection, Autumn/Winter 2001/02. SABS stands for 'see and be seen', and the collection protects from climate, surveillance and pollution. Protection of head and face from wind and rain when cycling must not impede peripheral vision. For this reason, the hood in the jacket has a clear panel. Technical textiles are used, such as Corwool (a blend of Cordura by DuPont and wool) lined with an Outlast phase-change material for thermal regulation and 3M reflective fabric.

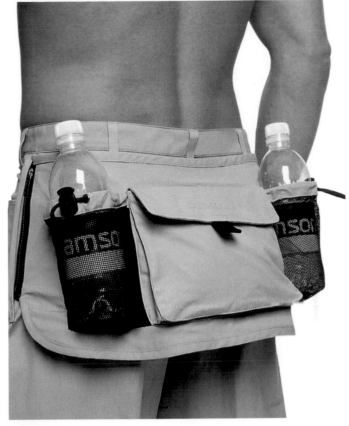

Samsonite Blacklabel, Travel wear Collection, Spring/Summer 2001. These travel trousers are made in a stretch textile with a detachable bag for storage of essential items, such as water in hot climates.

Samsonite Blacklabel, Travel wear Collection, Spring/Summer 2001. This sports vest top is made of Cordura (DuPont). It is cleverly designed so that an integrated backpack can simply pull out of a zipped pocket. Storage for essential items leaves the hands free.

Liza Bruce, Cruise/swimwear 1995. Liza Bruce often uses synthetics with a high percentage of Lycra (DuPont), and her swimwear is cut to be comfortable and to flatter the female form. A luxuriously soft pistachio sateen has 20% Lycra with 80% polyamide (below). The design has a scoop neck with lingerie-style finish and no elastication.

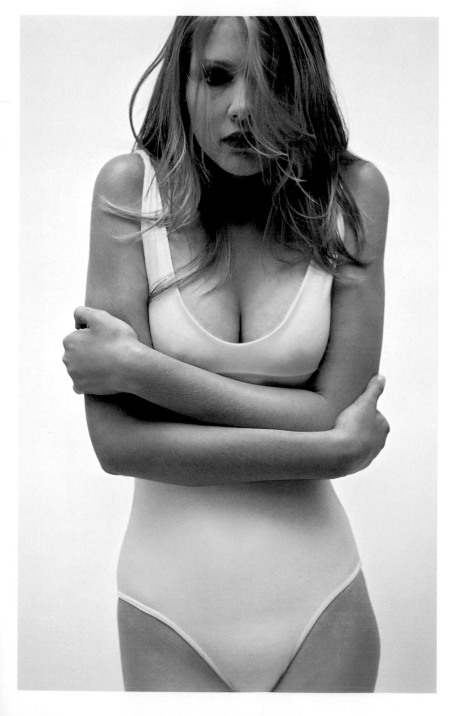

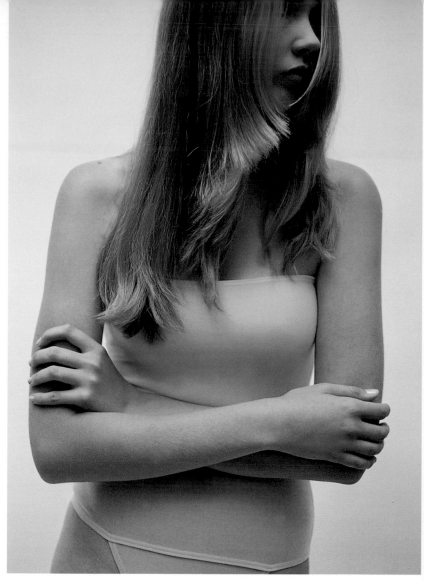

Designer fashion ranges are very influenced by the latest high-performance swimwear textiles – microfibres, and antibacterial and chlorine-resistant fabrics, for example. Aerodynamic cutting also comes from sports design, which is moving closer to everyday clothing as fashion borrows from vest-tops, shirts, shorts, skirts and tunics. There is even a growing market for vintage sports clothes and accessories, and old Nike, adidas, Fila and Champion are sought-after pieces.

The future of fashion and, indeed, sports clothing will lie in offering the customer specially made products. Body scanners record accurate body measurements with thermal imagery and ultrasound for a perfect fit. Mass production is going out of favour, and is being replaced by the desire to create individual statements.

Liza Bruce, Cruise/swimwear, 1995. A bandeau-top swimsuit (above) is made from polyamide blended with 10% Lycra (DuPont) and has a mesh-grain look. The almost transparent acid-yellow fabric is given a geometric cut.

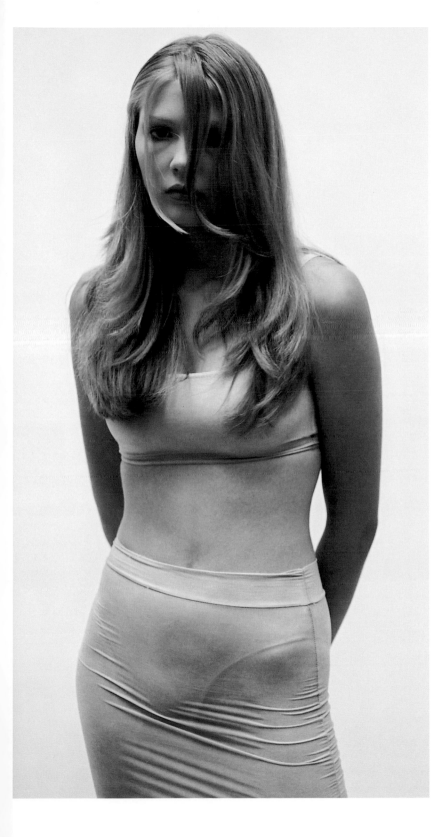

Liza Bruce, Cruise/swimwear, 1995. Polyamide with 10% Lycra (DuPont) blend is used for the skirted two-piece suit (left). Lilac, sheer, matt and almost transparent, the fabric is so light that despite the two layers it still clings to the body.

Liza Bruce, Cruise/swimwear, 1995. This two-piece swimsuit (below) uses two fabrics each made of polyamide and Lycra (DuPont); one having a 'leather' look and the other a contrasting matt appearance. This gives an effect of punk-meets-Catwoman.

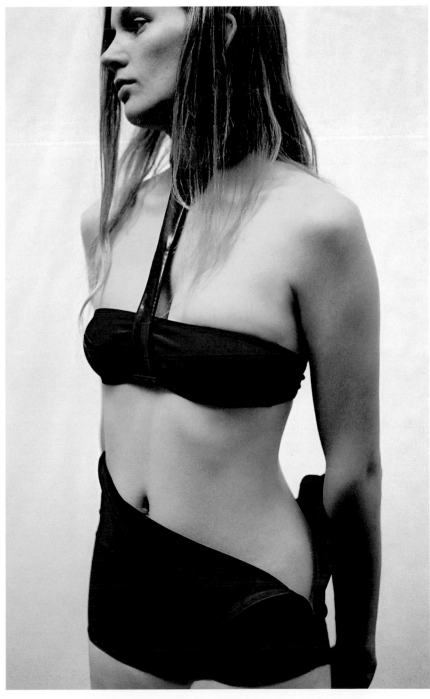

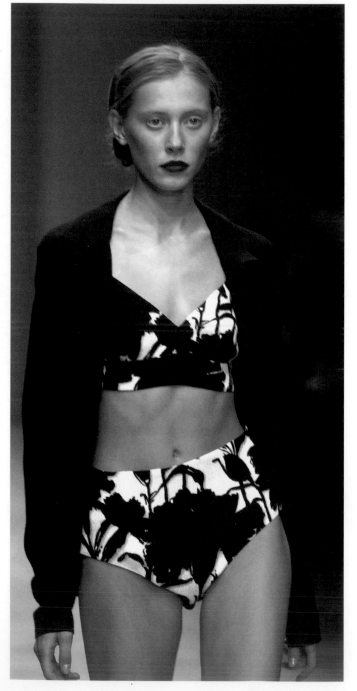

Prada, Spring/Summer 2001.
Swimwear in bold prints conjures
up the 1950s, and is shown here
with a jacket to make swimwear-
inspired separates into daywear.

Freedom is a key word in today's highly mobile society, and the clothes we choose to wear need to express this. Varying silhouettes and versatile detailing provide both function and comfort. Removable elements make for adaptable, multifunctional garments for different environments. Garments can be lengthened or shortened, made narrower or wider – trousers zip-off to turn into shorts, and sleeves to switch from long to three-quarter to short, or to be removed altogether; and there are sleeves that can be shortened by being rolled up and buttoned. Slits or side-zip openings on tops and trouser hems give extra width for increased movement. Tape adjusters at the ankle, adjustable cord at hem, waist and neckline give both style and protection; retractable flaps and detachable hoods are part of this functional style.

Reversible clothing with relaxed cutting and sports-styling can be both functional and decorative. Reversibility is a practical way of making a garment highly versatile; coats can even become sleeping bags or shelters. Form no longer follows function as textiles can adapt. Multi-purpose clothing uses high-performance textiles and new lightweight composites with different faces. Reversible garments are, in effect, two garments sewn together back-to-back, but this makes them more expensive. Nonetheless, their versatility is proving attractive in the fashion market.

Urban streetwear, especially for men, takes its active and armoured look from the clothes and accessories pioneered by extreme sports. It makes use of inventive pattern-cutting, with panels for a fitted or a more relaxed look. The gentler sports also influence fashion, and pleating borrowed from tennis clothes gives extra width where needed. Thighs, knees, elbows, ankles and the seat of garments are often articulated and reinforced (using Kevlar or double cloth, for example) for greater flexibility and protection. Padded collars, synthetic textiles or hard plastics (for calf guards, shoulder and back shielding), and reflective tape trim are all in fashion.

Underarm panels can be made from power-stretch, meshed or ultra-absorbent textiles when flexibility, ventilation and moisture-control are required. Elastic-stretch side-panels or raglan-style sleeves can also be used for maximum arm movement. In places where a special material creates more bulk, ease of movement can be retained by using another textile – for example, knitted wool sleeves can be used to reduce underarm bulk in a thickly padded nylon parka.

Vent openings can help keep the temperature of the body constant, and vented knees and elbows (sometimes with mesh inserts) allow for maximum movement and ventilation,

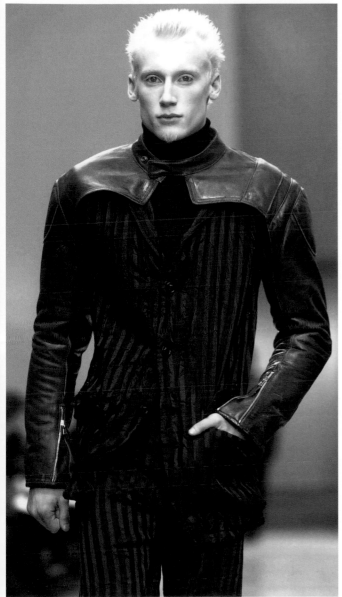

Jean Paul Gaultier, Autumn/ Winter 2001/02. Jean Paul Gaultier combines the look of a city suit with the rebellious look of distressed black leather used to protect the shoulders and arms. The result is alternative yet functional urban dressing.

Vexed Generation Clothing Limited, Stealth Utility Collection, Spring/Summer 2001. The concept is that the high-performance qualities should be subtle. This coat is made of Corwool (a blend of Cordura by DuPont and wool) with a waterproof, breathable laminate. It is lined with Outlast phase-change material. Different ways of styling are used, including built-in vents and cutting to keep the fabric away from the body so that perspiration does not make the wearer uncomfortable.

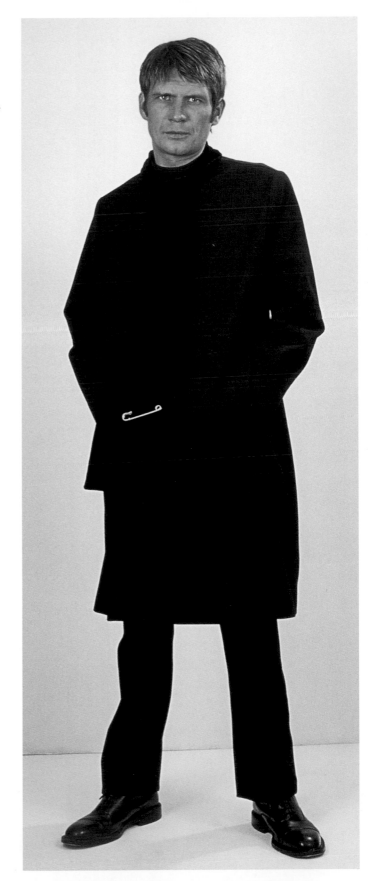

while snug funnel necks keep the wearer warm. For wet and windy weather conditions, inner and outer neck sealing can provide protection, and some garments even have built-in internal drainage channels. The need for all-round vision influences the design and cut of a hood.

The latest menswear collections use utilitarian cutting and detailing. Purists distil the influence to its essence – no logos, hoods, toggle fastenings or zips, but easy-fitting, over-sized cutting for pull-over, comfortable tops that are half-sweater and half-jacket.

In the styling, what dictates the final look includes ergonomics, safety concerns and the comfort of the wearer. Our bodies are curved, and our clothes and accessories should also be. Performance cutting means that the garment will follow the body contours but will not necessarily be figure-hugging, because ease of movement is essential. Ergonomic garment cutting is new in contemporary styling. Flex joints at armpits, crutch and across the shoulders are often incorporated. The knees of trousers can be darted. Pre-bent knees on trousers and elbows on sleeves, curved darts, seams

Samsonite Blacklabel, Travel Wear Collection, Autumn/Winter 2001/02. Many layers are shown here, with the coat offering a warm protective outer shell. The concealed zip with buttons provides windproofing, and the deep pockets are very practical. A sports influence is apparent, and warm, natural fabrics give a sensuous feel.

Junya Watanabe, Autumn/Winter 2001/02. Always avant-garde, this Japanese designer often uses advanced fabrics and inventive cutting techniques. Here, the padded collar gives protection on the shoulders and upper chest (opposite, left). The main body of the dress is in a thick fleecy fabric. Ample cutting allows the body free movement.

Chanel, Autumn/Winter 2001/02. This all-in-one padded outfit is part-sleeping-bag and part-duvet-coat (opposite right). Zipped seams allow ease of movement, and the wearer can fasten up completely for ultimate warmth and protection. Karl Lagerfeld at Chanel continues the Coco Chanel tradition, taking many influences from sports clothing.

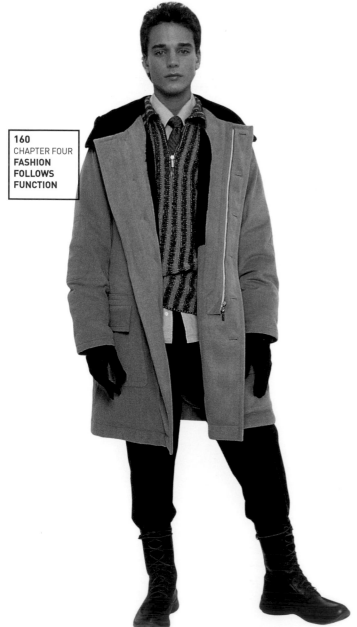

and scooped hems create a body-conscious look, with a softer aesthetic. Curvilinear cutting allows unrestricted movement and curvaceous but lean forms.

The concept of layering has come from sports clothes into many sports-inspired fashion collections. Layering can affect the success or failure of a high-performance textile. The basic idea is to keep the wearer warm, dry and comfortable by keeping out the elements and expelling body-moisture.

Featherweight padding, quilting and bonding also provide protection for people on the move, whether in the sports arena or on the city streets, and has made a strong impact on the look of urban fashion. Wadding traps air as insulation, and for padding and quilting is now ultra-soft, extremely flat and super-lightweight, making clothes for both sports and fashion that are comfortable, flexible and non-bulky. Airy synthetics and traditional goose down are both good choices as materials for wadding. Duvet coats and down-filled jackets are very popular on city streets in winter. High-necked, sleeveless, padded gilets (bodywarmers) are particularly versatile, and can be worn under jackets, over thin T-shirts and thick sweaters, or on their own – a garment for all seasons.

Some clothes are shallow-padded throughout, which is made possible through the use of ultra-lightweight textiles. Alternatively, padding can be used in certain places where the garment has to be specially protective or durable, for example, knees, elbows, seat, shoulders and back – sometimes this takes the form of double-face fabric constructions or synthetic foam inserts. An additional advantage of padded and quilted fabrics is that they do not crease or wrinkle readily. Accessories – bags and backpacks, hats, shoes and gloves – are frequently padded as well.

Jackets and overcoats made from the latest techno textiles can be worn over T-shirts, sweaters or evening wear – meaning that they can be either dressed up or down. In the same way as for sports clothes, detachable linings for jackets or overcoats can provide an extra layer of protection from the weather. Attached with internal zips, they might be made of densely woven microfibre fabrics or synthetic fleeces. Linings of polyester mesh are lightweight and insulating – they help to disperse perspiration and can also give a look that is subtly casual. Synthetic mesh or fleece linings are sometimes used for men's business suits to give a sporty edge.

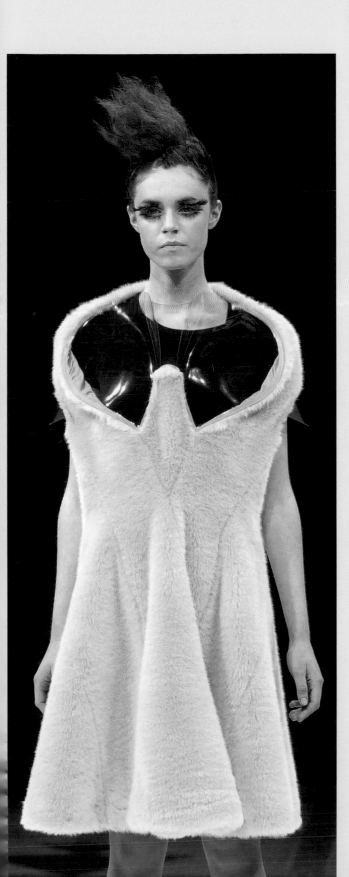

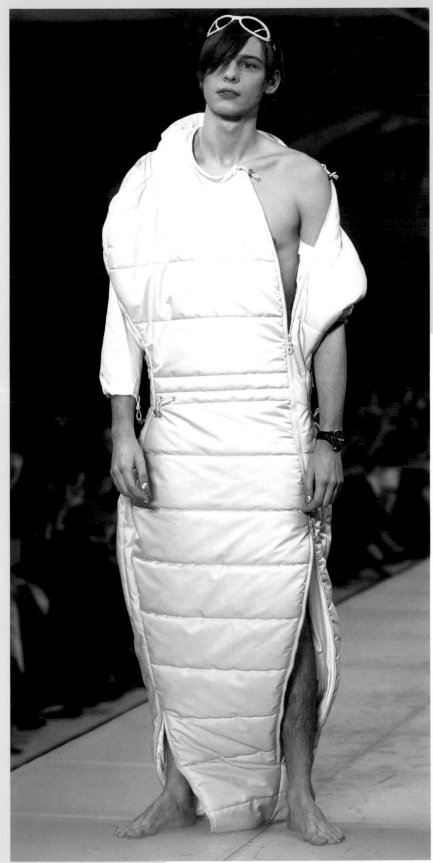

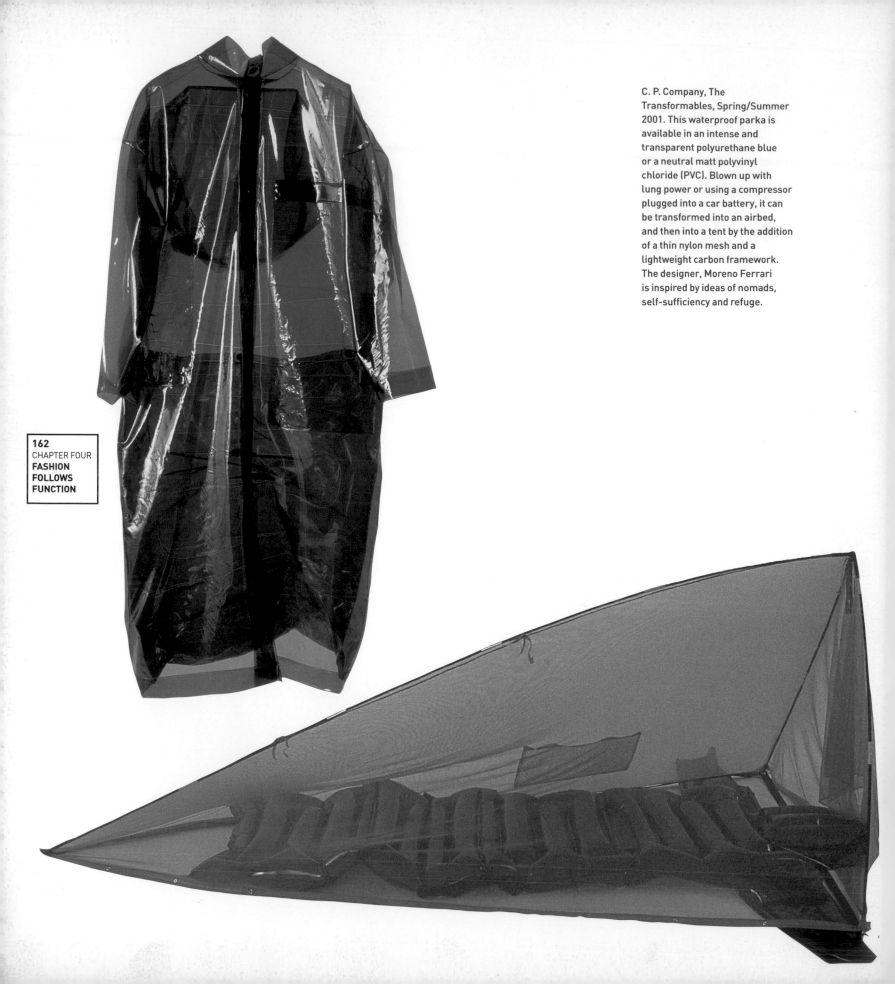

C. P. Company, The
Transformables, Spring/Summer
2001. This waterproof parka is
available in an intense and
transparent polyurethane blue
or a neutral matt polyvinyl
chloride (PVC). Blown up with
lung power or using a compressor
plugged into a car battery, it can
be transformed into an airbed,
and then into a tent by the addition
of a thin nylon mesh and a
lightweight carbon framework.
The designer, Moreno Ferrari
is inspired by ideas of nomads,
self-sufficiency and refuge.

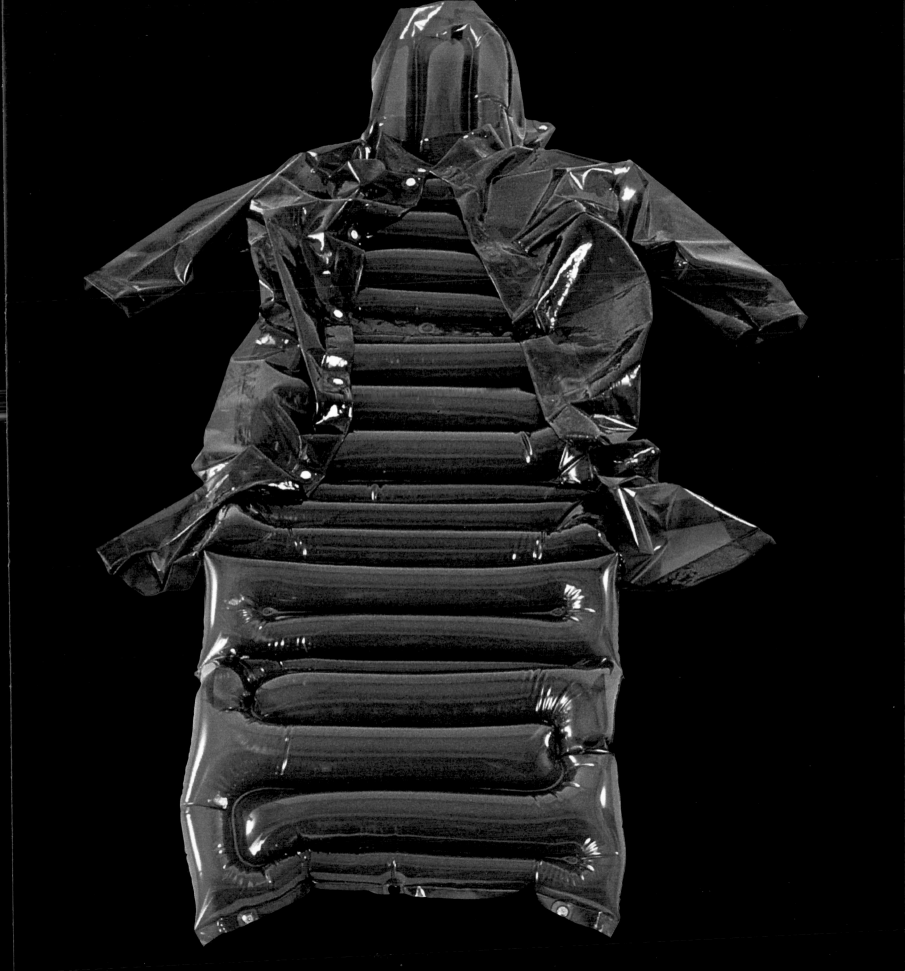

DieselStyleLab, Autumn/Winter 2001/02. DieselStyleLab is the experimental line of the Italian fashion company Diesel, which uses unusual fabrics and innovative cutting, styling and detailing. An asymmetric-cut skirt has a frill-edged frayed denim detailing and is worn with a denim waistcoat with a fake fur collar (right). A printed bomber jacket with fake fur collar and denim mini skirt (below right) are worn here with leg warmers which are reminiscent of protective wear and ski boots. The collection was inspired by nomadic bikers and survivors.

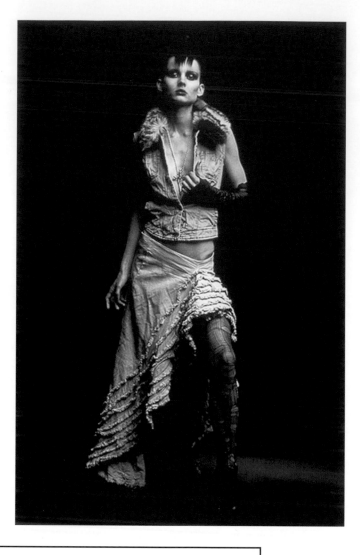

'S MaxMara, Autumn/WInter 1999/2000. Two In One But Tailored, and Doubled With Stretch Details. 'S MaxMara's designs are minimalist, and often make use of high-tech materials. A wool blend treated with Teflon (DuPont) is used for the coat (opposite left) with nylon padding and stitch-finishing detail. It has a concealed front fastening and the pockets are set into the seams to keep the silhouette streamlined. The hooded jacket (opposite right) is made from stretch nylon, padded for protection.

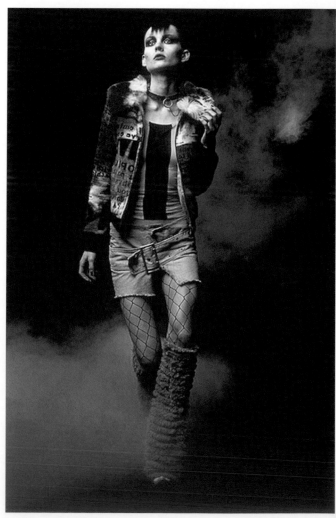

DETAILS

Seaming inspired by sports clothes is often meant to be seen as a main feature in a fashion design. Flatlock seams lie neatly and do not cause friction to the wearer; machine-stitched hems and cuffs make reference to utilitarian dressing; while welded seaming can be important for total wind-, and rain- and snow-protection. Waterproof clothes that feature laminates and coatings require careful and often sophisticated assembly so as not to lessen performance, and special seaming is a crucial requirement. Stitched and glued flat, seams give a body-conscious look, and covered and sealed seams protect the

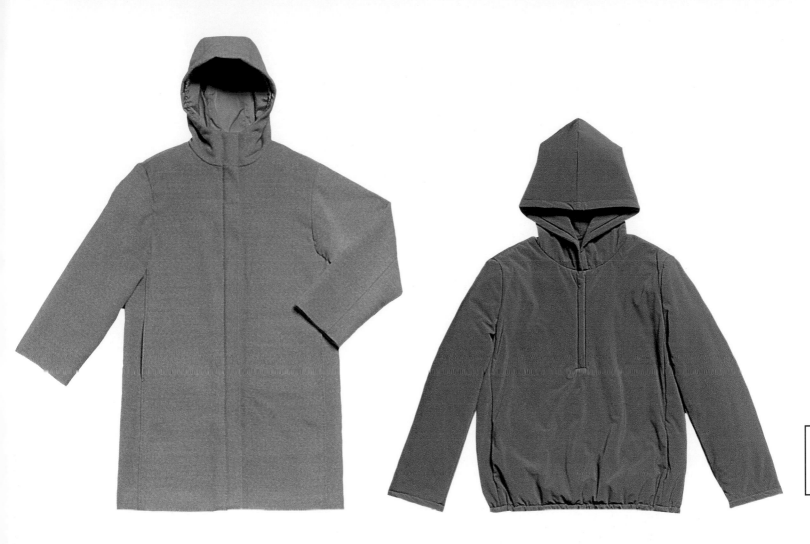

stitching from abrasion and weather. Seams in contrasting colours, inside-out seams and double-stitched seams can add a decorative element. Twisted seams and curved seams avoid straight lines to follow the body's natural form, and fabric can also be pre-shaped to give a contemporary look with increased fit and comfort. Levi's Engineered Jeans collection (launched in early 2000) features 'twisted-to-fit' clothing where seams are twisted and fabric is pre-shaped to emphasize form and function.

The construction of clothing has significantly developed – laser and sonic cutting (generally used on synthetics) fuse the edges and prevent fraying so there is no need for overlocking. Garments can be moulded with shapes 'carved' from closed-cell synthetic foams. In this way, seams can be avoided, and cloth can be joined with heat, chemical bonding and, more recently, ultrasound.

The distinct advantages of seamless clothes is that they are lighter in weight and totally weatherproof – there is no stitching to puncture the textile, with the added risk of tearing along the stitching as if on a perforated line. Since rain beats down most heavily on the shoulders, it is a particular advantage for wet-weather clothes to have no seams on the shoulders. Another advantage is that the bulk of the seam allowance can be dispensed with, and this makes for ultra-streamlining. The garment joins will not chafe or cause friction but will feel smooth next to the skin. Very suitable for sports clothes, seamless construction is also practical for underwear and body-hugging looks without visible lines. This seamless moulding method has revolutionized pattern-cutting and construction techniques. Many designers are using it because it gives a new look, increased comfort and high performance.

Styling details of urban streetwear are frequently borrowed from the technical sports sectors – ample pockets; easy-to-operate, visible fastenings; storm cuffs; detachable hoods that emerge from rolled collars. Drawing inspiration from prosthetics where maximum support is necessary, fashion designers have combined hard and soft materials to create eye-catching sculptural designs – hoods, for example, that frame the face in an attractive way while giving protection, and protective peaks that are wired so that they stay in place without flapping and obscuring the vision. Hidden compartments in clothing help keep safe precious possessions, such as mobile telephones and mini-computers. Latex moulded feet that are part of the garment give increased wind- and water-protection, and even this highly functional design has been appropriated by fashion designers with trouser-sock-boot integrated wear giving new meaning to the 'all-in-one'.

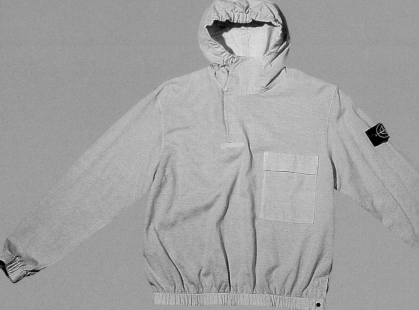
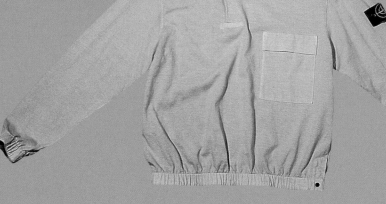

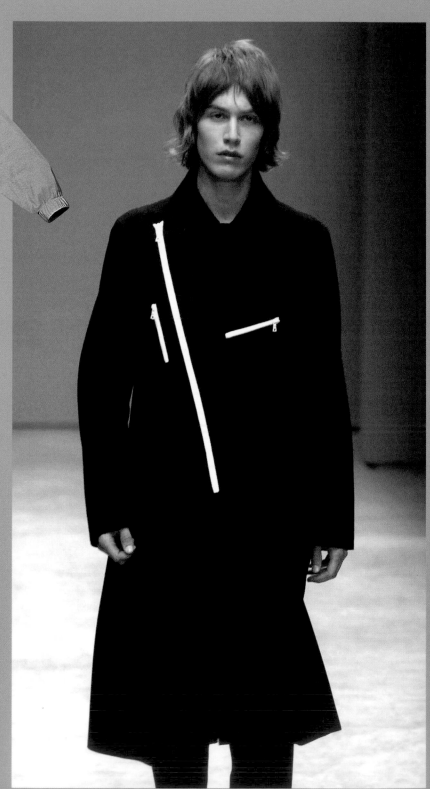

Stone Island, Spring/Summer 2001. The hooded sweatshirt (above) has asymmetrical Velcro fastenings that lead up to a high collar with hook-closure. The small front pocket also has a Velcro-secured flap. The hood is lined with thermo-taped cotton and nylon, and both hem and cuffs are elasticated

Miu Miu, Autumn/Winter 2001/02. Miu Miu is Prada's diffusion line. Outerwear (right) can offer protection but still look stylish. The diagonal front and pocket zips, prevent wind and rain penetration, and the angled opening gives easy access to the pockets.

Fastenings can help to prevent wind - and water-penetration. Some garments incorporate cleverly designed closure systems at the openings for head, neck, arms and legs. Tunnel strings, elastic drawstring closures at collar, cuff, waist, and hem help to keep the clothing close to the body and shield from the elements. Fastening details can be practical, easy to operate and clearly visible, and emphasize a utilitarian aesthetic for clothes, shoes and accessories.

Zipper detailing is often highly functional in fashion designs. It imparts a particular look, alluding to active and casual dressing. There are many different types of zips available, and a sports detail frequently taken up by fashion is the use of 'pullers', often in colours contrasting with the clothes to make them even easier to see and operate; zipped pockets on jackets

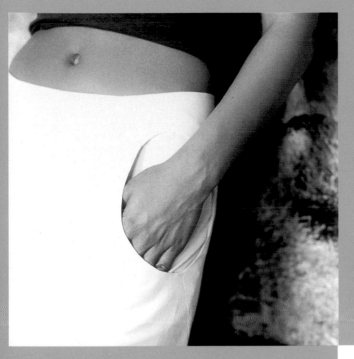

Mandarina Duck, Egg Skirt, Spring/Summer 2000. Fiberduck is used for a skirt with egg-shaped pockets. The patented pocket is an expandable cell, an idea which is adapted for different collections using various materials and shapes. Ergonomic cutting follows the body silhouette. Research into unusual fabrics for protective clothing or sports exemplifies the fabric-centred approach of Italy's designers.

Samsonite Blacklabel, Travel Wear Collection, Spring/Summer 2001. The cotton sweater has a special safety pocket, ideal for passport, air tickets and other travel documents. The garment takes its relaxed cut and practical detailing from sports clothes.

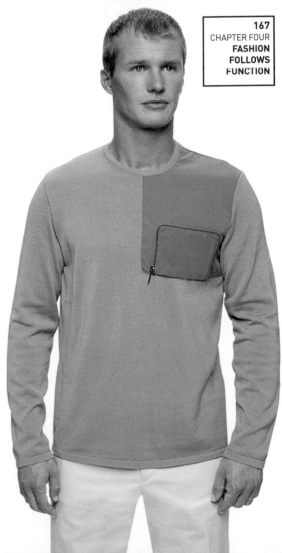

and overcoats can be opened and closed even while wearing gloves. Side and underarm openings can be unzipped when the wearer is active, and needs ventilation. Full-length two-way zip fastenings speed up putting on or removing clothing, and vertical zips from the ankle to the knee on close-fitting trousers make sports or fashion footwear easy to put on and off, while wrist zips give maximum protection, but are easy to open for ventilation or when dressing. Jackets that zip up the front often conceal the zip under storm flaps, sometimes on the diagonal, to prevent water and wind penetration.

Concealed fastenings – buttons hidden behind plackets for a streamlined look, drawstrings with cord-lock ends – are seen in many collections. Magnet fastenings, snap fastenings at the hem, square and over-sized popper fastenings are also highly fashionable, and locking toggles are not limited to duffle coats but are also seen on wrap-over skirts and lightweight shirts. Fastenings made of Velcro need only one hand to open or close them.

Pockets feature strongly in fashion, from practical sealed, windproof and self-draining pockets to internal, concealed (or with flaps), zipped or Velcro-fastened. Mesh pockets made from DuPont's CoolMax are lightweight and have good moisture-management, while those made from net allow the contents to be seen at a glance. Ultra-lightweight mesh-lined pockets give both reinforcement and insulation. Fleece-lined 'handwarmer' pockets are popular both in extreme environments and on cold city streets. Large pockets (circular, semi-circular or oval) give easy access and allow storage of valuables or of balls for racket sports. Pockets with side gussets, or 'bellows', and 'apron' skirts are very roomy. Such 'stash' pockets can hold communication systems – mobile phones, mini-computers – and also food and water. Pockets come in all shapes and sizes, including kangaroo, pouch and cargo.

Pockets can be set at an angle to allow better access. Taking inspiration from cycling, pockets are seen on the back of garments; pockets on sleeves and sited low down on trousers borrow from functional and technical wear. Pockets that are detachable at the waist or hip, fastened with buttons or Velcro, can be attached when needed and removed when not.

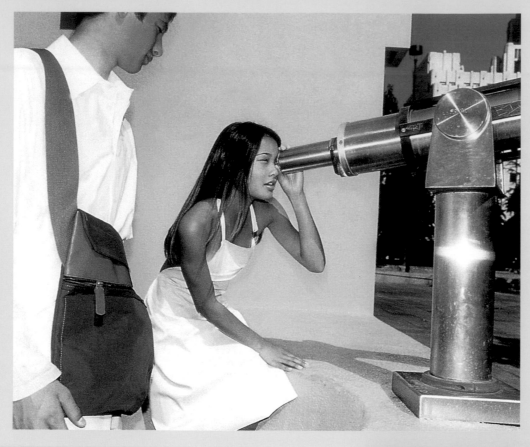

Mandarina Duck, Spring/Summer 2000. The woman wears a rubberized cotton 'apron' dress and the man a cotton shirt and trousers (left). Slung around his body is a Basis Bag made of a strong nylon that looks like cotton, with a polyvinyl chloride (PVC) interior. An electro-soldered band of rubber makes every bag more durable as well as distinctive.

Mandarina Duck, Spring/Summer 2000. The multifunctional Task Bag lies close to the body (below). It comes in various designs and has several different compartments. It is made of a synthetic which has been given a polyurethane coating that imparts a dull finish, and is lined in a coated mesh fabric. The shoulder strap is leather and injected rubber. A black Fiberduck jacket is worn with a white 'Egg' Fiberduck skirt.

ACCESSORIES

Accessories utilize the latest materials, such as microfibre fabrics and advanced finishing treatments, employing them for their good looks and interesting textures as much as for their performance. Elastic is used for flexible accessories; bags, for instance, are often made from combinations of leather and elastic. T-shirts and even jackets can fold into detachable bags or pockets. The idea of an accessory as part of the garment has been around for a while and is very practical; there are integrated bags and backpacks that wrap around and follow the shape of the body. These can often look stylish while also giving an outfit many extra pockets. 'Accessory as clothing' is useful for busy urban people as well as those engaged in sports.

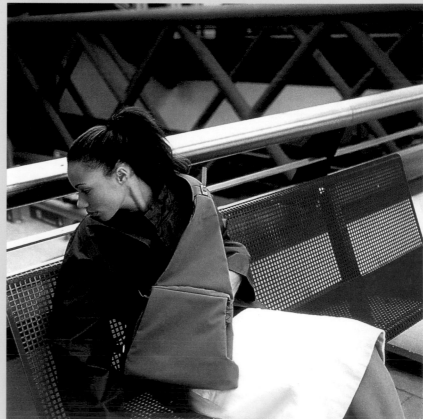

Mandarina Duck, Autumn/Winter 2001/02. The jacket (below) is made of Light Fiberduck, a patented parchment-like material, similar to the original Fiberduck but less dense and so more luminous in appearance. The Work Bag is made from a blend of two synthetics which make it waterproof and dirt-resistant.

C. P. Company, The Foldaway Hammock jacket, Spring/Summer 2001. For people on the go, this jacket (right), with its built-in hammock to tie between trees, could be fun and useful.

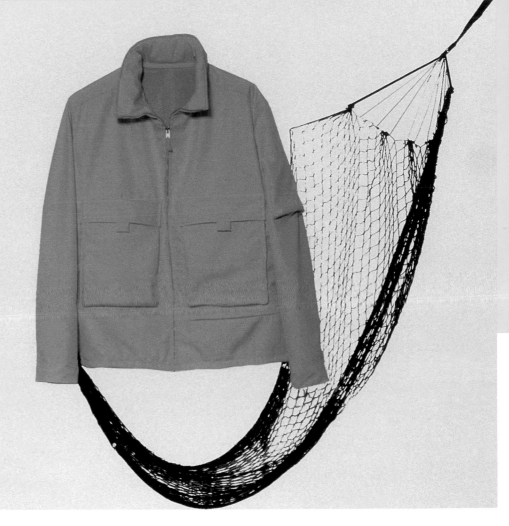

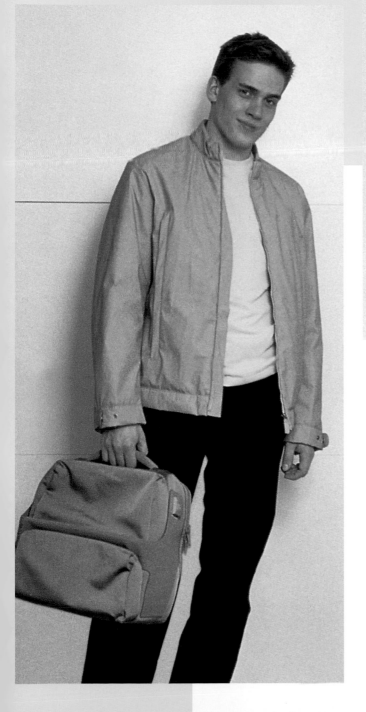

Headgear, gloves and footwear are all being rethought and redesigned in terms of the choice of textile and style. Since much of our body heat is lost through the head, wearing a hat or a hood can significantly reduce this loss while also giving protection. Fleece-lined waterproof hats and hoods are efficient (with hats generally giving better all-round vision). Some bicycle helmets still look very traditional, while others are designed to look like hats; covered in canvas they conceal a helmet underneath – an example of fashion influencing functional sportswear. Hoods with drawstring closures at the back need only one action and have no strings hanging around the face, which makes them useful for sports and for people with active lives. Ear flaps of all kinds have become particularly fashionable.

Sports gloves have also made an impact on urban fashion accessories. They are often made from synthetics, such as polyester microfleece and polyamide mesh. Soft linings can provide further comfort by preventing wind, rain and snow penetration. Leather, suede and DuPont's Kevlar are used on the palms and thumbs of sports gloves to give improved grip, and this detailing has been assimilated into fashion gloves. Skiers with microchips inserted into their gloves can pass their hand in front of a scanner for entry to ski lifts without removing their gloves – the urban equivalent might be gloves with microchips to open the door of your house, car and garage.

Footwear influences how we move and reflects our lifestyle. Specialist sports shoes enable adidas, Scalar, Autumn/Winter 2001/02. This is an off-road running shoe which is extremely light. The eye-catching three chrome straps of Velcro give support and hold the foot in place. adiPRENE (registered trademark) technology uses a cushioning material under the heel which reduces any effects of repetitive impact.

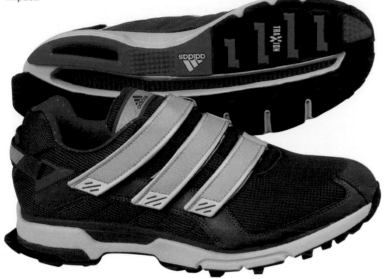

the foot to function quickly and safely, and this in turn has inspired and influenced the designers of contemporary fashion shoes and boots, who now use the latest technology and sophisticated materials. Sports references are seen everywhere in urban footwear, including the top end of the market.

The human foot supports the whole weight of the body and is extremely well designed, but it is delicate, making protection and comfort vital. During activity only certain areas of the foot actually touch the ground, and the footwear designer has to consider carefully where support is needed. Materials used to protect, cushion and absorb impact and shock include polyurethane foams and gels; Nike have even put an inert gas in a polyurethane membrane for a bounce effect when running. Originally developed for specialist sports footwear, these are now often used in fashion footwear. Shoes can be padded throughout and some can even massage the wearer's feet for

'reflexology on the move'. New synthetic materials and treated leathers are lightweight and flexible while still offering protection; cork is also used in combination with other materials, as it is soft and readily absorbs shock. Unusual materials include Flextech, which is made of copper and is used for ultra-lightweight soles for which both adidas and Bally have exclusive world rights; this revolutionary material offers protection and shape-retention. Solid carbon plates can be inserted into shoes, as demonstrated by adidas's ProPlate technology, which is an alternative to the bounce concept. This means that the foot will flex less, and energy is not lost but used more effectively for faster running. Such technology will, no doubt soon filter down to the shoes and boots designed for everyday wear.

Chroma polyurethane materials which use light-interference pigments create interesting effects when the colours change according

adidas, Oberon, Autumn/Winter 2001/02. This distinctive running shoe gives cushioning and support. The upper is made of a lightweight and durable silver-coloured mesh. The carbon and rubber outsole is extremely tough in areas that get the most wear, and adiPRENE (registered trademark) technology is also employed here for a cushioning material under the heel.

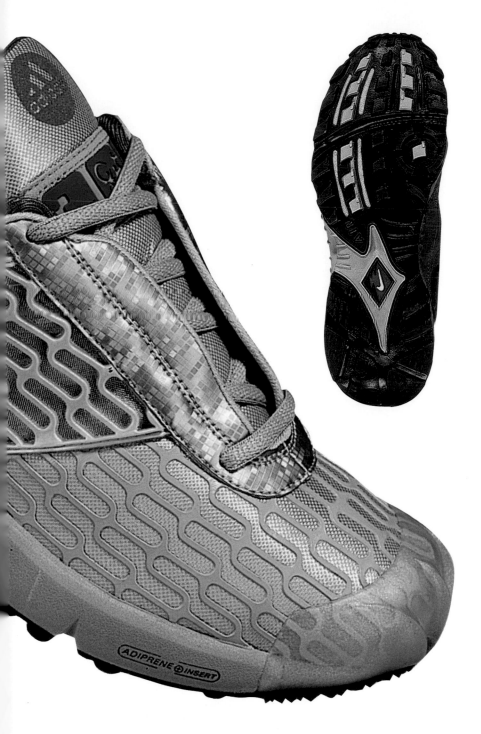

Nike Air Terra Humara. Terra is Latin for earth, and the Humara were a Native American tribe known for their sustained running. This shoe (above) is from the Nike Air Range in which an inert gas in a tough polyurethane membrane absorbs shock.

Nike Air Zoom Drive. This shoe (right), also from the Air Range, has a seamless upper, which eliminates one source of the formation of blisters – from the foot rubbing against seams. The sole has a 'waffle-fill' for extra grip even in the pouring rain. The functional shock-absorbers can be seen in the transparent area under the heel.

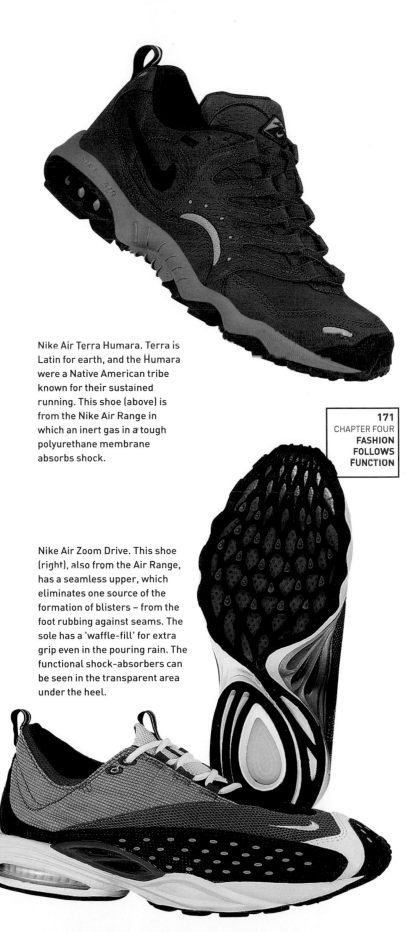

to the viewer's angle. Transparent elements can be used in the lower part of the shoes to show such internal mechanisms as functional shock-absorbers under the heel – first seen on sports footwear, they are now worn on international catwalks. Even the soles of shoes can be both functional and decorative – rubber suction spots underfoot allow for superior staying power, and are being used for evening footwear. Carbon and rubber outer soles with raised treads or tough ridges give good grip, but in neon colours with dramatic, aerodynamic patterns they can also make a bold statement.

Training shoes (known in the UK as trainers, and in the USA as sneakers) are a powerful symbol of youth culture, and often a signal of belonging to a particular group or gang. 'Brown shoe goods' – hiking or walking boots – are an alternative to trainers, and they demonstrate how sports-inspired boots combine protection with urban style. Brands such as Timberland and Caterpillar also secure a strong cult following.

There is a huge increase in the sports footwear market, and limited editions

The Converse Skate Team, Chany Jeanguenin (right). Converse footwear is popular with skateboarders and, as with basketball, this company collaborates with the top performers in the field. Skateboard sneakers receive a lot of wear, and footwear must be abrasion-resistant and durable.

Converse All Star Core Hi. Converse made the first basketball boot. The classic All Star established in 1921 is still going strong (below). It offers function with its traction and ankle support, together with good looks, and is frequently worn as a fashion statement.

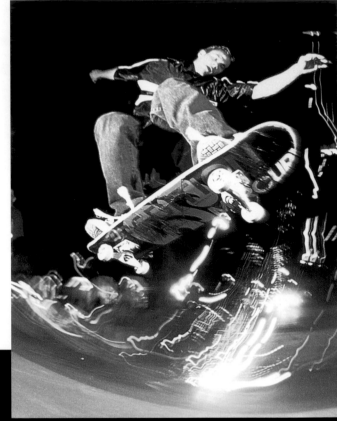

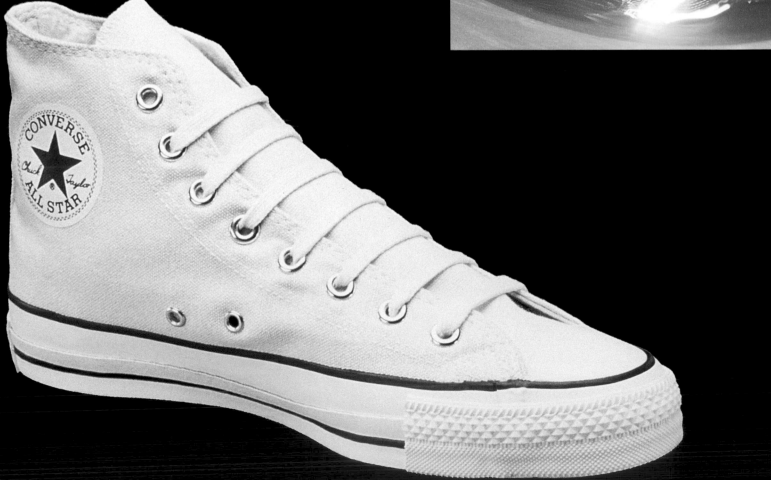

Samsonite Blacklabel, Footwear Collection, Autumn/Winter 2001/02. The Tour line on the left is influenced by a sole used for running shoes. The Details line on the right has rubber winter-tread soles which are in four sections relating to the main areas needing support. The uppers of both are made of soft calfskin.

Prada Pre-Collection, Spring/ Summer 2001. Shoes by Prada (below), made of calfskin, have a functional, drawstring fastening.

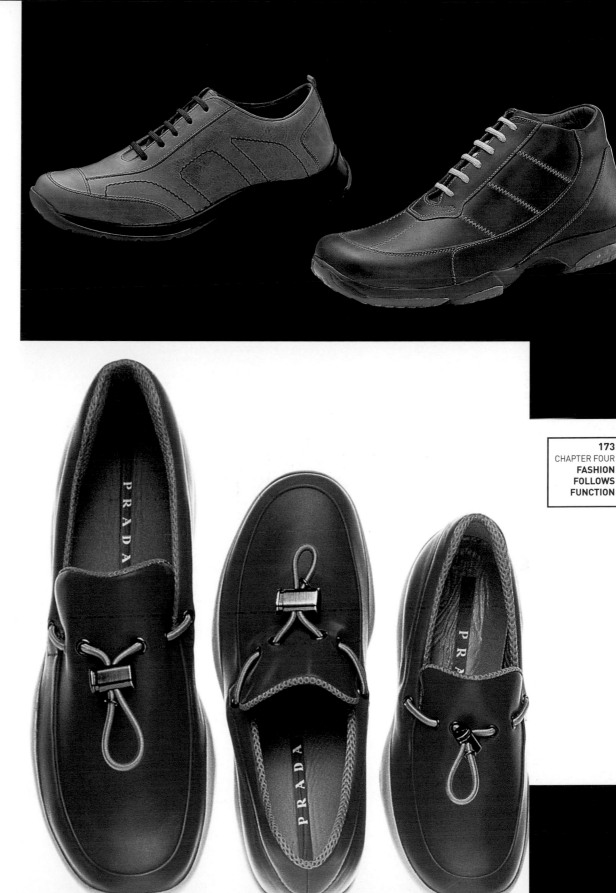

and customization are highly prized. Customized shoes and boots are given bright colours and bold designs – the sports world influences the choice of materials, the basic colours and highlights, soles and graphics. Functional detailing makes the shoes even more distinctive. Many wear high-performance footwear as part of their daily look, and it is one of the most exciting and constantly changing areas of design. As noted in Chapter 1, it is calculated that only one in five, or even as few as one in ten pairs of sports shoes are bought for sporting activities, and that the rest are worn as a fashion statement.

Sporty styling in shoes is popular in all seasons from high, chunky boots in the winter, to yachting deck shoes and de luxe sports sandals in the summer. Most contemporary footwear is relaxed and has a 'lounging-at-home' look – easy to slip on and off. 'Two-in-one' trainers have a softer shoe inside a tougher outer shoe, so that the wearer can move easily from the studio or gym to the home. In contrast, sports soles on evening shoes create a fusion between elegance and function (glamour above and utility below), or sports-styled uppers can be combined with glamorous lowers, such as very high heels. Another new development is 'skate trainers' – footwear for multifunctional fashion – one click and the wheels in the soles of the shoes unfold so the wearer can fly along the street.

The skates fold back to give way to soles with an excellent grip. There are also extensions to footwear which give a very fashionable futuristic look – calf, knee and shin protectors with some strapping to the leg, for example.

If style and detailing in footwear are generally forward-looking, so, too, is the choice of materials. Flexible and soft, the new materials allow ease of movement and provide shock-absorption. The properties of the new synthetics make them serious alternatives to leather. Footwear is made up of smaller and smaller components, which means that unusual materials, such as metals, can be chosen for decorative and protective purposes.

Leather, the traditional material for shoes, is still significant (calfskins and lambskins are supersoft), but, blended with the new materials and new finishes, can combine high function with up-to-the-minute looks and textures. Denim, heavy drill and many synthetics are combined with leather for both outerwear and footwear, and leather and foam mixes give protection and support.

To make leather more waterproof, it is coated with dubbin, a greasy preparation that closes the pores and makes the surface less absorbent yet leaves leather's texture visible, These days, however, there are new methods of tanning leather to prevent water-absorption. There are also simulated or synthetic leathers made from microfibres, with a varied surface for an authentic look – some have two-tone finishes that look completely natural.

Mesh and polyamide mixes for uppers and as inserts are seen in performance footwear, high-tech athletic sandals and urban streetwear, because they are lightweight and can provide ventilation; they also have the advantage of drying very quickly. Lycra and other stretch textiles are used both for uppers and fastenings for sports and fashion footwear. Synthetic rubber is no longer confined to wet-weather footwear – rubber shoes and boots, with their snug fit and waterproof and super-light properties, feature on international catwalks, and burnished rubber is particularly popular. Neoprene has been borrowed from surf and diving gear to be mixed with fabrics for fashion footwear. Reflective fabrics, borrowed from the industrial sector by sports designers, are now frequently used for fashion shoes. These thermoplastics can be used for seamless footwear which is comfortable and provides a new aesthetic.

Mountaineering and climbing footwear is constructed with waterproof, breathable membranes and heat-sealed seams, and linings are often made from materials with antibacterial or absorbent properties. These are all functions that the world of fashion is also finding very desirable. Ultra-fine membranes used as linings, however, must be kept clean or the pores become blocked and will not function as intended. The fully-gusseted tongue construction and high lacing are borrowed from these functional boots because they give efficient support and protection. In specialist sports footwear, cushioning and support are generally built in, and some designs also have drainage systems; there are often rubberized toe overlays to prevent scuffing – and these have all now become fashionable.

Many fastening devices for shoes are taken from technical footwear, and function is therefore being made stylish. Loops are also used, Velcro strap closures are ever-popular, as are drawstring closures and asymmetric side-lacing; traditional lacing if used can be concealed.

Several companies who started by creating specialist sports footwear have branched out into fashion lines. The big names in footwear now have their own collections for both men and women (some lines are unisex), and they build on their technical expertise for multifunctional fashion. Technical textiles, utilitarian styling and practical detailing abound.

Chanel, Autumn/Winter 2001/02.
The House of Chanel introduced
skiwear into its collections in
2000. This end-of-show duo
illustrates 'de luxe sportswear',
mixing glamour and sport (in
this case, snowboarding and
snowblading). Padding, both
for protection and support, are
demonstrated in the menswear
all-in-one, and the womenswear
outfit has a hooded cape
to protect the shoulders.
Accessories include the
snowblades and logo'd
snowboard and muff.

THE FUTURE

The sports world has had a major impact
on contemporary fashion, and the latest
technological advances in fibres and fabrics
have had a positive influence on the clothing
we buy and on our lifestyles. Most designers
and companies seek a synthesis between
past, present and future, selecting both
traditional and highly technical materials,
as well as mixing old styles with new
methods of cut, construction and detailing.

Since the new materials are seen as the
way forward in the worlds of sports, textiles
and fashion, designers are increasingly
knowledgeable about these materials and
their applications. Both avant-garde and
mainstream clothing have been affected
by the revolution in specialist high-
performance fabrics, and it is predicted
that this process will only accelerate.
The future promises totally new looks,
sophisticated textures and ever-more
advanced performance capabilities.
Our active lives will surely register a growing
sports influence as international fashion
designers send models down the catwalk
in luxurious sports-inspired clothes that
are supremely functional and stylish, and
highly desirable.

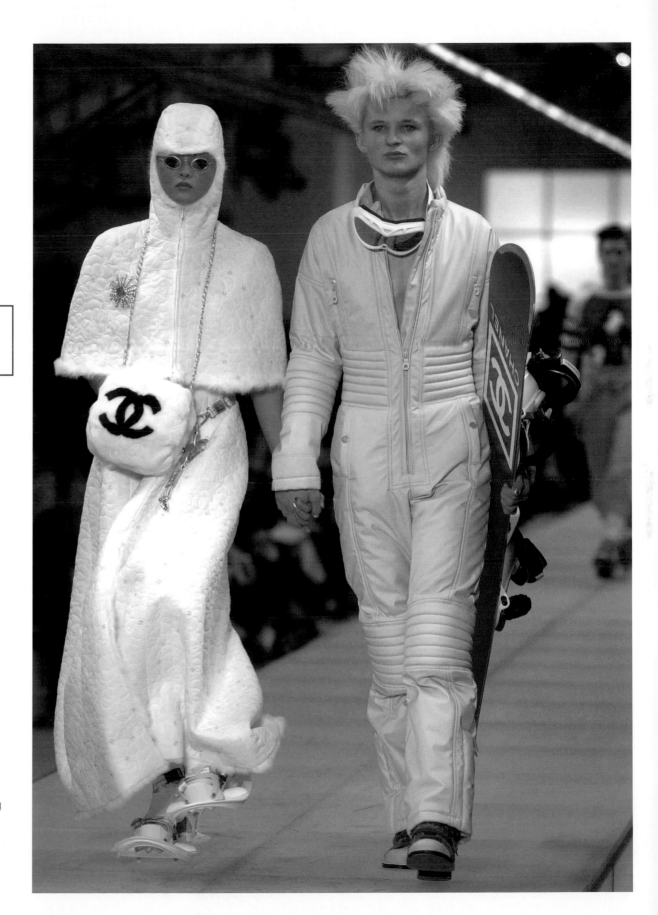

GLOSSARY OF TECHNICAL TERMS AND PROCESSES

aerodynamic Describing fabrics designed and clothes cut so that the air flows freely over the body with as little resistance as possible.

anthropometry The measurements of the human body.

antibacterial Describing a textile that inhibits the growth and spread of bacteria, and remains fresh-smelling and hygienic.

anti-chlorine Describing a material that prevents deterioration and loss of stretch properties when the fabric is frequently exposed to chlorine, e.g. from a swimming pool.

antimicrobial Describing a property, in-built or in a finish, that controls the growth of bacteria and fungi for a fresh-smelling textile that prevents infection.

aramid A **polyamide** engineered at molecular level to produce a structure that is exceptionally strong. It is used in protective clothing as a lightweight and more flexible alternative to metal. DuPont's Kevlar is one of the most common brands.

articulated As applied to a garment, cut and constructed to allow for greater movement and flexibility, e.g. by folding or pleating fabric.

backing A lining that is attached directly to the reverse of the face fabric either by sewing, or by using heat or chemicals. The textiles 'become one' and are usually treated as such during the construction of the garment.

BASE jumping BASE is an acronym for Building, Antenna, Span and Earth, the various structures that BASE jumpers launch themselves from, releasing their parachutes as near to the ground as possible. Jumpers usually have some experience of sky-diving. BASE jumping is generally illegal.

bodywarmer A close-fitting sleeveless garment that provides warmth and yet allows ease of movement. Also known as a gilet.

bonded As applied to layers of material that are joined using, for example, heat, glues, chemicals or ultra-sound.

breathable Describing a property that allows perspiration to pass through the fabric to the outside environment. This helps maintain an even body temperature.

bungee jumping A variation of a Polynesian tribal ritual. Bungee jumpers launch themselves from high places while attached to an elastic rope.

cagoule A pull-on hooded outer garment, frequently made of waterproof, lightweight synthetics.

cashmere A soft yarn from the cashmere goat. It is expensive because of the amount needed to make a garment (approximately four fleeces for a sweater).

cellulose Textile fibres derived from plants, e.g. cotton and linen.

closed-cell foam A type of construction of a synthetic textile which results in an airy, lightweight, flexible material.

coating A layer, usually on one side of a fabric with a performance property such as wind- or water-resistance, or that changes the look or texture.

cocoon Describing a garment cut to wrap around the body.

composite A combination of two or more identifiable materials usually with improved performance characteristics, each of which contributes a specific benefit.

corduroy From the French, *corde du roi*, a pile fabric, usually in cotton and generally associated with casual clothing, but also available in other yarns, such as silk.

darts A tapering fold of fabric sewn (usually right sides of fabric together) and leading to a point of fullness. Darts shape the fabric to the body.

diffusion line A relatively inexpensive line of clothing using simpler cutting and styling than the fashion designer's main line collection, and different materials.

elastane fibre The international abbreviation for this elastic **polyurethane** is EL. It is usually blended with other fibres, natural, regenerated or synthetic, to give clothes a stretch property, which is very important in sports.

engineered print A print whose position on the garment works with the silhouette, seaming and other construction details. Also known as a placement print.

face fabric The topmost fabric.

fibrillating The splitting up of fibrils (small fibres). See also **pilling.**

flatlock seam A seam that is very flat on both the right side and the wrong side of the garment. This produces streamlined, close-fitting garments without the friction caused by bulky seams.

funnel neck A funnel-shaped garment-neck that covers the neck in a smooth line from the shoulder.

fused Of materials, melted together using, for example, heat, glue, chemical or ultra-sound.

gamma rays Very short wavelength X-rays caused by radiation.

haute couture Custom-made high fashion clothes, as distinct from **prêt-à-porter** (ready-to-wear). These are generally made from more expensive fabrics, have more complicated cut, construction and detailing, often with hand-finishing and decoration. The main centres are in Paris and Rome (where it is known as *alta moda*).

heat-moulding The process of shaping certain materials (synthetics and wool) by reconfiguring the molecular structure which becomes fluid when heated. Both surface interest and fully dimensional forms can be achieved.

heat-reactive The property of a chemical that, printed or painted on a textile, will swell when subjected to heat, creating a surface texture ranging from subtle to extreme.

heat-transfer A method of using heat to transfer an image from paper to textile.

heli-skiing Skiing from remote mountain places, inaccessible by ski-lift and reached by helicopter.

hollow fibre Ultra-lightweight fibre with no core. The fibre makes textiles that have volume and good insulating properties, as they trap air.

hydrophilic Water-attracting.

hydrophobic Water-repelling.

kite-surfing Surfing using a kite for airlift to jump above the waves and perform various acrobatics on and above the water.

knitting A form of fabric construction where a single length of yarn is taken and interlinked with itself, each row being dependent on the last.

laser-net A fabric made into a net by a laser cutting out pieces of fabric and leaving behind a mesh.

leggings Close-fitting, footless garments for the legs generally made of a high-stretch textile. They were originally used for dancewear and became fashionable in the 1980s.

leno A type of weave that has a special twisted warp thread allowing the weft to be spaced to create an open effect. Leno weaves are often used to 'show off' an unusual weft yarn.

liner Removable layer, for example, in a shoe, and which can be made from **antibacterial**, antifungal and other special materials.

lining A layer of material applied to the inside of a garment. The lining and garment are made separately, and generally sewn wrong sides together. Lining fabrics are usually thinner than the top fabric, except for those chosen for warmth and softness, such as fleece.

loden A dense wool fabric, traditionally used for outerwear, as it is strong, durable and warm, protecting the wearer from wind and rain.

luge A sport which uses a light toboggan for one or two people.

membrane A very thin layer of material, generally synthetic, that is attached at the garment seams as a liner, or laminated to the whole fabric as a finishing treatment, or between the **face fabric** and a **lining**. Advanced membranes can have such characteristics as wind- and water-resistance, and many are **breathable** for comfort and protection.

mercerized As applied to cotton, treatment with a caustic alkali, which gives increased strength and a characteristic sheen.

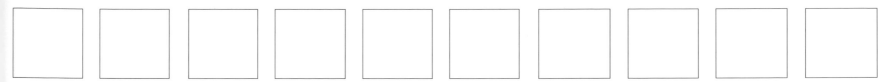

mesh An open knit/woven/interlaced fabric.

microclimate With reference to clothing this means the climate enclosed by the wearer's garment. For optimum performance in sports, the body's temperature must be kept constant.

microencapsulation The process by which substances are encased in a bubble-like structure and incorporated into a fabric or applied to the surface as a coating. In some instances the chemical (perfumes, vitamins, etc.) can be released when subjected to pressure, while in others (**phase-change materials**) the chemical remains trapped and alters its structure when subjected to stimuli, such as temperature change.

microfibre An extremely fine fibre – up to sixty times finer than the average human hair. A microfibre can have a range of specifically engineered characteristics. Usually made of either **polyester** or **polyamide**, microfibres can be woven or knitted to make high-performance textiles. Microfibres are chosen for next-to-skin base layers for their **moisture-control and management**, for insulating layers for their good thermal regulation, or for outer layers for wind/water/snow protection and look.

micron One millionth of a metre.

microporous Describing very absorbent textiles that have tiny pores making them **breathable**, and that also protect the wearer from wind, rain and snow.

moisture-control and management Property of a textile that absorbs sweat and **wicks** it quickly away from the skin to the outer layer where it can evaporate. This ensures that the wearer stays warm and dry, and can prevent overheating and chilling after activity.

motocross High-speed biking on a closed course.

neoprene A synthetic rubber obtained by the polymerization of chloroprene.

nonwoven A material that is usually made by laying down a web of fibres and then fusing them by heat-treatments, water jets, friction, interlacing or 'needle-punching' (needles without thread take fibres from the top layer through to the bottom to make the cloth), or a combination of any of these.

oleophobic Oil-repelling.

padding A layer with volume, lightweight if made with advanced materials. Padding is capable of absorbing shock, preventing friction and protecting the wearer.

PCR fleece A fleece-like fabric made from polyester obtained from post-consumer recycled plastic bottles.

pedal-pushers Trousers that finish somewhere between the knee and the ankle.

performance-cut A specific type of cutting and shaping so that the garment follows the body's curves closely to allow maximum movement and comfort.

phase-change material (PCM) A material that changes its state, e.g. from liquid to solid. Some PCMs, like paraffin wax, respond to changes of atmospheric or body temperature, liquefying during activity by absorbing excess heat, and solidifying afterwards to release stored heat.

physiology Science of the functions of living organisms (here, the human body).

pile The surface on a fabric that is raised and plush, for example a velvet or **terry towelling** – this can be a cut or uncut pile where the raised yarn is left in loops. Such fabrics tend to be very absorbent and insulating.

pilling When short fibres build up on the surface of a fabric, usually in blended textiles, the tougher fibres cut and trap the softer ones to give an unsightly 'bobbly' appearance. This is also known in the industry as **fibrillating**.

piqué A cotton fabric with a textured appearance achieved by certain weave structures, such as honeycomb or waffle. It is commonly used in sports clothes as it is very absorbent.

pleating Folded and sewn fabric which creates an area that allows more movement. There are various types of pleats, a box pleat where two folds face each other; an inverted pleat where two folds face away from each other; knife pleats where a series of single pleats face in the same direction; and sun-ray pleating where the whole fabric is pleated.

polyamide The international abbreviation of this a synthetic **polymer** is PA. It is also known as nylon, and is a fibre that is quick-drying, lightweight, abrasion-resistant, durable and easy-care. It can be specially engineered to take on a variety of appearances and surface effects, e.g. matt or lustrous, and smooth or textured. Polyamide is available as a **microfibre**, and a version of it, Polyamide 6.6, is used as the basis for many microfibres.

polyester The international abbreviation of this a synthetic **polymer** is PES. It is versatile and very suitable for sportswear. It is lightweight, abrasion-resistant, quick-drying, durable and easy-care. It can give different looks and handling properties, and is available in a range of weights, and as a **microfibre**.

polyethylene A **polymer** based on oil (also called polythene).

polymer A natural or synthetic compound with large molecules made up of many simple repeating units.

polyurethane A synthetic resin whose **polymer** units are linked by urethane groups. It is often used as a coating to protect from wind and rain.

polyvinyl chloride (PVC) A tough synthetic resin which is resistant to most chemicals.

pre-formed/pre-shaped As applied to sections of a textile which have been heat-moulded to follow the concave or convex shape of a part of the human body (such as the elbow or knee).

prêt-à-porter Otherwise known as ready-to-wear, emerging in the 1960s to offer collections, distinct from haute couture, of more wearable, everyday garments.

racing silks The bright and contrasting coloured and patterned shirts worn by racing jockeys to make identification of their mounts easier.

raglan A type of sleeve which is cut so that its seams run either side of the shoulder from neckline to underarm rather than on the shoulder – roomy and practical for outdoor wear.

recovery The ability of a textile to return to its original shape.

retroreflective Reflecting light back along the incident path, regardless of the path's angle of incidence.

ribbed A structure with a ridged or raised pattern of lines. In a knitted fabric this is achieved by alternating plain and purl stitches; in a woven cloth by use of a heavier yarn. This generally gives a more durable and flexible fabric and is used either as an edge at cuffs and collars or throughout the body of the garment.

ripstop A special textile, usually made of nylon, with a grid-like construction that prevents rips from spreading. A thick yarn used with a thin one gives it its characteristic checked appearance. It is lightweight and has great strength and resistance. Applications include sports outerwear, linings and equipment.

seam-sealing A technique for making a high-performance waterproof garment. Methods vary, and include heat-sealing or the application of a special adhesive tape on sewn seams to cover puncture holes made by the needle. The tape has to be very durable and is usually a synthetic.

self-curing Describes a material that will harden and turn brittle over time.

shape memory alloys (SMAs) Known in the USA as Memory Metals, these belong to a group of materials referred to as Smart Materials and Systems. They are most commonly used as a nickel and titanium alloy in wire form, and less commonly as sheets. The alloy is malleable, but has the ability to return to its 'memorized' form when subjected to heat above a specified temperature.

silicon A non-metal element found in the earth's crust which exists primarily as oxides and silicates. Silicon has semi-conducting properties.

silicone A synthetic **polymer** composed of repeating **silicon** and oxygen atoms with organic groups attached to the silicon. Silicone typically has low-resistance properties and is water-repellent. Most types are also insensitive to temperature change and many chemicals. This polymer is used to make plastics and rubbers.

sky-diving Jumping from an aeroplane and descending some way before opening the parachute.

sky-surfing Sky-diving with a special board (not unlike a surfboard) that allows the diver to perform tricks while in mid-air.

'smart' fabrics Textiles capable of sensing and responding to external stimuli, such as changes in lighting and temperature.

snowboarding 'Surfing on snow' – the feet are strapped to a large board to manoeuvre down snow-covered mountain slopes. It has attracted a different crowd from skiing – younger and 'cooler'.

speed-skiing Skiing very fast on a specially constructed ski slope.

sportswear In the UK this term refers to specialist clothes and accessories specifically designed for a particular sport, and also informal clothing derived from sports in term of style, fabric and cut. In the USA it more usually refers to casual wear.

stretch A highly elastic property in yarns or fabrics commonly used in sportswear to allow ease of movement and thereby enhance comfort. This is usually achieved through the use of an elastic yarn, such as DuPont's Lycra brand, though it can also be produced by a high twist in the yarn or in the fabric structure (e.g. knit is inherently more flexible than weave). Bi-stretch runs parallel with both **warp** and **weft** of a woven material, while a three-dimensional stretch runs in all directions.

strip Distinctive team clothes worn by footballers (and their supporters) in both soccer and Rugby.

substrate The underlying surface, textile or otherwise.

technology transfer The transfer of technology from one sector to another, often resulting in a new material. Technical materials originally developed for industry, for instance, are being used as fashion fabrics.

techno-naturals Most are natural materials blended with synthetics or using finishing treatments to give them enhanced performance while retaining a natural look and texture. Some, however, are totally natural but manufactured in new ways.

terry towelling A thick, soft absorbent cloth, usually cotton or cotton blend, with raised, uncut looped threads on both surfaces giving it a **pile**, used primarily for towels (variation of 'terret', meaning a loop).

thermochromic The ability to change colour in response to variations in temperature.

thermoplastic Synthetics and wool have this property, which means that they can be reshaped using heat. The textile's molecular structure breaks down and becomes fluid when heated and can then be re-ordered for surface texture or three-dimensional form. The result is permanent and cannot be reversed unless the temperature at which the fabric was set is exceeded.

thermoprinting Printing using heat to transfer and set the design. This is often capable of high fidelity, picking up on minute texture and image.

three-layer system This can greatly enhance an athlete's performance. A good base-layer fabric is breathable and **wicks** moisture (perspiration) quickly to the air outside the garment. Next is an insulating layer, trapping air, that is **breathable**, soft and warm. Finally there is a breathable and weatherproof layer.

tow-surfing Surfing while being towed through the water by speedboat. The higher speed catches bigger waves.

trainer Term in common use in the UK for soft or flexible training shoe, sports shoe or running shoe, referred to as a sneaker in the USA.

trial-riding Biking over barrels, rocks and other obstacles.

Velcro The trademark for a 'loop and fasten' material for fastenings. One surface has loops and the other needles; when pressed together they form a temporary bond, and the process is fully reversible.

ventilation Free circulation of air around the inside of a garment. Cool air is allowed to pass in and carry away warm air (produced by activity) to maintain a stable body temperature and prevent overheating.

vest Next-to-skin layer of underwear for torso in the UK, but in the USA describes a garment like the UK waistcoat, sleeveless and buttoned down the front, worn over a shirt and sometimes under a jacket.

wadding A very airy, soft, light material generally used between face fabric and lining to give warmth.

wakeboarding Water-skiing with a board instead of skis to allow jumps and tricks.

warp The vertical threads of a woven fabric that run parallel to the selvedge (the edge of the fabric, often more tightly woven). They are usually made of strong, durable yarn.

water-repellent Describes a textile resistant to water but not totally waterproof.

weaving An interlacing fabric construction where **warp** and **weft** threads cross over and under each other to form a cloth.

weft The horizontal threads of a woven fabric that run at right angles to the selvedge (the edge of a fabric, often more tightly woven). Yarn for the weft can be more experimental than that of the **warp**.

wicking The ability for a fibre or fabric to transmit moisture; for example, sweat from the skin to the air outside the garment, where it evaporates.

zorbing Rolling down a slope strapped into a huge transparent plastic ball.

BIOGRAPHIES

Acordis

Acordis is a group of fibre-manufacturing companies based in Arnhem, The Netherlands, formed after the takeover of Courtaulds by Akzo Nobel in 1998. Akzo Nobel had been manufacturing technical textiles since the 1930s and became known for nonwovens, aramids, carbon fibres, and for creating the breathable microfibre membrane, Sympatex. Courtaulds was founded in the UK in the early nineteenth century and manufactured the first regenerated cellulose fibre, viscose rayon, in 1904. Cellulosic fibre innovation, research and development are a large part of Acordis's business, and trademark fibres include Amicor, Viloft and Courtelle, all of which are used for sports attire and sports-inspired fashion.

adidas

The sportswear company, adidas was founded in Germany by Adi Dassler. Although he was making shoes in the 1920s, the company was not registered until 1949. The trademark three stripes were initially designed to give support at the sides of the shoes but have become a very successful logo, recognizable worldwide. Other adidas logos are the trefoil and the name 'adidas'. All are registered trademarks. The design HQ is in Herzogenaurach in Germany where a team of specialists works on the development of new high-performance materials. They analyse the design of the human foot to give it protection, support and shock absorption. Performance clothing and street wear are now also produced by adidas. The first collection was launched for Autumn/Winter 2001/02.

Maria Blaisse

Born in The Netherlands in 1944, Maria Blaisse studied textiles at the Gerrit Rietveld Academie in Amsterdam, and then worked for the Jack Lenor Larsen Design Studio. From 1974–87 she was Professor of Textile and Flexible Design at the Gerrit Rietveld Academie, and since 1982 has been an international guest lecturer. Trained as a weaver, she has been working with industrial materials, such as synthetic rubbers, closed-cell foam and nonwovens, for a number of years. She employs such techniques as laminating and vacuum-moulding that exploit the thermoplastic properties of these materials. She uses circles, squares, rectangles and triangles as the base-shapes for her wearable art works. Maria Blaisse also stages performances with dancers and musicians.

Liza Bruce

Born in New York in 1955, she is now based in London. Designer Liza Bruce creates swimwear, cruise wear and a range of fitness and leisure wear using high quality techno-stretch textiles. Sport has influenced her designs, which are minimalistic, futuristic and use graphic shapes, yet are cut to flatter the female form.

Burberry

The British company Burberry was founded in 1856 by Thomas Burberry who, in 1880, invented gabardine cloth – a tough, water- and windproof fabric – that was used for the famous trench coat. Burberry coats were initially worn for mountain sports and Burberry is also known for its signature red, tan, black and white plaid. Its clothing was a precursor of the modern sporty look. In 1997 the Italian designer Roberto Menichetti was brought in as creative director (he had previously worked with Jil Sander and Claude Montana). The new collections for Spring/Summer 1999 were called Burberry Prorsum ('prorsum' is 'forward' in Italian). Many of the pieces made reference to sports, for example, motorcycle clothing. The Spring/Summer 2000 collection featured the first Burberry bikini in the traditional plaid, and in Spring 2001 the first swimwear line was launched. Roberto Menichetti has since left Burberry, and Christopher Bailey, who previously worked with Gucci, succeeded him as designer.

Burton

Burton, the first company to design clothing specifically for snowboarding, was started in 1977 by Jake Carpenter, and has its corporate headquarters in Burlington, Vermont. It produces a wide range of snowboarding footwear, inner and outerwear, accessories and snowboards. High-performance fabrics feature strongly in all Burton products. Lines now include Burton, Red, Gervis and Junkyard. Burton's 'Chill' programme helps underprivileged city teenagers learn how to snowboard.

Cannondale

Cannondale started in a crowded loft above a pickle factory when it introduced the bicycle industry's first bicycle trailer in 1971. The Connecticut-based company soon added clothes, accessories and a bicycle to its range of products. It regularly sponsors athletes, and in 1999 the Saeco/Cannondale Team had five stage-wins in the Tour de France. Innovations in clothing include the Oslo Fleece pullover and Thermal Jacket, both of which use Polartec fleece fabric from Malden Mills.

Chanel

Born in Saumur, France in 1883, Gabrielle 'Coco' Chanel originated the de luxe sportswear aesthetic. She moved to Paris in 1909 and began making hats for friends, then in 1912 established 'Chanel Modes' on the rue Cambon in Paris, with boutiques in Deauville and Biarritz. She designed her first swimsuit in 1914, and she herself pioneered the suntan. In the early 1920s she made trousers for women fashionable, and her relaxed clothing revealed a distinct sports influence. 'Mademoiselle', as she was known to her colleagues, put the emphasis on fabric in her collections. Softness, fluidity and drape were all-important, suggesting informality and effortless, elegant dressing. She was the first to utilize jersey for women's fashion. Chanel retired in 1939 and went to live in Switzerland, but in 1954 reopened the rue Cambon House of Chanel. She continued to influence the fashion world with her modern, classic clothing. She died in Paris in 1971.

Since 1983 Karl Lagerfeld has been head designer, and collections continue to show strong sports influences.

Converse

Converse, based in the USA, manufactures athletic footwear and clothes for basketball. The company was founded as the Converse Rubber Shoe Company in 1908, and since then has made functional and stylish footwear for court and street. In 1915 it launched the first basketball boot, and in 1920 professional basketball player Chuck Taylor endorsed this product (and restyled it slightly). It became known as the All Star. Chuck Taylor joined Converse in Chicago as part of its sales team, and promoted the footwear throughout the USA. In 1940 he recruited an Olympic basketball player, Grady Lewis, and during the 1960s they made Converse a household name. Other players who have endorsed this product include Julius Erving and Dennis Rodman. The Converse All Star model has become a Converse trademark and is still popular. The company has also worked with top skateboarders to create tough and stylish new skateboard footwear.

C. P. Company

The Italian company, C. P. Company, founded in 1975, has made an impact on menswear, especially in the area of fabric innovation and street wear. Since 1994 C. P. Company have also produced womenswear high-performance clothing. Designer Moreno Ferrari, born in La Spezia near Genoa, shows his sophisticated active clothes in collections influenced by military uniforms and workwear. He likes to use technical textiles, including some researched for and borrowed from motorcycle wear. Sportswear Company, based in Milan, owns, produces and distributes the C. P. Company label. It invests in technology, and research into exclusive fabrics and the making of clothes.

Dainese

In 1972 Lino Dainese set up a company to make motorcycle wear. This was partly because of his own interest in the sport and also from a realization that, despite Italy's reputation for high-quality leather, all Italy's motorcycle clothing was imported. The first product was a pair of trousers designed for motocross. In the 1970s, the company became involved in sponsorship and collaboration with motorcyclist Barry Sheene, with whom it developed new ideas for protective clothing, launching the first back-protector in 1983. It is now applying its knowledge of designing protective clothing to other sports, including in-line skating and snowboarding.

Derby, University of

The MA in Performance Sportswear Design, the first Masters programme to specialize in sportswear, started at the University of Derby, UK, in 1996. Jane McCann, the programme leader, trained in Fashion Design at Belfast College of Art, then at the Royal

179
BIOGRAPHIES

College of Art, London. She worked for Relations Textiles, a Paris-based fashion-prediction studio, and made promotional garments for the International Wool Secretariat, Courtaulds, ICI, DuPont (working on the fibre Tactel) and prototype garments for ISPO and Première Vision. McCann has worked as a design consultant for Event Sportswear, Ultimate Equipment, Speedo Europe, Nevica Contracts and the team uniform of Visa International, a major sponsor of the Winter Olympics at Lillehammer, Norway. Her interest in sustainability in design led to the founding of the label Any Mountain. Graduates of the MA are employed by Berghaus, Karrimor, Rab, Puma, Philips Design, Fila UK, and there are many professional links with such companies as DuPont and Patagonia. Each student works with the very latest textiles, including synthetics and techno-naturals, to make clothes and accessories, including footwear, for climbing, racket, snow and scooter sports, etc.

Diesel
The Italian company Diesel was founded by Renzo Rosso in 1979 and soon became known for its utilitarian clothing. The 55 DSL clothes range is often made from technical fabrics, and DieselStyleLab, a more experimental line, was launched in 1998. The company uses the latest developments in technical textiles (most originally intended for sports) and advanced finishing treatments, and its fabrics are often made especially by textile mills. These are used with natural and traditional fabrics for innovative street wear that often has an industrial reference. Its womenswear, menswear and accessories are inventive not only in the choice of cloth but also in the futuristic cut and styling.

Christian Dior
Christian Dior, born in 1905 in Granville, France, worked as a dress designer with Robert Piguet, and then in 1941 for Lucien Lelong where he made his mark. The House of Dior was founded in Paris with funding from Marcel Boussac, who was involved in the cotton business. Christian Dior is perhaps most famous for his first collection, launched in 1947 – its New Look emphasized the female shape – narrow waist, rounded hips and very full three-quarter-length 'A'-line skirts, revolutionizing fashion and making newspaper headlines, especially after the austerity of wartime when textiles and clothing were severely rationed. Yves Saint Laurent started working for Dior in 1953, and took over as artistic director when Dior died in 1957. In 1960, when Yves Saint Laurent went to serve in the Algerian war, Marc Bohan became head designer, a position that John Galliano now holds.

DuPont
The multinational company was founded as E.I. du Pont de Nemours and Co. in 1802 in Wilmington, USA. It has been researching synthetics since the late 1930s, and is known for such high-performance textiles as polyamide, which often have sports applications. In the 1970s it developed a PTFE (polytetrafluoroethylene) resin that contained tiny glass beads and is used as a coating on many fabrics to give a durable finish to withstand extreme weather conditions. Its research in the mid 1980s led to Tactel (a microfibre brand name), which adapted polyamide for sportswear textiles. It has invented many revolutionary fibres including Lycra, Kevlar, Teflon, Dacron, Supplex, CoolMax, Thermastat, Thermolite Active, Cordura, and the nonwovens Tyvek and its Neotis label (formerly Inova). Teflon is used as a coating on many fabrics to make them stain-resistant and waterproof. Lycra, developed in 1959, became very popular in the 1980s, affecting the techniques and look of tailoring. From January 2001 DuPont's fibres Lycra, Tactel, Cordura, Dacron and CoolMax have been known as Apparel and Textiles Sciences in order to focus on this particular market.

ElekSen
Founded in 1998 as ElectroTextiles by Chris Chapman and David Sandbach, this UK company is interested in interactive materials, and manufactures fabrics that respond to touch and other stimuli. It develops and licenses the ElekSen technology, and works with other companies to create products that are flexible, soft and highly functional. ElekSen Limited employs the latest technologies, such as micro-electronics and in-built sensors. Its market sectors include sports and leisure wear, healthcare and mobile communications, and among its products are a soft keyboard, soft remote controls, conference telephone and wrist-phone. ElekSen products were included in the exhibition 'Workspheres' at the Museum of Modern Art, New York, February 2001.

John Galliano
John Galliano, born in Gibraltar in 1961, moved to London with his family when he was six. He studied fashion at London's Central Saint Martins, and did placements with such designers as Stephen Marks (French Connection) and Tommy Nutter (the late Savile Row tailor). John Galliano's graduation show in 1984 'Les Incroyables' was given the windows of Browns in London as a showcase, and this influential fashion store bought his entire collection. While at college, he experimented with bias-cutting, and he still often uses this for romantic clothing. He was appointed head designer for Givenchy in 1995, and then for Dior in 1996.

Jean Paul Gaultier
Fashion designer, Jean Paul Gaultier, born in 1951 in Arcueil, France, worked for Pierre Cardin, Jacques Esterel and Jean Patou before showing his first collection in 1977. He takes his inspiration from a variety of sources, successfully mixing cultures and streetstyles, and his past collections have fused bohemia with sport. He became internationally known for his underwear as outerwear when Madonna wore his corset with the exaggerated conical breasts as part of her 'Blond Ambition' tour in 1990. Past collections have included skirts for men (he frequently challenges ideas of gender), and clothes with competitive swimwear references, such as racing-style 'T-backs'. He now has his own couture label.

Helly Hansen
In 1875 in Norway, Helly Juell Hansen, tired of being wet and cold at sea, asked his wife to make durable, waterproof clothes. The early ones were made of coarse linen waterproofed with linseed oil, and, although they were produced for Hansen's own use, they were also sold to others. Hansen formed a company in 1877, exhibiting his clothes the following year at the Paris Expo, where he was awarded a Diploma for Excellence. Today the company designs and produces hardwearing, breathable, waterproof clothing for workwear, outdoor wear, winter sports and watersports. This includes clothing for skiing, snowboarding, mountaineering and sailing and, more recently, aerobics. Helly Hansen clothing has been used in the Whitbread Round the World races at sea, the Olympics and for climbing the world's highest mountains.

Holland & Holland
This London house, founded in 1835 has a look that evokes an English heritage and the country sports of hunting, shooting and fishing. The French designer, José Levy worked with the company as a designer in the late 1990s. He used cashmere jerseys and silks in combination with heavier fabrics, such as coated cottons and linens, and his silhouettes were functional and intended for outdoor wear and urban fashion, combining their very traditional image with style. A team of designers now works on the collections. Holland & Holland have moved away from 'fashion' collections to concentrate on its original and classic sports clothes – separates for country sports reinvented with a contemporary urban feel – both practical and good-looking.

Joelynian
Joelynian is a London-based fashion design duo – Joely Davis was born in the USA in 1971, and Nian Brindle was born in the UK in 1969. Both worked for Liza Bruce before setting up their own label in 1996. Joely Davis studied at the University of Georgia, USA, and has worked as a stylist in Japan. She then studied at Central Saint Martins, London, and at the University of Westminster. Nian Brindle studied at the University of Manchester. Joelynian uses high-performance textiles with streamlined silhouettes and aerodynamic cutting. The Spring/Summer 1999 collection launched the 'Trikini' as three-piece swimwear made of a polyamide stretch textile with a high percentage of Lycra. Recent collections have included designer swimwear in the latest technical textiles and a swimwear collection for the UK chainstore BhS in 1999. This collaboration included the 'Trikini' concept and gave it mass-market appeal. Since April 2000 Joelynian has specialized in designer swimwear.

Calvin Klein

Born in 1942 in New York, Calvin Klein graduated from the Fashion Institute of Technology, New York, in 1962. He founded his business at the end of the 1960s, and during the mid-1970s became known for his clean lines and relaxed tailoring. He makes reference to American sports clothes, but also acknowledges fashion influences from the Japanese avant-garde and ideas from Europe. In the 1970s he produced his famous designer jeans, and his range now includes underwear. His empire includes his CK line for both men and women.

Michiko Koshino

Michiko Koshino is one of three sisters (Junko, Hiroko and Michiko), born in Osaka, Japan, all now fashion designers. Michiko Koshino first worked in her mother's boutique, then came to London in 1973 and worked for Stirling Cooper, setting up her own company in 1975. She is based in London and has shown at London Fashion Week since it began in the early 1980s. She is known for her inventive cutting techniques for functional, experimental but wearable clothing. She uses a range of textiles from naturals to the highly technical, and past collections have included reflectives, neoprenes and inflatable garments (which began as an economy travelling idea and became very fashionable in the 1990s). Michiko Koshino has three fashion collections – the mainline collection, the 100s line (a limited edition with a military influence for urban clothing) and Yen Jeans (a denim line).

Kuraray

The Japanese textile manufacturer Kuraray Co. Ltd was established in 1926 to produce viscose rayon. Its product range was soon extended to include research and development in polymers, synthetics and chemical engineering. Today the company produces resins, chemicals, nonwovens, synthetic leather, laser discs and medical products. Innovative highly engineered fibres and fabrics remain central, including Kuralon (a polyvinyl alcohol fibre) and Clarino (synthetic leather). In 1965 a European office was established in Germany, initially in Hamburg but now based in Düsseldorf.

René Lacoste

René Lacoste, French tennis star (born in Paris in 1904), won the Davis Cup against the USA in 1927. In 1933, René Lacoste and André Gillier (owner and president of a large French knitwear manufacturer) set up a company to make tennis and golf shirts. The first Lacoste shirt was made from a light knitted cotton piqué fabric and was a welcome alternative to the starched woven shirts worn at the time. The embroidered 'alligator' logo was used from the start. The company went from strength to strength, with exports to Italy and the USA, and launched a children's collection in 1959, shorts and striped Lacoste shirts in 1960, and tracksuits in 1966. In 1963 Lacoste

invented the first steel tennis racket, and in the same year his son Bernard Lacoste became chairman of the company. In 1985 Lacoste tennis shoes were launched, followed by boat shoes in 1986 and walking shoes in 1988. Lacoste now supplies clothing for a wide range of sports, and is a major international brand. René Lacoste died in 1996. The designer Christopher Lemaire was appointed to the company in 2000, taking over from Gilles Rosier. He is Creative Director of Lacoste clothing lines for Devanlay S. A., and oversees the styling of other Lacoste brands for La Chemise Lacoste. His first Lacoste clothing collection was launched for Spring/Summer 2002.

Ralph Lauren

Ralph Lauren, born in New York in 1939, epitomizes the American sporty look in his fashion collections. He is, however, also inspired by the traditional British look. His collections frequently make references to sports in choice of fabric, cut, style, detail and finish – even the photographic locations. He built his empire in the 1960s on ties, and then became famous for his shirts embroidered with the polo player. In 1968 a menswear collection was formed first with the label Polo Ralph Lauren, and then, in the early 1970s, womenswear. There are now many different lines, including Polo Sport Ralph Lauren established in 1987 that offers fashionable clothing for explorers, travellers, and sports people. The RLX label for active wear uses performance textiles, such as high-stretch and reflectives.

Julien Macdonald

Fashion knitwear designer, Julien Macdonald was born in 1972 in Merthyr Tydfil, Wales. Even before graduating from the Royal College of Art in London in 1996 his knitwear had been used in the collections of Alexander McQueen, Antonio Berardi and Koji Tatsuno. His degree show caught the attention of Karl Lagerfeld, and he subsequently worked as a knitwear designer for Chanel in 1996. His own first collection was in 1997. Julien Macdonald concentrates mainly on fine-gauge knitwear and produces elegant, modern fashion. He has worked with a wide range of textiles including fluorescent yarns and the antibacterial fibre, Amicor by Acordis, generally used in sports clothes, underwear and shoes. Julien Macdonald has been head designer at Givenchy since 2001.

Malden Mills

Malden Mills, founded in the 1906 by Henry Feuerstein, is based in Lawrence, Massachusetts. The company is best known for its collaboration with the sports clothing company Patagonia in developing a recycled fleece made from waste plastic bottles. The company now produces Polarfleece and Polartec, high-performance synthetic variations that provide moisture-management and thermal insulation. The company has mills in the USA and Germany, and holds more than thirty trademarks and twenty patents worldwide.

Mandarina Duck

In 1968 the two founders, Paola Trento and Piero Mannato set up the first manufacturing unit called Plastimoda to create heat-set products (mainly plastic and rubber). Mandarina Duck was established in 1977 and takes its name from the bird with water-repellent plumage. Colour and properties of materials receive great attention from this Italian-based company, and it quickly became famous for its luggage and accessories. Mandarina Duck prefers materials that combine naturals with the latest developments in technological textiles. In 1997 the Mandarina Duck 'Apparel Project' was launched, which includes high-tech clothing and bags. In the first collection, the patented paper-like fabric called Fiberduck, made from a material originally used in the automobile industry, was introduced. A less dense version, Light Fiberduck filters light to give a luminous effect. Mandarina Duck works with international artists and designers.

MaxMara

The MaxMara company, founded in 1951 by Achille Maramotti, is now run by his son Luigi Maramotti as Chairman. The company factory is in Reggio Emilia, Italy, and the MaxMara textile mills research and manufacture new textiles, involved in both fabrics and garments. The MaxMara group can follow through from fabric to finish. It now has many collections and brands, including MaxMara (the main label), Sportmax, Sportmax Code, Marella, I Blues, Marina Rinaldi, Marina Sport, Weekend by MaxMara and 'S MaxMara. Sportmax was established in the late 1960s and features clothing with a definite sports influence, as does Sportmax Code (launched in 1999). The 'S' in 'S MaxMara stands for space, simplicity, style and synthesis, and its clothes offer minimalist designs, often using technical materials. Different designers have worked for MaxMara, including Dolce & Gabbana and Karl Lagerfeld.

Mizuno

The Japanese Mizuno Corporation, founded in 1906, established an American operation, Mizuno USA Inc., in 1982 to manufacture and distribute golf, baseball, softball, running, track and field, and volleyball equipment, clothes and footwear for an international market. The company has been responsible for a number of innovations in sports apparel and shoes, such as the Wave technology designed for more ergonomic footwear. In 2001 Mizuno became an official sponsor of USA Volleyball, making it the official footwear and apparel supplier for the US men's and women's Olympic teams.

Musto

Keith Musto and Edward Hyde founded the partnership Musto and Hyde Sails in 1965 in the UK, and this became a limited company in 1971. Musto and Hyde developed their 3-layer Clothing System for sailors in 1979, and the following year decided to concentrate on clothing. Since the mid-1980s Musto clothing has featured in all the world's major sailing events including the America's Cup and the Whitbread Round the World Race. The company's range includes Musto HPX Ocean and HPX Offshore foul-weather gear, and Musto Stretch HPX Offshore (with 30 per cent elasticity) all of which use Gore-Tex waterproof, breathable technology.

Nike

The Nike company, called after the Greek personification of victory, was founded by Bill Bowerman and Phil Knight. Bowerman, a track coach at the University of Oregon, USA, made the first lightweight soles for sports shoes from rubber and leather which he glued together using a waffle iron. In 1964 he formed a partnership with Phil Knight, one of his former athletes, to manufacture and promote these shoes with the unusual soles. In 1967 he initiated development of the Marathon, a lightweight nylon running shoe. The Nike company was founded in 1972 and its Swoosh logo is instantly recognizable worldwide. Nike is now one of the largest sports gear manufacturers, making footwear ranging from performance sports shoes (running, turf-training, basketball) to casual wear (boots, shoes and sandals for hiking and general streetwear), and also clothes. Nike launched its first range of snowboard wear in 1999 and also has a clothing line called ACG (All Conditions Gear) which uses advanced performance textiles (often developed by Nike) with simple styling for sports-inspired garments.

The North Face

The North Face was founded in 1966 by two hiking enthusiasts who opened a small retail shop in San Francisco. The company began designing and producing its own range of clothing, and was soon named after the most difficult mountain face for climbers in the northern hemisphere – the North Face of Everest. With headquarters now in San Leandro, California, it produces technically advanced clothes and footwear for climbers, mountaineers, extreme skiers and explorers. Expedition System, HydroSeal, Steep Tech, Tekware, Vaporator, Hydrenaline, Hydrenalite, Micronamics, UltraWick and X-2 and The North Face logo are its registered trademarks.

Nylstar

Nylstar was formed in 1994 when the French company Rhône-Poulenc (now Rhodia) and the Italian company, Snia Fibre (now Snia SpA) merged. Both have been involved in synthetic textiles since the start of the twentieth century, and they amalgamated to use their respective expertise in polyamide polymers and textile fibres. Nylstar has expanded to become one of the biggest European manufacturers of synthetic yarn, manufacturing performance textiles for extreme sports and more general purposes. Its registered trademark Elité uses modified polyester for sophisticated yarns for many applications. The Meryl (registered trademark) range of speciality yarns uses ultra-fine polyamide

fibres for superior performance for swimming, sailing and athletics. Meryl was used in the BT Global Challenge race. For this around-the-world race, undergarments in knitted Meryl are made by Musto, Usa Pro, Fit Kit (UK), Medico, Bruno Bunani (Germany) and Pompea (Italy).

O'Neill

The O'Neill story began when surfer Jack O'Neill opened a surf shop in California in the 1950s. Attempting to keep warm while surfing, he experimented with different materials, and it was his discovery of neoprene as an appropriate material for wetsuits that led to his big breakthrough. He sold his first neoprene wetsuit in 1952 and the company has continued to refine the wetsuit designs for diving, water-skiing, wakeboarding and triathlon events ever since. The company has also expanded its range to include waterproof breathable outerwear and fleeces for snow sports, leisure wear and accessories.

Lucy Orta

Lucy Orta, born near Birmingham in 1966, has been based in Paris since 1991. She originally trained in fashion and textiles, and now makes art that often blurs the distinction between clothing and architecture while also commenting on contemporary social and political issues. She frequently uses the latest high-tech fabrics originally developed for extreme sports. Her works include *Refuge Wear* (1992–94), multifunctional, transformable clothing/sleeping bags/tents; *Survival Kits* (1993), garments and accessories with detachable kits that contained life jackets, water reserves and food; *Modular Architecture* (1996), sculptural forms between clothing and architecture; *Collective Wear* or *Nexus Architecture* (1997), prototype garments/shelters that can accommodate up to sixteen people; and *Urban Life Guards* (2000) which was specially commissioned by Expofil, Paris. Lucy Orta exhibited at the 1995 Venice Biennale and at the second Johannesburg Biennale in October 1997. Since 1993, she has also staged public performances and installations.

Outlast Technologies, Inc.

Co-founded by Ed Payne and Bernard Perry in 1990 as Gateway Technologies, Inc., it became Outlast Technologies, Inc., in 1995 in order to have the same name as its successful branded product, the phase-change material Outlast. It is based in Boulder, Colorado, USA, and first developed this product for NASA in the late 1980s. Neither of the founders trained in science and technology but are entrepreneurs who funded their own idea for the first few years before attracting outside investment in 1993. This phase-change material uses paraffin wax inside a shell that can be incorporated into an actual textile as a fibre, fabric or a foam. Various outer surfaces or linings can be used with Outlast for different visual and tactile effects as well as for high-performance properties.

Patagonia

The company, based in California, started up in 1957 when Yvon Chouinard decided to make his own climbing gear. Today it is most associated with environmental issues, to which it takes a holistic approach that affects every aspect of the business, from the production of raw materials to the funding of local environment action groups. Best known for its fleece using recycled plastic bottles, Patagonia has also developed a number of high-performance fabrics based on ethnic garments. The clothing range includes high-performance and leisure inner and outerwear for adults and children.

Fred Perry

Tennis star Fred Perry is one of many players to set up their own sports clothing label. In 1934 Perry was the first Englishman to win the men's singles at Wimbledon, winning again in 1935 and 1936. Widely regarded as the best dressed player of his day, Perry developed the business by launching Fred Perry sports shirts. His laurel-wreath symbol was adopted by the All England Club for use on Wimbledon sportswear, but the classic Fred Perry look has always appealed beyond tennis itself, and in the 1960s was a favourite with the British Mods. More recently it has come back into fashion as part of London's East End look, appearing in such magazines as *i-D*. Managing Director Jon Kalupa says that the company strives for a 'sports-authentic' look. The clothing range includes tennis and polo whites, knits, jackets and outerwear.

Philips Design

Based in The Netherlands, the research laboratories of Philips Design investigate and invent the latest in wearable electronics. In 1997 they started looking at consumer applications and undertook the Wearable Electronics project in Redhill, UK. The team uses fashion designers, industrial design engineers, software engineers, as well as trend analysts and socio-cultural researchers. They devise garments and accessories with integrated communication, information and entertainment systems, and use Body Area Network technology (originally known as Personal Area Network) that was pioneered by MIT. Philips Design use very sophisticated textiles and combine these with conductive yarn, concealed wiring and various devices for products claimed to enhance our present and future lifestyles. Some have direct relevance to sporting activities as they monitor heart and pulse rates and body temperature. Philips Design collaborated with Levi's to create the Industrial Clothing Division in 2000, whose aim is to integrate clothing and technology.

Prada

This company was formed in 1913 by Mario Prada, and became famous for its traditional leather goods. Miuccia Prada, born in Milan in 1950, and granddaughter of Mario Prada, joined the company in the late 1970s and transformed it; she launched the first ready-to-wear collection in 1985, and turned matt, black nylon into the famous and coveted Prada bag. The range offered by Prada includes womenswear and menswear, footwear and other accessories; there is also a diffusion line called Miu Miu. In 1999 Prada Sport was launched as a luxurious sports line combining the aesthetics of sports and glamour. Miuccia Prada uses synthetics and advanced finishing treatments for a contemporary, minimalist look, using many fabrics originally intended for skiing, snowboarding and watersports. She dressed the team for the Prada Challenger 2000 in the America's Cup. The first Prada Sport boutique was opened in the summer of 2000 on the fifth floor in Harrods store, London.

Quiksilver
Quiksilver – The Boardriding Company specializes in surf and beachwear and was founded in Torquay, Australia, 1969 by two surfers, Alan Green and John Law. In 1976, world champion Jeff Hakman and Bob McKnight founded Quiksilver USA, and then Quiksilver Europe was formed in 1984. It organizes and sponsors many surf and snow competitions and events, including the Quiksilver Grommet Tour, 2001. It works closely with boardsport athletes. Its clothing for surfers combines function and fashion, and it now also caters for the snow- and skateboard markets. Quiksilver uses advanced fabrics, and styling is kept simple. Its clothes, both for specific sports and streetstyle, have a cult following. In 1991 it launched Roxy for female boardriders, and it also has a very successful womenswear line for sports and swimming; in 1999 this became Roxy Life in Europe. In 2000 the Teenie line was aimed at girls (6–14), and was directly inspired by the Roxy label, whereas Alex Goes is aimed at the slightly older (25–40) active, sporty woman. This contemporary label by Lissa Zwahlen includes functional, fashionable clothing with luggage and other accessories, and is aimed at the US market.

Reebok
In the 1890s Joseph William Foster made the first known running shoes with spikes. He went on to make shoes by hand for top athletes, and formed J. W. Foster and Sons. Almost half a century later, in 1958, two of the founder's grandsons started a sister company called Reebok after the African gazelle. The company's big breakthrough came in 1982, when Reebok designed the first sports shoe especially for women for the new fitness craze – aerobics. The Reebok International group of brands includes Reebok, Rockport and Weebok for children, and Ralph Lauren Footwear.

Reflec Technology
Reflec Technology is a division of Reflec plc. and is based in Winsford, Cheshire, UK. Founded in 1993, it started trading 1995/96. This division works with reflective technology, manufacturing products for sports and safety wear. The technology was originally developed for Reflec's textile printing inks, used by Nike, adidas, Polo Ralph Lauren and other big names

in sports and fashion. Available as textile inks or as tape fabrics/films, the advanced technology reflects light back to its original source. A graphic transfer system is used for reflective tape on footwear – a highly reflective carrier paper is printed with a hot-melt adhesive which transfers the reflective property to fabric or product to give logos and emblems with high visibility. There is also a colour-print transfer system which uses special inks with reflectors coated with aluminium. Adhesives are applied to transfer paper, and are then printed and heat-treated on to sports and urban clothing. Reflec Technology also has its own clothing range. It has an international distribution with offices in the USA and Hong Kong.

Rhovyl
In 1948 the French Rhône-Poulenc group formed Rhovyl to make a PVC-based chlorofibre. Alain Regard bought Rhovyl in 1992, and it is now a world leader in chlorofibre manufacturing. This fibre, known for its performance properties, has been used in the Tour de France on several occasions. Between 1978 and 1988 Rhovyl concentrated on technology, and from 1988 to 1998 on ecology. The synthetic fibre, Rhovyl is versatile, and there are many different types. It is very suitable for sports clothes as the fibre manages moisture well, and its antibacterial properties ensure that the textile smells fresh even after strenuous activity.

Effi Samara
Fashion designer, Effi Samara, was born in 1970 in Athens, and the family moved to England in 1984. She is particularly interested in the equestrian look, and her work is often a cross between sports-inspired and formal clothing. She has explored a wide range of materials, including polyethylene and stretch textiles.

Samsonite
The Samsonite Corporation was founded in Denver, USA, in 1910 by Jesse Shwayder, and became known for its traditional and dependable luggage. The Samsonite 'Travel wear' collection is a new venture. Within this the Samsonite Blacklabel, launched in 1997, was developed by Samsonite and the Florence-based Lineapiù Group who manufacture the fibres and fabrics. Neil Barrett (formerly of Prada and Gucci menswear) designed some of the first collections. He likes gadgetry, and his designs featured temperature-control systems and secret compartments in jackets containing such things as a compass. Gigi Vezzola (previously with Dolce & Gabbana) now designs for the Samsonite range.

Schoeller
Established in Switzerland in 1968, Schoeller Textil AG is famous for its technological fabrics, and has won several awards, including the Design Prize in Switzerland (in 1997 for fire-fighters' clothing). In the mid-1980s the company stated as its main aim 'the development and production of special fabrics for sport,

leisure-time and occupational safety'. In the 1990s it concentrated on multifunctional fabrics with diverse applications, developing adaptable textiles by exploring new flexible fabric finishes. Its textiles frequently offer high-performance properties and are used widely in sports – they include advanced woven fabrics, stretch textiles and technically finished cloth with metallic, reflective and pearlescent effects. The textiles, highly functional as well as beautiful, have been used by Nike, adidas and Puma as well as by such fashion designers as Donna Karan, Thierry Mugler, Prada and Versace.

Spartan
Spartan Limited was established in 1958 and is based in the UK. It designs and manufactures wetsuits, controlling the operation from beginning to end. This company has used a special type of neoprene from Yamamoto (who have manufactured neoprene for over forty years) called 3-DIS (3-Dimensional Intelligent Skin) that ensures comfort and high performance. Seams are chemically bonded to ensure that they are waterproof. In 1991, Spartan developed its two-layer system – an undersuit and a thinner outer suit. The layering concept is one that is widely used in performance sportswear, and in a wetsuit it allows for increased thermal insulation as well as flexibility. Spartan produce wetsuits for both men and women, and a range of accessories, including hoods and gloves.

Speedo
Speedo was established in Sydney at the MacRae Knitting Mills, which originally manufactured underwear. In 1928 the company produced its first swimsuit, the Racerback; it was made from silk at a time when other companies still used wool. The Racerback was immediately adopted by world champion swimmer Arnie Borg, and his success helped to establish Speedo as one of the world's leading swimwear brands. In 1957 the company began to use nylon, and mixed nylon with Lycra in the 1970s. Speedo's ergonomic Fastskin swimsuit, based on sharkskin, dominated the swimming events at the 2000 Olympic Games.

Stone Island
Stone Island, like C. P. Company, is owned, produced and distributed by Sportswear Company, based in Milan. This label began in 1981 with the aim of making innovative sports clothes. The main designer, Paul Harvey (a graduate of Central Saint Martins, London), favours highly technical textiles, often those developed for other industries. Materials such as glass, ceramic, metal and carbon fibre have all been used, as well as nonwovens and the new smart fabrics, for fashionable urban streetwear that is very influenced by sports. Stone Island is interested in fabric finishes, and experiments with new printing techniques. It was also the first company to dye Kevlar (DuPont) by giving it a polyurethane coating. Other techniques

include spattering on microfibre fabric using a Japanese 'vacuum chamber' and the more traditional bleach printing. Stone Island's men's urban fashion makes use of new materials and relaxed, comfortable cutting, fuller shapes and ergonomic styling.

Sam de Terán

Sam de Terán is a fashion sports clothes designer, born in Spain and now London-based, who makes swimwear and clothes for diving, exercising, skiing and tennis. Her ski wear is worn by such celebrities as 'Bond' girl Sophie Marceau. Her first collection, in 1993, showed swimwear with bi-stretch properties that allowed the garment to follow the body contours. Past collections have shown functional, streamlined garments and accessories that are elegant and suitable for the city streets. She uses the latest textiles, including those by the Swiss textile companies Schoeller and Jakob Schlaepfer. Her clothes are both good-looking and tough.

3M

3M was founded in 1902 at the Lake Superior town of Two Harbors, Minnesota, when five businessmen agreed to mine a mineral deposit for grinding-wheel abrasives. But the deposits proved to be of little value, and the new Minnesota Mining and Manufacturing Company moved to nearby Duluth to focus on sandpaper products. In the early 1920s the company produced the first waterproof sandpaper, which eased the health problem of dust created by sanding. This company produces everything from Scotch tape and Post-it notes to reflective tapes and printing inks. Their retro-reflective Scotchlite fabric, tapes, printing inks and sewing thread provide protection by making wearers visible under artificial light. This technology is used in every aspect of sports clothing and equipment from shoes to outerwear. The company also produces Thinsulate, a lightweight non-woven insulation fabric for clothes, and Hydroweave, a layered and quilted fabric that keeps the wearer cool for long periods.

Toray

Toray Industries, Inc., is based in Shiga, Japan, and was founded in 1926 as Toyo Rayon Co., Ltd, changing its name in 1970. It produces fibres, textiles, plastics, chemicals and advanced composite materials. It produces textiles based on the three important synthetics: nylon, polyester and acrylic. Its high-performance synthetics have many uses, including general and extreme sports clothes.

Dries Van Noten

The Belgian fashion designer, Dries Van Noten, born in Antwerp in 1958, graduated from the Antwerp Academy in 1981, famous for its avant-garde fashion designers. He started in 1985 first selling his collection from a small shop in Antwerp, and then showing menswear with the Antwerp Six. He soon branched out with his own label. In 1991, he had his first catwalk show in Paris for menswear and in 1993 for womenswear. In 1996, he added children's wear. The Far East and the Middle East are both strong influences on his choice of textiles and colour.

Vexed Generation

Vexed Generation Clothing Limited was established by Adam Thorpe and Joe Hunter in 1994. Adam Thorpe, had worked as a design consultant for sports clothes. Joe Hunter studied Graphic Design and had created a recycled fashion collection. Their clothing makes reference to the urban environment, and their collections aim to be of social and environmental significance, demonstrating an awareness of the need for protection against urban pollution and surveillance. They use the latest textiles which are often industrial and technical and which were originally designed for space programmes or for the military. The styling may be functional, and draws inspiration from extreme sports and even survival wear. Their work has been included in several exhibitions, including the British Council exhibitions 'Lost and Found' (1999) and 'Fabric of Fashion' (2000).

Junya Watanabe

Born in Japan in 1961, Junya Watanabe studied at the famous Bunka Fashion Institute in Tokyo before working for Rei Kawakubo of Comme des Garçons, as her protégé, since 1984. He worked on the Comme des Garçons Tricot line, where he became the main designer in 1987. In 1992 Junya Watanabe launched his own label, Junya Watanabe for Comme des Garçons. In 1993 he was given the Mainichi award for young designers and also showed in Paris. His collections often use the very latest technical fabrics including bonded materials and padded fabrics, while his garment cut has shown 'robotic' styles with jointed seams, allowing maximum movement and a close fit.

W. L. Gore and Associates

W. L. Gore and Associates was set up by Bill and Vieve Gore in the USA in 1958 with the intention of exploring the market for fluorocarbon polymers, and polytetrafluoroethylene (PTFE) in particular. The company is best known for its waterproof breathable fabric, Gore-Tex, which was first marketed in 1976 under the slogan 'guaranteed to keep you dry'. Since then it has continued to refine the technology, keeping a watchful eye on licensee production standards. It has also added a Windstopper fabric to its range of products, which provides insulation against wind while remaining breathable and a pure PTFE fabric.

The Woolmark Company

The Woolmark Company operates in 65 countries; its main offices are in the UK, Italy and Australia. Its trademarks include the Woolmark (launched in 1964), Woolmark Blend and Wool Blend. Recently it has expanded its product range and developed Sportwool and Sportwool PRO, high-tech fabrics for active wear and sports. Research into Sportwool began in the early 1990s in collaboration with the Commonwealth Scientific and Industrial Research Organization (CSIRO). This is a blend of Australian merino wool and polyester, and offers high-performance properties such as moisture-control, thermal insulation and breathability. Sportwool has been used for cycling, and with Cloverbrook, a UK-based company, a fabric for footballers has been produced. The Woolmark Company has also collaborated with the US company Cargill Dow to research into merino wool combined with resins from renewable sources. The resulting fabrics are absorbent and capable of wicking perspiration quickly away from the skin; they are also crease-resistant and durable. Jackets for the New Zealand team in the America's Cup 2000 used New Zealand merino wool for Loro Piana's 'Storm System' fabric, which gives high protection in extreme weather conditions.

DIRECTORY OF ADDRESSES

Acordis (UK) Limited, (Amicor)
Westcroft, Saint Street
Bradford BD7 4AD, UK
Acordis (UK) Limited, (Viloft)
PO Box 5, Spondon
Derby DE21 7BP, UK
Acordis Acrylic Fibres
Faserwerk Kelheim
Regensburger Strasse 109
93309 Kelheim / Donau, Germany
www.amicor.co.uk
www.acordis.com

adidas (Germany)
Adi-Dassler-Strasse 2
91074 Herzogenaurach, Germany
adidas International
541 N.E. 20th Suite 207
Portland, OR 97232, USA
adidas (USA)
PO Box 4015,
Beaverton, OR 97076, USA
adidas (Italy)
Manifattura Colombo M&C SpA
via Olimpia 3
20052 Monza, Italy
adidas (UK) Limited
The adidas Centre
PO Box 39, Pepper Road
Hazel Grove, Stockport SK7 5SD, UK
adidas (Ireland) Limited
Elm House
Unit 4 Leopardstown Business Park
Sandyford Industrial Estate
Dublin, Ireland
www.adidas.com
www.adidas.co.jp

Maria Blaisse, Flexible Design
Bickersgracht 55
1013LE Amsterdam
The Netherlands

Luigi Botto SpA
via Roma 99, 13825 Vallemosso
Biella, Italy
Luigi Botto UK Ltd
Suffolk House, Whitfield Place
London W1T 5JU, UK

Liza Bruce
9 Pont Street, Belgravia
London SW1X 9EJ, UK
Liza Bruce
80 Thompson Street, SoHo
New York, NY 10012, USA

Burberry
21–23 New Bond Street
London W1S 2RE, UK
Burberry
131 Spring Street
New York, NY 10012, USA

Burberry
9560 Wilshire Boulevard
Beverly Hills, CA 90212, USA
Burberry
55 rue de Rennes
75006 Paris, France
Burberry
Kurfürstendamm 183
10707, Berlin, Germany
Burberry
8 rue Ceard
1204 Geneva, Switzerland
www.burberry.com

Cannondale
Available at:
City Bicycle Works
2419 K Street
Sacramento, CA 95816, USA
Lombardi Sports
1600 Jackson Street
San Francisco, CA 94109, USA
Big Mountain Sports
3808 Big Mountain Road
Whitefish, MT 59937, USA
Larry And Jeff's Bicycles Plus
1400 3rd Avenue, 79th–80th St
New York, NY 10021, USA
Rijwiel Express
Hessenbrug 2
Antwerp 2000, Belgium
Bikepark Covent Garden
11–13 Macklin Street
Covent Garden
London WC2B 5NH, UK
www.cannondale.com

Chanel
31 rue Cambon
75001 Paris, France
Chanel
278–280 Brompton Road
London SW3 2AB, UK
Chanel
15 East 57th Street
New York, NY 10022, USA
www.chanel.com

Converse Inc.
1 Fordham Road
North Reading, MA 01864, USA
Converse UK
Gilbert Pollard Sports
Focal Point – North Longwood Road,
Paddock, Huddersfield HD3 4EY, UK
Converse, Conquest Sports Australia
28–36 Terra Cotta Drive
Blackburn 3130, Victoria, Australia
Converse, Itouchu Japan
1–3 Kutaro machi, 4-chome
Chuo-ku, Osaka 541 8577, Japan
www.converse.com

C. P. Company
Products of C. P. Company and Stone Island
corso Venezia 12
20121 Milan, Italy
Products of C. P. Company and Stone Island
106 Wooster Street, SoHo
New York, NY 10012, USA
Products of C. P. Company and Stone Island
46–48 Beak Street
London W1R 3DA, UK
www.cp.company.com

Dainese Pro Shop
via Tertulliano 3
20145 Milan, Italy
Dainese Pro Shop
via Sammartino 91b
90141 Palermo, Italy
Dainese Corner
Koenigin Elisabeth Strasse 9
14059 Berlin, Germany
Dainese Pro Shop
Bachlechner Strasse 31a
6020 Innsbruck, Austria
P + H Motorcycles Dainese Corner
112–113 Lewes Road
Brighton BN2 3QB, UK
Also available at:
Cheung's Motorcycle
G/F 40–42 Sa Po Road
Kowloon, Hong Kong
Monza Imports
2–24 Vaughan Terrace
3051 North Melbourne
Victoria, Australia
Extreme Motor Sports
41 West Sunrise Highway
Freeport, NY 11520, USA
KC International
15555 Tradesman Drive
San Antonio, TX 78249, USA
www.dainese.it

University of Derby
MA Performance Sportswear Design
School of Design, Jacksons Mill
37 Bridge Street
Derby DE1 3LB, UK

Diesel Headquarters
Staff International SpA,
via del Progresso 10
36025 Noventa Vicentina, Italy
Diesel UK Limited
55 Argyle Street
London WC1H 8EF, UK
Diesel
770 Lexington Avenue, 9th Floor
New York, NY 10021, USA
Diesel
26 rue de la Reynie
75001 Paris, France

Diesel
Kunsgatan 3
11101 Stockholm, Sweden
www.diesel.com
Diesel SpA
via dell'Industria 7
36060 Molvena (Vicenza), Italy
DieselStyleLab
12 Floral Street
London WC2E 9DH, UK
DieselStyleLab
416 West Broadway
New York, NY 10012, USA
www.dieselstylelab.com

Christian Dior
30 avenue Montaigne
75008 Paris, France
Christian Dior
31 Sloane Street
London SW1X 9NR, UK
Christian Dior
21 East 57th Street
New York, NY 10022, USA
Christian Dior
230 North Rodeo Drive
Beverly Hills, CA 90210, USA
www.dior.com

DuPont Tactel
Industrie Street 1
Werk Ostringen
76684 Ostringen, Germany
DuPont
94 Regent Road
Leicester LE1 7DJ, UK
www.dupont.com/tactel

ElekSen Limited
Pinewood Studios, Pinewood Road
Iver Heath, Buckinghamshire SLO 0NH, UK
www.eleksen.com

Jean Paul Gaultier
Galerie Gaultier
30 rue du Faubourg Saint-Antoine
75012 Paris, France
Galerie Gaultier
171–175 Draycott Avenue
London SW3 3AJ, UK
Jean Paul Gaultier
759 Madison Avenue
between 65th and 66th Streets
New York, NY 10021, USA
Jean Paul Gaultier
5–2–28 Jingumae
Shibuya-ku, Tokyo, Japan
www.jpgaultier.fr

Griffin
297 Portobello Road
London W10 5TD, UK
www.griffin-studio.com

Helly Hansen
3326 160th Avenue Southeast
Suite 200
Bellevue, WA 98008, USA
Also available at:
YHA Adventure Shop
152–160 Wardour Street
London W1F 8YA, UK
www.hellyhansen.com

Holland & Holland
31–33 Bruton Street
London W1J 6HH, UK
Holland & Holland
50 East 57th Street
New York, NY 10021, USA
Holland & Holland
9 avenue Victor Hugo
75116 Paris, France

IDEO Europe
Whitebear Yard
144a Clerkenwell Road
London EC1R 5DF, UK
www.ideo.com

Joelynian
Spring House, 10 Spring Place
London NW5 3BH, UK

Donna Karan
819 Madison Avenue
New York, NY 10021, USA
Donna Karan
19 New Bond Street
London W1Y 9HF, UK
Donna Karan Italy Srl.
via Seanato 14–16
20121 Milan, Italy
www.donnakaran.com
DKNY
655 Madison Avenue
New York, NY 10021, USA
DKNY
27 Old Bond Street
London W1X 3AA, UK
DKNY
76–80 King Street
Manchester M2 4NH, UK
www.dkny.com

Calvin Klein
654 Madison Avenue
New York, NY 10021, USA
Calvin Klein
100 Highland Park Village
Dallas, TX 75205, USA
Calvin Klein (cK)
53–55 New Bond Street
London W1Y 9DG, UK
Calvin Klein (cK)
via Roma 354
10121 Turin, Italy

Calvin Klein (cK)
Red Square 3, GUM
Moscow, Russia
Calvin Klein (cK)
Bur Juman Centre, Dubai
United Arab Emirates
Calvin Klein
Schloss-Aoyama 4-21-26
Minami-Aoyama, Minato-ku
Tokyo 107, Japan

Michiko Koshino
59 Broadwick Street
London W1F 9QQ, UK
www.michikokoshino.co.uk
www.michikokoshino.co.jp

Lacoste
rue du Faubourg Saint-Antoine
Paris 75012, France
Lacoste
20 Brompton Road
London SW1X 7QN, UK
www.lacoste.fr

Ralph Lauren
867 Madison Avenue
New York, NY 10022, USA
Ralph Lauren
1 Magnificent Mile
750 North Michigan Avenue
Chicago, IL 60611, USA
Ralph Lauren
143 New Bond Street
London W1S 2TP, UK
Ralph Lauren
2 place de la Madeleine
75008 Paris, France
www.polo.com

Julien Macdonald (Studio)
65 Golborne Road
London W10 5NP, UK

Malden Mills
46 Stafford Street
Lawrence, MA 08141, USA
www.polartec.com

Mandarina Duck Headquarters
Plastimoda SpA
via Don Minzoni 36
40057 Cadriano di Granarolo Emilia
Bologna, Italy
Mandarina Duck
219 rue Saint Honoré
75001 Paris, France
Mandarina Duck
16 Conduit Street
London W1S 2XL, UK
Mandarina Duck
Kurfürstendamm 36
10719 Berlin, Germany
www.mandarinaduck.com

MaxMara
corso Vittorio Emanuele
20121 Milan, Italy
MaxMara
31 avenue Montaigne
75008 Paris, France
MaxMara
153 New Bond Street
London W1S 2TY, UK
MaxMara
813 Madison Avenue
New York, NY 10021, USA

Microthermal Systems
Stomatex House, Bodmin Business Park
Launceston Road
Bodmin, Cornwall PL31 3AR, UK

Mizuno UK
Mizuno House
612 Reading Road, Winnerash
Berks RG41 5HE, UK
www.mizunousa.com

Musto
Christy Way, Laindon
Essex SS15 6TR, UK
Also available at:
Captain O. M Watts
5–7 Dover Street
London W1S 4LD, UK
Kap Horn Sportswear
Handvaerkervej 12
4000 Roskilde, Denmark
Nippgen Bootszubehör
Hauptstrasse 92
12159 Berlin, Germany
Boat Locker
1543 Port Road East
Westport, CT 06880, USA
Chandlery
132B Harbor Way
Santa Barbara, CA 93109, USA
Whitworths Nautical World Crows Nest
49 Alexander Street
Crows Nest NSW 2065, Australia
The Whitworths Nautical World Queensland
55 Balaclava Street
Woolloongabba QLD 4102, Australia
www.musto.co.uk

Nike World Headquarters
1 Bowerman Drive
Beaverton, OR 97005–6453, USA
Nike European Headquarters
Colosseum 1
1213 Hilversum, The Netherlands
Nike (UK) Limited
1 Victory Way
Doxford International Business Park
Sunderland, Tyne & Wear SR3 3XF, UK
www.nike.com

The North Face
2013 Farlawn Drive
San Leandro, CA 94577, USA
The North Face
180 Post Street
San Francisco, CA 94108, USA
The North Face
1023 1st Avenue
Seattle, WA 98104, USA
The North Face
2490 S, Colorado Blvd
Denver, CO 80222, USA
The North Face
875 N, Michigan Ave
Chicago, IL 60611, USA
Also available at:
Bikepark Covent Garden
11–13 Macklin Street, Covent Garden
London WC2B 5NH, UK
Peak
Wilhelminenhofstrasse 88
12459 Berlin, Germany
Basecamp
Gaissacherstrasse 18
81371 Munich, Germany
The Outdoor Shop
2/F Silvercord
30 Canton Road, Tsimshatsui
Kowloon, Hong Kong
La Montagna Sport Sas
Di P, Garavaglia & C
via Lazzaretto 14
20124 Milan, Italy
Carl Denig Bv
Weteringschans 113–115
1017SB Amsterdam
The Netherlands
www.thenorthface.com

Nylstar (Headquarters)
via Friuli 55
20031 Cesano Maderno
Milan, Italy
Nylstar Inc. USA
496 Gallimore Dairy Road – Suite A
Greensboro, NC 27409, USA
Nylstar Asia Pacific
Manulife Tower 18/F
169 Electric Road
North Point
Hong Kong
Nylstar
PO Box 253
Bury, Lancs BL8 2FE, UK
Nylstar France
BP 19 avenue de l'Ermitage
62051 St Laurent Blangy Cedex, France
Nylstar Germany
Postfach 10 03 03
79122 Freiburg, Germany
www.nylstar.com

O'Neill
1071 41st Avenue
PO Box 6300
Santa Cruz, CA 95063, USA
O'Neill
9–15 Neal Street
London WC2H 9PW, UK
Also available at:
Laguna Surf & Sport
1088 S. Coast Highway
Laguna Beach, CA 92651, USA
B.C. Surf & Sport
1495 North Federal Boulevard
Fort Lauderdale, FL 33305, USA
Paragon Sporting Goods
24 East 18th Street
New York, NY 10003, USA
www.oneill.com

Lucy Orta
Studio Orta, 42 boulevard de Bercy
75012 Paris, France
orta@imaginet.fr

Outlast Technologies Inc.
6235 Lookout Road
Boulder, CO 80301, USA
Oulast Technologies
PO Box 3258
Brighton BN2 5WJ, UK
www.outlast.com

Patagonia
259 West Santa Clara Street
Ventura, CA 93001, USA
Also available at
YHA Adventure Shop
152–160 Wardour Street
London W1F 8YA, UK
www.patagonia.com

Fred Perry
547 West 27th Street
New York, NY 10001, USA
www.fredperry.com

Philips Design
PO Box 218
5600 MD Eindhoven, The Netherlands
Philips Design
Cross Oak Lane
Redhill, Surrey RH1 5HA, UK
www.philips.de/prm

Prada
via Andrea Maffei 2
20135 Milan, Italy
Prada Sport
Fifth Floor, Harrods, Brompton Road
London SW1X 7XL, UK
Prada
Madison Avenue 57th Street
New York, NY 10022, USA
www.prada.com

Quiksilver Europe (Headquarters)
Z. I. de Jalday, BP119
64501 Saint Jean de Luz, France
Quiksilver Boardrider Club
30–32 avenue des Champs-Elysées
75008 Paris, France
Quiksilver Boardrider Club
Thomas Neal's Centre
Earlham Street
London WC2H 9LD, UK
Quiksilver Boardrider Club
55 Piazza Kennedy, CC. Kennedy
1901 La Spezia, Italy
Quiksilver USA (Paragon Athletic)
24E 18th Street
New York, NY 10003, USA
Quiksilver USA (Paragon Athletic)
867 Broadway
New York, NY 10003, USA
www.quiksilver.com
www.quiksilver-europe.com
www.usa.quiksilver.com

Reebok
1895 J. W. Foster Boulevard
Canton, MA 02021, USA
www.reebok.com

Reflec Technology Limited
Road 1, Winsford Industrial Estate
Winsford, Cheshire CW7 3QQ, UK
Reflec USA Corp.
200 Homer Avenue
Ashland, MA 01721–1717, USA
Reflec Asia Ltd
RM 1403–1405 Beverley House
93–107, Lockhart Road
Wanchai, Hong Kong
www.reflec.co.uk

Rhovyl
BP 99
55310 Tronville en Barrois, France
www.rhovyl.com

Running Bare Australia PTY
City South Business Park
Unit 10, 26–34 Dunning Avenue
Rosebery, NSW 2018, Australia

Effi Samara
15 Dover Street/7A Stafford Street
London W1X 3PG, UK

Samsonite Blacklabel
via S. Pietro all'Orto angolo
corso Matteotti
20121 Milan, Italy
Samsonite Blacklabel
49–50 New Bond Street
London W1S 1RD, UK
Samsonite Blacklabel
Shinsegae Kangham, Seoul, Korea
www.samsonite.com

Schoeller Textil AG
Bahnhofstrasse
9475 Sevelen, Switzerland
www.schoeller-textiles.com

Sofinal
Textielstraat 20
8790 Waregem, Belgium
www.sofinal.be

Spartan
PO Box 211, Nazeing
Waltham Abbey EN9 2HE, UK
www.spartan.uk.com

Speedo
150 Columbus Avenue
New York, NY 10023, USA
Speedo
Mall of America,131 West Market Street
Bloomington, MN 55425, USA
Speedo
1 Embarcadero Center
San Francisco, CA 94111, USA
Speedo
Century City Shopping Center
10250 Santa Monica Boulevard
Los Angeles, CA 90067, USA
www.speedo.com

Sportswear Company
via Bramante 8
20154 Milan, Italy

Stone Island
see C. P. Company
www.stoneisland.com

3M
Building 225–IS–15
St Paul, MN 55144, USA
www.3m.com

Tencel Limited
The Acordis Group
Sager House
50 Seymour Street
London W1H 7JG, UK
www.tencel.com

Sam de Terán
25 Aldridge Road Villas,
London W11 1BN, UK

Toray Industries Inc.
Toray Building
2–1 Nihonbashi-Muromachi
2-chome, Chuo-ku
Tokyo 103–8666, Japan
Toray Europe Limited
3rd Floor, Old Park Lane
London W1K 1AD, UK
Toray Deutschland GmbH
Hugenotten Allee 171
63263 Neu-Isenburg, Germany

Toray Capital (America), Inc.
5th Floor, 600 Third Avenue
New York, NY 10016, USA
www.toray.co.jp
www.entrant.net

Vexed Generation Clothing Limited
Unit 46, Regents Studios
8 Andrew's Road
London E8 4QN, UK
www.vexed.co.uk

W. L. Gore
PO Box 729
Elkton, MD 21922, USA
www.gore-tex.com

The Woolmark Company
Valley Drive,
Ilkley, West Yorkshire LS29 8PB, UK
The Woolmark Company Srl
corso Matteotti 3
20121 Milan, Italy
The Woolmark Company
Wool House, 369 Royal Parade
Parkville, Victoria 3052, Australia
www.woolmark.com

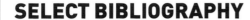

SELECT BIBLIOGRAPHY

Books

Andrew, Susan, *Winning: The Design of Sports*, London, 1998

Antonelli, Paola, *Mutant Materials in Contemporary Design*, New York, 1995

Braddock, Sarah E., and Marie O'Mahony, *Techno Textiles: Revolutionary Fabrics for Fashion and Design*, London and New York, 1998

Busch, Akiko, (ed) *Design for Sport*, London and New York, 1998; Cologne, 2000

Corbman, Bernard P., *Textiles: Fiber to Fabric*, (6th edn), London, 1983

Frost, Louise, and Alistair Griffiths, *Plants of Eden*, Cornwall, 2001

Handley, Susannah, *Nylon: The Manmade Fashion Revolution*, London, 1999

New Nomads: An exploration of wearable electronics by Philips, Rotterdam, 2000

Orta, Lucy, *The Process of Transformation*, Paris, 1998

Rivers, Victoria Z., *The Shining Cloth*, London, 1999; Rotterdam, 2000

Seeling, Charlotte, *Fashion: The Century of the Designer 1900–1999*, Cologne, 2000

Tucker, Andrew, *The London Fashion Book*, London, 1998

Van Beirendonck, Walter, and Luc Derycke (ed.), *Fashion2001 Landed*, Antwerp, 2001

Varjola, Pirjo, *The Etholen Collection: the ethnographic Alaskan collection of Adolf Etholen and his contemporaries in the National Museum of Finland*, Helsinki, 1990

Watkins, Susan M., *Clothing: The Portable Environment*, Iowa, 1995

Catalogues and Conference Proceedings

The Animal Construction Company, The Hunterian Museum and Art Gallery, Glasgow, 1999

Braddock, Sarah E., and Marie O'Mahony, *Edge: the Influence of Sportswear*, Copenhagen, 2001

Guillaume, Valérie, *Mutations//Mode 1960–2000*, Musée de la Mode de la Ville de Paris, 2000

O'Mahony, M., and S. E. Braddock (eds), *Inspiration and Innovation in Sportswear*, Interstoff, Messe Frankfurt, 1999

O'Mahony, Marie, and Sarah E. Braddock, (exhibn cat.), *The Fabric of Fashion*, Copenhagen), 2000

Visions of the Body: Fashion or Invisible Corset, The National Museum of Modern Art, Tokyo and the Kyoto Costume Institute, 1999

Magazine Articles

Bailey, Liz, 'Be a very smart dresser', *The Times*, London, 26 Feb 2001

Barrington, Anna, 'Profiles in fabric', *Sportswear International*, North America, Dec 1998/Jan 1999

Bartley, Luella, 'Death of the Trainer', *Vogue*, London, Aug 1998

Blanchard, Tamsin, 'DieselStyleLab: diffuse upwards', *Textile View*, Amsterdam, No. 48, Winter 1999

Buttolph, Angela, 'Watergate', *Vogue*, London, Jan 1999

'Building the Elite Athlete: science and the technology of sport', *Scientific American*, Volume II, No. 3, 2001

Cook, Richard, 'Zip Codes', *Line*, London, Spring 2000

Cosgrave, Bronwyn, 'Work it out', *Vogue*, London, March 2000

——, 'Club scene', *Vogue*, London, June 2001

Czeisler, Margaret Tully, 'Active Support', *Line*, London, Spring 2000

Dyson, Jenny, 'Check it out', *Elle*, London, Feb. 2001

Ellis, Kristi, 'Quiksilver Leaves the Beach With New Line', *Women's Wear Daily*, New York, 2 Aug 2000

Ewen, Lara, and Nancy MacDonell Smith, 'The history of fashion sport 1900–2000', *Sportswear International*, North America, Dec 1998/Jan 1999

Foster, Linda, 'Going Techno', *Textile View*, Amsterdam, No. 49, Spring 2000

——, 'View on Denim', *Textile View*, Amsterdam, No. 50, Summer 2000

——, 'That 80s Feeling', *Textile View*, Amsterdam, No. 52, Winter 2000

——, 'Fibres and fabrics', *Textile View*, Amsterdam, No. 53, Spring 2001

Gunn, Molly, 'Out of the bag', *Sunday Telegraph*, London, 8 Oct 2000

Hillier, Bevis, 'Exuberant minimalism', *World of Interiors*, London, May 1998

Holgate, Mark, 'Working Wardrobe', *Vogue*, London, Feb 1999

——, 'Multiple choice', *Vogue*, London, March 1999

——, 'American Classic', *Vogue*, London, May 1999

——, 'Into the Future', *Vogue*, London, Aug 1999

Huckbody, Jamie, 'Say It Loud', *i-D*, London, Jan/Feb 2000

Irvine, Susan, 'Elastic Fantastic', *The Sunday Telegraph*, London, 25 April 1999

Jones, Barbara, 'Light Fantastic', *International Textiles*, London, No. 818, Dec 2000,

Lalanne, Olivier, 'Sport et Mode Passent un Pacs', *Vogue*, Paris, Feb 1999

MacLeod, Rosalind, Hélène Martinez and Maria Cristina Pavarini, 'Street poets', *Sportswear International*, North America, No. 2, 1999

McDonell, Terry, 'Le Look Surfer', *Vogue*, Paris, Feb 1999

Myers, Coco, 'Brave new world', *Elle*, New York, Sept 1999

——, 'The comfort class', *Elle*, New York, Sept 1999

O'Donnell, Kate, 'High style', *Vogue*, London, Nov 1999

Quick, Harriet, 'The Max factor', *Vogue*, London, March 2001

Rawsthorn, Alice, 'Bravo for Burberry', *Vogue*, London, Nov 2000

Stegemann, Dirk, 'Athletes in motion', *Sportswear International*, North America, No. 2, 1999

Street, Julie, 'Fibre with rosie', *Wallpaper**, London, April 2000

Sultanik, Edina, 'On vented knees', *Sportswear International*, North America, Dec 1998/Jan 1999

Watson, Linda, 'Check mate', *Harpers & Queen*, London, March 1999

'Who's Who 2002 in the North American Sportswear Market', *Sportswear International*, 2001

Wilson, Eric, 'Sneaker Dresses Get on the Right Track', *Women's Wear Daily*, New York, 16 Feb 1999

Winwood, Lou, 'Fast masters', *Guardian Weekend*, London, 20 Feb 1999

PICTURE CREDITS

Page numbers of illustrations are in bold
a = above, **b** = below, **c** = centre, **l** = left, **r** = right, **t** = top
1: Schoeller. **2–3**: Rens van Mierlo, Korff & van Mierlo with photography art direction by Marion Verbücken, Philips Design. **8**: Tim Griffiths. **9**: Mizuno. **10**: Darren England/Allsport. **12l**: Olympia Film (courtesy Kobal). **12r** Katharine Hepburn (courtesy Kobal). **13a**: Columbia (courtesy Kobal). **13b**: MGM (courtesy Kobal). **15**: Gary M Prior/ Allsport. **18**: Simon Bruty/Allsport. **19a**: Lou Ferriago (courtesy Kobal). **19b** Concord/Warner Brothers (courtesy Kobal). **20a**: Nick Wilson/Allsport. **20b**. Adam Pretty/Allsport. **21**: Allsport UK/Allsport. **22**: Darren England/Allsport. **24**: Donald Christie. **26–27**: Alexander Boxill. **29**: Patagonia. **30**: Clive Brunskill/Allsport. **31a**: Brian Bahr/ Allsport. **31b**: Tom Hauck/Allsport. **32a**: Doug Pensinger/ Allsport. **32b**: Simon Bruty/Allsport. **36**: Jamie Squire/Allsport. **38**: Anna Beeke. **40**: Kappa. **41**: Jamie Kingham. **42, 43a & b**: Schoeller. **44a**: DuPont International. **44b**: Arena. **45**: adidas. **46**: Pete Webb. **47**: Anna Beeke. **48**: Pierre Mignot. **49**: Le NY. **50, 51a & b**: Jamie Kingham. **52a & b, 53l**: Nylstar laboratory.

53r: Triumph. **54, 55l**: Schoeller. **55r**: Outlast Technologies. **56t**: Schoeller. **56b & c**: Nylstar laboratory. **57**: adidas. **58, 59**: The Woolmark Company. **60**: Schoeller. **61**: Le NY. **62**: Horst Diekgerdes. **63, 64, 65b**: Tencel Ltd. **65t & c**: Acordis. **67**: Schoeller. **69**: Le NY. **70l, 71r**: Dave Wilcox. **70r, 71l**: Schoeller. **72**: Toray Industries, Inc. **73l & r**: Le NY. **74, 75**: Schoeller. **77**: Le NY. **78**: Chris Bracewell. **79**: Schoeller. **80al & ac**: Richard Davies. **80ar**: (image created by) Hoop Associates. **80b, 81a & b, 82l & r & rb, 83**: Rens van Mierlo, Korff & van Mierlo with photography art direction by Marion Verbücken, Philips Design. **85**: Le NY. **86**: Mike Cooper/Allsport. **89b**: Schoeller. **90**: Nathan Bilow/Allsport. **91**: Helly Hansen. **93**: Musto. **94l**: Patagonia. **95t**: Donald Christie. **97**: Mike Cooper/Allsport. **100–101**: Vent Design/O'Neill. **104–105**: Mizuno. **106**: Patagonia. **108–109**: Design Works/Vanson. **110**: Helly Hansen. **111**: Musto. **112l** Toyobo; **112r**: Patagonia. **113**: Toyobo. **114**: Schoeller. **117**: Aquatex Industries. **118**: Pascal Rondeau/Allsport. **120**: Ironman. **121**: Chris Cole/Allsport. **123**: Alex Williams/Microthermal. **124**: Nick Wilson/Allsport. **125**: Science Photo Library. **126, 127**: Nike. **128**: Shaun Botterill/Allsport. **130**: Chris Moore. **132l & r**: Ian Jones.

133l: Daniel Swallow. **133r, 134**: Jeff Hornbaker/Quiksilver. **135**: Holland &Holland. **136, 137l**: Chris Moore. **137ra & rb**: Oleg Micheyev. **138l**: Samsonite Blacklabel. **138r**: Sorin Morar. **139a**: Toni Campo & Roby Ventura. **139bl & br**: Samsonite Blacklabel. **140**: Sabastiano Pavia. **141l & r**: Samsonite Blacklabel. **142l**: Holland & Holland. **142r**: Chris Moore. **143**: Jeff Hornbaker/ Quiksilver. **144l**: David Tsay. **144r**: Chris Moore. **145l & r**: David Slijper. **146, 147l & r, 148l & r**: Chris Moore. **149a & b**: Lacoste. **150l**: Jane McCann. **150r**: Mari Mattila. **151t & c & b**: (graphics by) Nike. **152l & c & r, 153l & r**: Chris Moore. **154l & r, 155l**: H. Hannes. **155ra & b**: Samsonite Blacklabel. **156l & r, 157l & r**: Nicholas Alvis Vega. **158, 159l**: Chris Moore. **159r**: H. Hannes. **160**: Samsonite Blacklabel. **161l & r**: Chris Moore. **162a & b, 163**: Gabriele Balestra. **164l & r**: Eric Nehr. **165l & r**: Lucio Gelsi. **166l**: Sorin Morar. **166r**: Chris Moore. **167l**: Sabastiano Pavia. **167r**: Samsonite Blacklabel. **168a**: Mandarina Duck. **168b**: Sabastiano Pavia. **169l**: Olivier Ansellem. **169r**: Gabriele Balestra. **170l, 170–71**: adidas. **171a & b**: Nike. **172a & b**: Converse. **173a**: Samsonite Blacklabel. **173b**: Antonio Calabrese. **175**: Chris Moore.

INDEX